Imaging of Neurologic Complications in Hematological Disorders

Editor

SANGAM KANEKAR

HEMATOLOGY/ONCOLOGY CLINICS OF NORTH AMERICA

www.hemonc.theclinics.com

Consulting Editors
GEORGE P. CANELLOS
H. FRANKLIN BUNN

August 2016 • Volume 30 • Number 4

ELSEVIER

1600 John F. Kennedy Boulevard • Suite 1800 • Philadelphia, Pennsylvania, 19103-2899

http://www.theclinics.com

HEMATOLOGY/ONCOLOGY CLINICS OF NORTH AMERICA Volume 30, Number 4
August 2016 ISSN 0889-8588, ISBN 13: 978-0-323-45969-3

Editor: Jennifer Flynn-Briggs
Developmental Editor: Kristen Helm

Hematology/Oncology Clinics (ISSN 0889-8588) is published bimonthly by Elsevier Inc., 360 Park Avenue South, New York, NY 10010-1710. Months of issue are February, April, June, August, October, and December. Business and Editorial Offices: 1600 John F. Kennedy Blvd., Ste. 1800, Philadelphia, PA 19103–2899. Customer Service Office: 3251 Riverport Lane, Maryland Heights, MO 63043. Periodicals postage paid at New York, NY and at additional mailing offices. Subscription prices are $385.00 per year (domestic individuals), $707.00 per year (domestic institutions), $100.00 per year (domestic students/residents), $440.00 per year (Canadian individuals), $875.00 per year (Canadian institutions) $520.00 per year (international individuals), $875.00 per year (international institutions), and $255.00 per year (international and Canadian students/residents). International air speed delivery is included in all *Clinics* subscription prices. All prices are subject to change without notice. **POSTMASTER:** Send address changes to *Hematology/Oncology Clinics of North America*, Elsevier Health Sciences Division, Subscription Customer Service, 3251 Riverport Lane, Maryland Heights, MO 63043. Customer Service (orders, claims, online, change of address): Elsevier Health Sciences Division, Subscription **Customer Service, 3251 Riverport Lane, Maryland Heights, MO 63043. Tel: 1-800-654-2452 (U.S. and Canada); 314-447-8871 (outside U.S. and Canada). Fax: 314-447-8029. E-mail: journalscustomerservice-usa@elsevier.com (for print support); journalsonlinesupport-usa@elsevier.com (for online support).**

Reprints. For copies of 100 or more, of articles in this publication, please contact the Commercial Reprints Department, Elsevier Inc., 360 Park Avenue South, New York, New York 10010-1710; Tel.: 212-633-3874, Fax: 212-633-3820, E-mail: reprints@elsevier.com.

Hematology/Oncology Clinics of North America is covered in *MEDLINE/PubMed (Index Medicus), EMBASE/ Excerpta Medica, and BIOSIS.*

Contributors

CONSULTING EDITORS

GEORGE P. CANELLOS, MD
William Rosenberg Professor of Medicine, Department of Medical Oncology, Dana-Farber Cancer Institute, Boston, Massachusetts

H. FRANKLIN BUNN, MD
Professor of Medicine, Division of Hematology, Brigham and Women's Hospital, Harvard Medical School, Boston, Massachusetts

EDITOR

SANGAM KANEKAR, MD
Associate Professor, Departments of Radiology and Neurology, Hershey Medical Center, The Pennsylvania State University, Hershey, Pennsylvania

AUTHORS

AMIT AGARWAL, MD
Department of Neurology, Hershey Medical Center, The Pennsylvania State University, Hershey, Pennsylvania

WILSON ALTMEYER, MD
Assistant Professor, Department of Radiology, University of Texas Health Science Center at San Antonio, San Antonio, Texas

BARRY AMOS, DO
Department of Radiology, Hershey Medical Center, The Pennsylvania State University, Hershey, Pennsylvania

REZA ASSADSANGABI, MD
Neuroradiology Fellow, Department of Radiology, Children's Hospital of Philadelphia, Perelman School of Medicine at the University of Pennsylvania, Philadelphia, Pennsylvania

FALGUN H. CHOKSHI, MD, MS
Division of Neuroradiology, Department of Radiology and Imaging Sciences, Emory University School of Medicine, Atlanta, Georgia

DANIEL R. COURIEL, MD, MS
Professor of Medicine; Director, Blood and Marrow Transplantation Program, Huntsman Cancer Institute, University of Utah, Salt Lake City, Utah

IRINA FILATOVA, MD
Department of Radiology, Hershey Medical Center, The Pennsylvania State University, Hershey, Pennsylvania

DAVID FRAME, PharmD
Department of Pharmacy, University of Michigan Health System, Ann Arbor, Michigan

DHEERAJ GANDHI, MD
Professor of Radiology, Department of Diagnostic Radiology, University of Maryland Medical System, Baltimore, Maryland

MEHRDAD HAJMOMENIAN, MD
Research Fellow, Department of Radiology, Children's Hospital of Philadelphia, Perelman School of Medicine at the University of Pennsylvania, Philadelphia, Pennsylvania

ELLEN G. HOEFFNER, MD
Professor; Neuroradiology Fellowship Program Director, Department of Radiology, University Hospital, University of Michigan, Ann Arbor, Michigan

SANGAM KANEKAR, MD
Associate Professor, Departments of Radiology and Neurology, Hershey Medical Center, The Pennsylvania State University, Hershey, Pennsylvania

CATHERINE J. LEE, MD
Blood and Marrow Transplantation Program, Huntsman Cancer Institute, University of Utah, Salt Lake City, Utah

SOPO LIN, MD
Department of Radiology, Hershey Medical Center, The Pennsylvania State University, Hershey, Pennsylvania

SUYASH MOHAN, MD, PDCC
Assistant Professor of Radiology, Department of Radiology, Division of Neuroradiology, Perelman School of Medicine at the University of Pennsylvania, Philadelphia, Pennsylvania

SEYED ALI NABAVIZADEH, MD
Instructor, Department of Radiology, Division of Neuroradiology, Perelman School of Medicine at the University of Pennsylvania, Philadelphia, Pennsylvania

TAO OUYANG, MD
Department of Radiology, Hershey Medical Center, The Pennsylvania State University, Hershey, Pennsylvania

RITESH PATEL, MD
Department of Radiology, Hershey Medical Center, The Pennsylvania State University, Hershey, Pennsylvania

PUNEET S. PAWHA, MD
Assistant Professor; Associate Director, Department of Radiology, The Mount Sinai Hospital, Icahn School of Medicine at Mount Sinai, New York, New York

PRASHANT RAGHAVAN, MD
Assistant Professor of Radiology, Department of Diagnostic Radiology, University of Maryland Medical System, Baltimore, Maryland

TANYA J. RATH, MD
Assistant Professor, Department of Radiology, University of Pittsburgh Medical Center, Pittsburgh, Pennsylvania

HOLLY RICKER, MPAS, PA-C
Blood and Marrow Transplantation Program, Huntsman Cancer Institute, University of Utah, Salt Lake City, Utah

SHYAM SABAT, MD
Department of Radiology, Hershey Medical Center, The Pennsylvania State University, Hershey, Pennsylvania

ASHOK SRINIVASAN, MBBS, MD
Associate Professor, Division of Neuroradiology, Department of Radiology, University of Michigan Health System, Ann Arbor, Michigan

JOEL STEIN, MD, PhD
Assistant Professor of Radiology, Department of Radiology, Division of Neuroradiology, Perelman School of Medicine at the University of Pennsylvania, Philadelphia, Pennsylvania

MARY STEINBACH, DNP
Blood and Marrow Transplantation Program, Huntsman Cancer Institute, University of Utah, Salt Lake City, Utah

ANDREW STEVEN, MD
Assistant Professor of Radiology, Department of Diagnostic Radiology, University of Maryland Medical System, Baltimore, Maryland

LINDSAY L. STRATCHKO, DO
Department of Neurology, Hershey Medical Center, The Pennsylvania State University, Hershey, Pennsylvania

FAIZ I. SYED, MD, MS
Clinical Instructor, Division of Neuroradiology, Department of Radiology, VA Ann Arbor Health System, University of Michigan Health System, Ann Arbor, Michigan

ARASTOO VOSSOUGH, MD
Assistant Professor, Department of Radiology, Children's Hospital of Philadelphia, Perelman School of Medicine at the University of Pennsylvania, Philadelphia, Pennsylvania

Contents

Preface: Imaging of Neurologic Complications in Hematologic Disorders   xiii

Sangam Kanekar

Neurologic Manifestations of Blood Dyscrasias   723

Daniel R. Couriel, Holly Ricker, Mary Steinbach, and Catherine J. Lee

> Neurologic manifestations are common in blood diseases, and they can be caused by the hematologic disorder or its treatment. This article discusses hematologic diseases in adult patients, and categorizes them into benign and malignant conditions. The more common benign hematologic diseases associated with neurologic manifestations include anemias, particularly caused by B_{12} deficiency and sickle cell disease, and a variety of disorders of hemostasis causing bleeding or thrombosis, including thrombotic microangiopathy. Malignant conditions like multiple myeloma, leukemias, and lymphomas can have neurologic complications resulting from direct involvement, or caused by the different therapies to treat these cancers.

Imaging Manifestations of Neurologic Complications in Anemia   733

Ritesh Patel, Shyam Sabat, and Sangam Kanekar

> The hallmark signs and symptoms of anemia are directly related to a decrease in oxygen delivery to vital tissues and organs and include pallor, fatigue, lightheadedness, and shortness of breath. Neurologic complications are often nonspecific and can include poor concentration, irritability, faintness, tinnitus, and headache. If undiagnosed or untreated, anemia can progress to cognitive dysfunction, psychosis, encephalopathy, myelopathy, peripheral neuropathy, and more focal syndromes, such as stroke, seizures, chorea, and transverse myelitis. Imaging can play an important role in the early diagnosis and treatment of these neurologic and systemic complications associated with anemia, and hence, better outcome.

Central Nervous System Complications of Hemorrhagic and Coagulation Disorders   757

Irina Filatova, Lindsay L. Stratchko, and Sangam Kanekar

> Hematologic disorders affect the central nervous system in a variety of ways, producing a wide range of neurologic disturbances. Early identification of these complications allows for early intervention and better outcome. Cross-sectional imaging plays an important role in identifying brain abnormalities and helps the clinician in deciding appropriate course of action and treatment. This article discusses in short the basics of hemostasis including the coagulation cascade and the application of basic laboratory tests in evaluation of hematologic function. Imaging features of various neurologic disorders associated with these clotting and bleeding diatheses are discussed in detail with illustrations.

Neurologic and Head and Neck Manifestations of Sickle Cell Disease   779

Andrew Steven, Prashant Raghavan, Tanya J. Rath, and Dheeraj Gandhi

Sickle cell disease is a common, inherited disorder characterized by chronic hemolytic anemia with repetitive episodes of vasoocclusion resulting from deformed red blood cells. This article reviews the most significant neurologic and head and neck manifestations of this disease.

Neuroimaging in Central Nervous System Lymphoma   799

Seyed Ali Nabavizadeh, Arastoo Vossough, Mehrdad Hajmomenian, Reza Assadsangabi, and Suyash Mohan

Primary central nervous system lymphoma (PCNSL) is a rare aggressive high-grade type of extranodal lymphoma. PCNSL can have a variable imaging appearance and can mimic other brain disorders such as encephalitis, demyelination, and stroke. In addition to PCNSL, the CNS can be secondarily involved by systemic lymphoma. Computed tomography and conventional MRI are the initial imaging modalities to evaluate these lesions. Recently, however, advanced MRI techniques are more often used in an effort to narrow the differential diagnosis and potentially inform diagnostic and therapeutic decisions.

Neuroimaging in Leukemia   823

Seyed Ali Nabavizadeh, Joel Stein, and Suyash Mohan

Leukemias are a heterogeneous group of hematologic malignancies that result from uncontrolled neoplastic proliferation of undifferentiated or partially differentiated hematopoietic cells. Patients with acute leukemia can have a variety of craniocerebral complications, which can result from direct leukemic involvement, secondary to cerebrovascular or infectious complications of leukemia, or can be treatment related. Imaging plays a central role in evaluating the central nervous system during treatment in patients with leukemia. CT scan is usually considered an effective initial imaging modality to evaluate for cerebrovascular complications. MRI is considered the imaging modality of choice due to its versatility.

Imaging of Multiple Myeloma   843

Barry Amos, Amit Agarwal, and Sangam Kanekar

Multiple myeloma is the most common bone malignancy. Multiple myeloma and related plasma cell proliferative disorders have a diverse set of clinicopathologic findings and yet, at times, it may be challenging for clinicians to clinch the diagnosis. Imaging plays an important role in identifying the extent of the disease, guiding biopsies, and diagnosing associated spinal and intracranial complications. The purpose of this review article is to describe the imaging findings associated with common neurologic complications seen with multiple myeloma and related plasma cell proliferative disorders (PCPDs).

Venous Thrombosis: Causes and Imaging Appearance   867

Andrew Steven, Prashant Raghavan, Wilson Altmeyer, and Dheeraj Gandhi

Cerebral venous sinus thrombosis is an elusive diagnosis with profound potential neurologic consequences. Although there are numerous reported predisposing conditions, by far the most common is a prothrombotic hypercoagulable state. Recent advances in MRI and computed tomography have improved diagnostic accuracy for this increasingly recognized disorder. Familiarity with imaging techniques and potential pitfalls is essential for accurate diagnosis and management of these patients.

Central Nervous System Complications of Hematopoietic Stem Cell Transplant 887

Faiz I. Syed, Daniel R. Couriel, David Frame, and Ashok Srinivasan

Hematopoietic stem cell transplantation (SCT) is now commonly used to treat several hematologic and nonhematologic diseases. Central nervous system (CNS) complications post-transplantation occur commonly in the first year and result in increased mortality from infectious, toxic, metabolic, or vascular causes. Infections secondary to aspergillus, toxoplasma and viruses cause many of the complications. Drug-related toxicities arising from conditioning regimens and graft-versus-host disease prophylaxis, as well as intraparenchymal hemorrhage, are not uncommon and can result in increased morbidity. Secondary CNS cancers have a higher incidence 5 or more years after allogeneic SCT.

Central Nervous System Complications of Oncologic Therapy 899

Ellen G. Hoeffner

Traditional and newer agents used to treat cancer can cause significant toxicity to the central nervous system. MRI of the brain and spine is the imaging modality of choice for patients with cancer who develop neurologic symptoms. It is important to be aware of the agents that can cause neurotoxicity and their associated imaging findings so that patients are properly diagnosed and treated. In some instances, conventional MRI may not be able to differentiate posttreatment effects from disease progression. In these instances advanced imaging techniques may be helpful, although further research is still needed.

Imaging of Spinal Manifestations of Hematological Disorders 921

Puneet S. Pawha and Falgun H. Chokshi

Imaging manifestations of hematological diseases and their potential complications are broad, and there may be significant overlap in features of various disease processes. Knowledge of appropriate choice of imaging test, pertinent imaging patterns, and pathophysiology of disease can help the reader increase specificity in the diagnosis and treatment of the patient. Most importantly, we encourage readers of this review to engage their radiologists during the diagnostic, treatment, and management phases of care delivery.

Imaging of Bone Marrow 945

Sopo Lin, Tao Ouyang, and Sangam Kanekar

Bone marrow is essential for function of hematopoiesis, which is vital for the normal functioning of the body. Bone marrow disorders or dysfunctions may be evaluated by blood workup, peripheral smears, marrow biopsy, plain radiographs, computed tomography (CT), MRI and nuclear medicine scan. It is important to distinguish normal spinal marrow from pathology to avoid missing a pathology or misinterpreting normal changes, either of which may result in further testing and increased health care costs. This article focuses on the diffuse bone marrow pathologies, because the majority of the bone marrow pathologies related to hematologic disorders are diffuse.

Index   **973**

HEMATOLOGY/ONCOLOGY
CLINICS OF NORTH AMERICA

FORTHCOMING ISSUES

October 2016
New Anticoagulant and Antithrombotic Agents
Jean Marie Connors, *Editor*

December 2016
Aggressive B- Cell Lymphoma
Laurie Sehn, *Editor*

February 2017
Lung Cancer
Roy S. Herbst and Daniel Morgensztern, *Editors*

RECENT ISSUES

June 2016
Transfusion Medicine
Jeanne E. Hendrickson and Christopher A. Tormey, *Editors*

April 2016
Global Hematology
David J. Roberts and Sir David J. Weatherall, *Editors*

February 2016
Neuroendocrine Tumors
Jennifer A. Chan and Matthew H. Kulke, *Editors*

ISSUE OF RELATED INTEREST

Radiologic Clinics of North America, March 2016 (Vol. 54, Issue 2)
Topics in Transplantation Imaging
Puneet Bhargava and Matthew T. Heller, *Editors*
Available at: http://www.radiologic.theclinics.com/

THE CLINICS ARE AVAILABLE ONLINE!
Access your subscription at:
www.theclinics.com

HEMATOLOGY/ONCOLOGY
CLINICS OF NORTH AMERICA

Preface

Imaging of Neurologic Complications in Hematologic Disorders

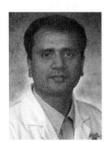

Sangam Kanekar, MD
Editor

Hematologic disorders often affect the central and peripheral nervous systems in a number of different ways, producing a wide range of neurologic symptoms. Some of these neurologic complications are well described, but others are less clearly defined and are mostly diagnosed on cross-section imaging like CT and MRI. Recent advances in oncology therapy have greatly improved the prognosis of patients with hematologic neoplasms. This has also resulted in an increased incidence of associated complications and toxic effects due to a longer term of survival of these patients.

Clinically, due to nonspecific presentation, central nervous system (CNS) complications are underdiagnosed. These complications may include hemorrhage; cerebral infarction; infiltration of the meninges, parenchyma, bone marrow, orbit, and spine. In addition, there may be CNS complications due to therapy; for example, radiation therapy–related white matter disease, mineralizing microangiopathy, parenchymal brain volume loss, radiation-induced cryptic vascular malformations, and secondary neoplasms.

I, along with my coauthors, present before you an issue of *Hematology/Oncology Clinics of North America* dedicated to "Imaging of Neurologic Complications in Hematologic Disorders." This issue has in total twelve articles, predominately dedicated to the imaging findings of neurologic complications in benign conditions and hematologic neoplasms. We conclude that imaging along with clinical suspicion plays an important role in early diagnosis of these complications and in turn will help in appropriate intervention.

I thank all the authors for their superexcellent contributions that make this issue an outstanding and extensive review on "Imaging of Neurologic Complications in Hematologic Disorders." I take this opportunity to thank Drs George P. Canellos, MD and H. Franklin Bunn, MD for accepting my idea and giving me an opportunity

Hematol Oncol Clin N Am 30 (2016) xiii–xiv
http://dx.doi.org/10.1016/j.hoc.2016.06.001
0889-8588/16/$ – see front matter © 2016 Published by Elsevier Inc.

hemonc.theclinics.com

to present this topic to a wider audience. I thank Kristen Helm for her continuous editorial support in completing this issue. Finally, I thank my wife, Revati, and my children, Samika and Rachita, for their support and love.

I hope you will enjoy reading this issue.

Sangam Kanekar, MD
Section of Neuroradiology
Departments of Radiology and Neurology
The Pennsylvania State University
Milton S. Hershey Medical Center and College of Medicine
500 University Drive
Hershey
PA 17033, USA

E-mail address:
skanekar@hmc.psu.edu

Neurologic Manifestations of Blood Dyscrasias

Daniel R. Couriel, MD, MS*, Holly Ricker, MPAS, PA-C, Mary Steinbach, DNP, Catherine J. Lee, MD

KEYWORDS

- Plasma cell • Dyscrasia • Myeloma • Neuropathy • Radiculopathy

KEY POINTS

- Neurologic manifestations are common in both benign and malignant disorders, and they can affect both central and peripheral nervous system.
- The most common neurologic manifestations in blood cell dyscrasias are those involving the peripheral nervous system.
- Anemias, particularly B_{12} deficiency and sickle cell disease, lymphomas, leukemias and myelomas are the diseases more frequently associated with neurological manifestations.

INTRODUCTION

Neurologic manifestations are common in blood diseases, and they can be caused by the hematologic disorder or its treatment.

This article discusses hematologic diseases in adult patients, and categorizes them into benign and malignant conditions. The more common benign hematologic diseases associated with neurologic manifestations include anemias, particularly caused by B_{12} deficiency and sickle cell disease, and a variety of disorders of hemostasis causing bleeding or thrombosis, including thrombotic microangiopathy (TMA). Malignant conditions like multiple myeloma (MM), leukemias, and lymphomas can have neurologic complications resulting from direct involvement, or caused by the different therapies to treat these cancers.

A classification of the most important hematologic conditions associated with neurologic complications or manifestations is presented in **Box 1**. This article gives a brief overview of these conditions, because they are developed in depth throughout this issue.

Blood and Marrow Transplantation Program, Huntsman Cancer Institute, University of Utah, 2000 Circle of Hope, Salt Lake City, UT 84112, USA
* Corresponding author. Huntsman Cancer Institute, University of Utah, 2000 Circle of Hope, Room 2151, Salt Lake City, UT 84144.
E-mail address: Daniel.Couriel@hci.utah.edu

Hematol Oncol Clin N Am 30 (2016) 723–731
http://dx.doi.org/10.1016/j.hoc.2016.03.001
0889-8588/16/$ – see front matter © 2016 Elsevier Inc. All rights reserved.

Box 1
Hematologic disorders

Benign hematologic conditions:

1. Anemias:
   a. B_{12} deficiency, folate deficiency
   b. Sickle cell disease
   c. Paroxysmal nocturnal hemoglobinuria

2. Disorders of hemostasis:
   a. Hemorrhagic disorders: hemophilia A and B, disseminated intravascular coagulation (DIC), thrombocytopenias, and disorders of platelet function
   b. Thrombotic disorders: antiphospholipid antibodies, inherited thrombophilia (eg, antithrombin III, protein C or S deficiency, factor V Leiden)
   c. Other: thrombotic microangiopathies (eg, thrombotic thrombocytopenic purpura, hemolytic-uremic syndrome)
      DIC

Malignant hematologic conditions:

1. Leukemia

2. Lymphoma

3. Myeloma

4. Treatment of hematologic conditions

BENIGN HEMATOLOGIC CONDITIONS
Anemias

Iron deficiency anemias are frequently associated with nonspecific symptoms like fatigue, weakness, irritability, dizziness, tinnitus, and headache. Pseudotumor cerebri and cerebral venous sinus thrombosis have also been associated with iron deficiency. However, thrombotic episodes are likely to be associated with the thrombocytosis that occurs in iron-deficient patients; this can sometimes be severe and cause cerebrovascular infarction or transient ischemic attacks (TIAs). In patients with preexisting severe vascular disease, anemia can contribute to cerebrovascular or cardiac events that usually reverse with an increase in hemoglobin.[1,2]

Vitamin B_{12} deficiency can cause neurologic symptoms even in the absence of appreciable alterations in peripheral blood and with normoblastic hematopoiesis. Furthermore, the size of the red cells can be within normal limits, because some of these patients have coexisting iron deficiency. Thus, methylmalonic acid and total homocysteine levels may be useful adjuncts in the diagnosis. Sensory peripheral neuropathy and myelopathy can occur because of loss of large, myelinated fibers, and axonal degeneration. Neuropathy usually has upper-limb onset and associated Lhermitte phenomenon. Myelopathy is accompanied by early and severe impairment of proprioception and vibration sense. Other less common forms of neurologic involvement, like sensory ataxic spastic paraparesis and optic neuropathy, have also been described. Encephalopathy with unspecified mental status changes or affective disorders have been found in about 20% of patients with B_{12} deficiency.[3,4] Folate deficiency is a more common cause of neurologic disease in children, in whom it typically presents with seizures, delayed motor and cognitive development, cerebellar ataxia, spasticity, and visual and hearing impairment. Subacute combined degeneration of the cord accompanying diet-induced folic acid deficiency may occur and can improve with replacement.[5,6]

Sickle cell disease is a frequent cause of neurologic symptoms, and about 25% of patients have some form of neurologic manifestation, most frequently cerebral infarction. Intracranial hemorrhage is much rarer, and usually subarachnoid and aneurysmal in cause.[7,8]

Paroxysmal nocturnal hemoglobinuria (PNH) is a stem cell disorder caused by mutations in the phosphatidylinositol glycan class A gene. This mutation results in a deficiency in the binding of several proteins that protect red cells from complement-induced hemolysis. Hemolysis is intravascular, and it occurs in the setting of hypercoagulability, which in these patients is multifactorial. The most common manifestation of this hypercoagulable state is large-vessel venous thrombosis, particularly in the brain and portal systems. Furthermore, a neurologic cause of death can be found in 10% of patients with PNH, including cerebral venous thrombosis, subarachnoid hemorrhage, and intracerebral hemorrhage.[9]

Disorders of Hemostasis

Hemorrhagic disorders

Hemophilias A and B have identical neurologic manifestations, which happen in the most severe forms of the disease. Peripheral nerve lesions are the most common complication, and they are usually related to muscular or joint bleeding. The iliac muscle is commonly involved, leading to femoral neuropathy. Severe hemophilic arthropathy of the elbow can sometimes lead to ulnar nerve palsy. Intracranial hemorrhage occurs in 2% to 14% of patients, and is the leading cause of death in these patients. Bleeding usually occurs in younger patients, and it can be subdural, epidural, subarachnoid, or intracerebral.[10,11]

Thrombocytopenias can lead to subdural, subarachnoid, and intracerebral bleeding, particularly during the first 2 weeks of onset, and at a platelet count of less than $20 \times 10^9/L$. A special case and the most frequent cause of drug-induced immune thrombocytopenia, heparin-induced thrombocytopenia, is paradoxically associated with thrombosis, including ischemic damage to limbs, central nervous system (CNS), myocardium, and lungs in up to 60% of cases.[12] Abnormal bleeding can result from disorders of platelet function, including adhesion, aggregation, secretion, and procoagulant activity. The most common causes are drug related, including aspirin, nonsteroidal antiinflammatory drugs, and ticlopidine.

Thrombotic disorders

Thrombosis may arise from abnormalities in the blood vessel wall, alterations in blood composition, and abnormalities in the dynamics of blood flow; the triad of Virchow. The list of well-recognized prothrombotic circumstances is extensive, and beyond the scope of this article. Thus, the focus here is on general aspects of the more common acquired and inherited disorders with neurologic manifestations.

The lupus anticoagulant and anticardiolipin are members of a group of antiphospholipid antibodies associated with venous and, to a lesser extent, arterial thrombosis. A diagnosis requires the combination of at least 1 clinical and 1 laboratory criterion that persist over time. In patients with lupus, predisposition to thrombosis is associated with antinuclear antibodies and antiphospholipid antibodies. The primary antiphospholipid syndrome is the association between arterial and venous thrombosis with the lupus anticoagulant, phospholipid antibodies, and a history of recurrent early miscarriage. Neurologic manifestations are common, and include migraine (20.2%), stroke (19.8%), TIA (11.1%), epilepsy (7%), amaurosis fugax (5.4%), and less frequently vascular dementia, transient amnesia, chorea, acute encephalopathy, optic neuritis, retinal artery thrombosis, cerebral venous sinus thrombosis, cerebellar ataxia, transverse myelopathy, and hemiballismus.

Inherited thrombophilias are a group of disorders with a defect or deficiency in the natural anticoagulant mechanisms that predisposes to the development of venous thrombosis. A genetic factor is identified in up to 50% of unselected patients with venous thromboembolism, and genetic or acquired factors in 80% of patients with cerebral venous sinus thrombosis. Antithrombin III, protein C, and protein S deficiencies; factor V Leiden mutations; the prothrombin G20210A gene mutation; and MTHFR C677T mutations (resulting in hyperhomocysteinemia) all predispose to thrombosis. Antithrombin III, protein C, and protein S deficiencies are rare, but pose the highest risk, with highly penetrant phenotypes that can lead to a 10-fold increase in risk for heterozygous carriers.[13,14]

Thrombotic microangiopathies

Thrombotic thrombocytopenic purpura (TTP) is a severe form of TMA that results from excessive systemic platelet aggregation caused by the accumulation of unfolded high-molecular-weight von Willebrand factor multimers in plasma. This failure to process von Willebrand factor into less adhesive forms is related to severe deficiency of ADAMTS13, a von Willebrand factor protease. TTP can be inherited or acquired, occurs most frequently in women between 20 and 50 years of age, and can have a high fatality rate depending on the cause and severity of the syndrome. Acquired cases are more frequently associated with pregnancy, hematopoietic stem cell transplantation, infection, and disseminated intravascular coagulation (DIC). Neurologic features are the most common presenting manifestations in TTP, occurring in about 60% of patients. As the result of involvement of any part of the CNS, there is a large variety of neurologic manifestations, typically transient and fluctuating, and frequently resembling a TIA. Posterior reversible encephalopathy syndrome is the most frequent brain imaging abnormality, along with microangiopathic hemolytic anemia, thrombocytopenia, hyperbilirubinemia, uremia, and bone marrow hyperplasia.[15,16] Hemolytic uremic syndrome (HUS), is the other form of TMA, typically presenting in children with a recent infection by organisms producing Shiga toxins such as Escherichia coli O157:H7 or Shigella. Therefore, diarrhea and abdominal pain frequently precede the onset of HUS. Deficiency of ADAMTS13 has not been shown in HUS, and, unlike TTP, most children survive with just supportive care. The most common neurologic manifestations are seizures, but behavioral changes and cerebral, cerebellar, and brainstem syndromes can occur.[17,18]

Disseminated intravascular coagulation

DIC should be considered an indication of the presence of an underlying disorder, and a manifestation of inappropriate thrombin activation. The coagulation system is activated by the rapid release of thromboplastic substances resulting in the production of fibrin. Clotting factors and platelets are consumed, and there is defective and activated fibrinolysis and impairment of the coagulation inhibition system. The clinical syndrome results from vascular obstruction from fibrin-rich thrombi. In contrast, the overwhelming consumption of alpha$_2$-antiplasmin and platelets, along with the anticoagulant properties of fibrin degradation products, can also result in bleeding. The list of causes that can lead to DIC is extensive, including tissue damage caused by burns, heat stroke, status epilepticus, severe infection, obstetric complications, and diabetic ketoacidosis. When the CNS is affected, the neurologic manifestations of DIC depend on the degree and location of the thrombotic and hemorrhagic events, as well as the primary disorder that triggered it. Any part of the brain can be affected, causing focal or generalized encephalopathic manifestations that can fluctuate markedly over time.[19]

MALIGNANT HEMATOLOGIC CONDITIONS
Leukemia and Lymphoma

In leukemias, involvement of the CNS is primarily caused by infiltration with leukemic cells, but it may also occur as a result of neurotoxicity induced by hemorrhage, infection, drugs, or radiation. Meningeal leukemia usually presents with headaches, nausea, and vomiting, sometimes associated with other symptoms like lethargy, irritability, neck stiffness, and photophobia. Papilledema is the most common sign, and leukemic deposits may compress or infiltrate the cranial nerves or spinal nerve roots. The diagnosis is confirmed on cerebrospinal fluid in about 90% of cases, and flow cytometric analysis has the highest diagnostic yield. When the leukemic deposits involve part of the CNS, manifestations are variable, depending on the specific location. For example, blindness may occur secondary to optic nerve and retinal infiltration; hypothalamic and pituitary dysfunction are well recognized and may be associated with hydrocephalus. Intracranial hemorrhage occurs in about 3% of patients with hematologic malignances, and more frequently in patients with intracranial lymphoma. Thrombocytopenia is a common feature of intracranial bleeding, but in cases like promyelocytic leukemia DIC may be the major contributor. Cellular hyperviscosity in patients with severe leukocytosis presents with somnolence, headaches, and impaired consciousness, and is more frequent in myeloid acute leukemias. Viral, bacterial, and fungal infections of the CNS can occur in patients with hematologic malignancies, and corticosteroids, chemotherapy, and broad-spectrum antibiotics are definite contributors.[20] In lymphomas, the CNS is involved through direct spread from primary nodal or extranodal sites. Occasionally, primary Hodgkin and non-Hodgkin of the CNS are seen. Spinal cord and meningeal involvement are common. Extradural deposits arise as the result of direct spread from the retroperitoneal or postmediastinal spaces via the intervertebral foramina from tumor growth along nerve roots, or by direct invasion from an affected vertebral body. Intramedullary metastases are rare and usually occur in lymphoblastic lymphoma. Intracranial involvement usually arises from infiltration of the skull base by direct extension from involved cervical lymph nodes, or lymphatic spread. Almost all cases of lymphomatous meningitis are found in lymphomas of diffuse histologies. In addition, primary CNS lymphomas account for 2.5% of brain tumors. All histologic subtypes can be observed, but 90% belong to the B-cell high-grade non-Hodgkin type. In general, these tumors are multicentric, and have an extremely poor prognosis, particularly in patients with immunodeficiencies, as can be seen associated with Epstein-Barr virus infection.[20,21]

Plasma Cell Dyscrasias

Malignant plasma cell dyscrasias are characterized by proliferation of a monoclonal population of plasma cells, manifested by a monoclonal immunoglobulin called paraprotein or M-protein. MM is the most frequent malignant plasma cell disorder, accounting for approximately 10% of all hematological malignancies. MM is defined by the presence of paraprotein in the serum and/or urine; at least 10% neoplastic plasma cells in the bone marrow or their presence in other tissue; and evidence of end-organ damage, related to the underlying plasma cell disorder, including hypercalcemia (C), renal failure (R), anemia (A), and bone lesions (B), commonly named the CRAB symptoms acronymically. Smoldering or asymptomatic MM is present when the same degree of paraprotein in serum and plasma cell infiltration of the bone marrow is not accompanied by CRAB symptoms. Of note, monoclonal gammopathy (monoclonal gammopathy of uncertain significance [MGUS]) is the most common and the most benign plasma cell disorder, comprising about two-thirds of all plasma cell dyscrasias. By definition, it is a laboratory abnormality describing a serum monoclonal protein level usually less than 3 g/dL, greater than 10% monoclonal plasma cells in the bone marrow, low or absent levels of mono-clonal protein in the urine, and no systemic or end-organ CRAB symptoms. Plasma-cytoma is defined by the presence of a localized plasma cell tumor without evidence of neoplastic plasma cells in bone marrow (<5%) and absence of other features of myeloma. Plasmacytoma most frequently occurs in bone, but can also be found outside bone in soft tissues. Plasmacytoma can present as solitary or multiple lesions, the latter more predictive of progression to myeloma. The POEMS (polyneuropathy, organomegaly, endocrinopathy, monoclonal gammopathy and skin changes) syndrome is a rare multisystemic disorder associated with the pres-ence of a plasma cell dyscrasia, usually osteosclerotic MM or MGUS. Neurologic complications are frequent during plasmacytoma and myeloma, and constitute the most frequent presenting symptom in MM, outside CRAB symptoms.[4,5] Peripheral neuropathies are common and are frequently associated with plasma cell dyscra-sias.[22,23] In a single-center study, about 10% of patients referred for idiopathic peripheral neuropathies had an associated monoclonal gammopathy. A third of pa-tients with MGUS have associated neuropathy.[22,24] Immunoglobulin (Ig) M MGUS comprises 17% of all paraproteinemias, and it is involved in more than 50% of all paraproteinemic neuropathies.[25,26] Peripheral neuropathy in MM can occur from disease, similar to MGUS neuropathy, or from treatment effects. The reported rates of polyneuropathy in MM are as high as 20%,[27,28] and the exact cause is still unknown.[29,30] Treatment-related neuropathies are more frequent than disease-related neuropathies, and they can affect up to 65% of patients.[24] The most common causes of treatment-related neuropathies are proteasome inhibitors (eg, bortezomib and carfilzomib), immunomodulatory drugs (mainly thalidomide), and chemotherapeutic agents more commonly used in the treatment of MM, such as vincristine and cisplatin.

Treatment-related neuropathies are usually symmetric, distal, progressive, sensory or sensorimotor; and with some differences depending on the offending agent. For example, bortezomib-related neuropathies can be milder, predominantly sensory, more reversible, and with a faster recovery than those related to thalidomide and vincristine.[28,31,32]

Radiculopathy is one of the most common forms of mechanical injury, usually caused by a vertebral plasmacytoma directly compressing nerve roots, and leading to radicular pain.[33] The incidence of cord compression as a complication has been declining in recent years, mostly because of the use of bisphosphonates. It is now seen in up to 5% of patients with myeloma, and is the presenting symptom in 3%.[34] The most common level of spinal cord involvement in these patients is the thoracic cord.[33]

Plasma cell dyscrasias can also compromise the CNS from direct compression, infiltration, or metabolic complications.[23]

MM can result in radiculopathy and/or spinal cord compression either from a local-ized plasma cell tumor (plasmacytoma) or a pathologic fracture from a lytic lesion,[29,35] and this was addressed earlier. Management of symptoms and pain may involve radiotherapy, high-dose steroids, and more recently percutaneous vertebroplasty has been shown to be safe and able to improve pain.[36]

Hyperviscosity syndrome describes a group of symptoms affecting the CNS and that are triggered by increased serum viscosity. In the case of plasma cell dyscrasias this most commonly occurs in WaldenstrÖm macroglobulinemia (WM) and IgM myeloma. WM is a low-grade lymphoma with IgM monoclonal gammopathy and bone marrow involvement of lymphoplasmacytic cells.[37] Hyperviscosity occurs 10% to 30% of the time in WM and only about 2% to 6% in IgG or IgA myeloma.[23] Symptoms include mucous membrane bleeding, visual disturbances, headaches, dizziness, ataxia, nystagmus, altered mental status, and stroke. Myelomatous meningitis (MyM) is a rare complication of MM. It is defined by the presence of neoplastic monoclonal plasma cells in the cerebrospinal fluid.[33,38] The incidence of MyM has been estimated to be around 1.0%.[39,40] It is unclear how leptomeningeal spread of plasma cells occurs, but one possible explanation is via hematogenous spread or direct extension from the affected bone.[41] The diagnosis of MyM is often delayed because of the nature of MM in that patients commonly have skull base and epidural involvement. Patients presenting with cranial nerve deficits involving cranial nerves II to VII, encephalopathy, radiculopathy, and or cauda equina syndrome should be evaluated for MyM.[39]

REFERENCES

1. Benedict SL, Bonkowsky JL, Thompson JA, et al. Cerebral sinovenous thrombosis in children: another reason to treat iron deficiency anemia. J Child Neurol 2004;19(7):526–31.
2. Leis AA, Stokic DS, Shepherd JM. Depression of spinal motoneurons may underlie weakness associated with severe anemia. Muscle Nerve 2003;27(1): 108–12.
3. Valente E, Scott JM, Ueland PM, et al. Diagnostic accuracy of holotranscobalamin, methylmalonic acid, serum cobalamin, and other indicators of tissue vitamin B_{12} status in the elderly. Clin Chem 2011;57(6):856–63.
4. Turner MR, Talbot K. Functional vitamin B12 deficiency. Pract Neurol 2009;9(1): 37–41.
5. Donnelly S, Callaghan N. Subacute combined degeneration of the spinal cord due to folate deficiency in association with a psychotic illness. Ir Med J 1990; 83(2):73–4.
6. Korenke GC, Hunneman DH, Eber S, et al. Severe encephalopathy with epilepsy in an infant caused by subclinical maternal pernicious anaemia: case report and review of the literature. Eur J Pediatr 2004;163(4–5):196–201.
7. Prengler M, Pavlakis SG, Prohovnik I, et al. Sickle cell disease: the neurological complications. Ann Neurol 2002;51(5):543–52.
8. Kirkham FJ, Hewes DK, Prengler M, et al. Nocturnal hypoxaemia and central-nervous-system events in sickle-cell disease. Lancet 2001;357(9269):1656–9.
9. Hill A, Kelly RJ, Hillmen P. Thrombosis in paroxysmal nocturnal hemoglobinuria. Blood 2013;121(25):4985–96 [quiz: 5105].
10. Knoebl P, Marco P, Baudo F, et al. Demographic and clinical data in acquired hemophilia A: results from the European Acquired Haemophilia Registry (EACH2). J Thromb Haemost 2012;10(4):622–31.
11. Baudo F, Collins P, Huth-Kühne A, et al. Management of bleeding in acquired hemophilia A: results from the European Acquired Haemophilia (EACH2) Registry. Blood 2012;120(1):39–46.

12. Pohl C, Harbrecht U, Greinacher A, et al. Neurologic complications in immune-mediated heparin-induced thrombocytopenia. Neurology 2000;54(6):1240–5.

13. Rosendaal FR, Reitsma PH. Genetics of venous thrombosis. J Thromb Haemost 2009;7(Suppl 1):301–4.

14. de Bruijn SF, Stam J, Koopman MM, et al. Case-control study of risk of cerebral sinus thrombosis in oral contraceptive users and in [correction of who are] carriers of hereditary prothrombotic conditions. The Cerebral Venous Sinus Thrombosis Study Group. BMJ 1998;316(7131):589–92.

15. George JN, Vesely SK. Thrombotic thrombocytopenic purpura-hemolytic uremic syndrome: diagnosis and treatment. Cleve Clin J Med 2001;68(10):857–8, 860, 863–4 passim.

16. Vesely SK, George JN, Lämmle B, et al. ADAMTS13 activity in thrombotic thrombocytopenic purpura-hemolytic uremic syndrome: relation to presenting features and clinical outcomes in a prospective cohort of 142 patients. Blood 2003;102(1):60–8.

17. Sakakibara R, Hattori T, Mizobuchi K, et al. Axonal polyneuropathy and encephalopathy in a patient with verotoxin producing *Escherichia coli* (VTEC) infection. J Neurol Neurosurg Psychiatry 1999;67(2):254–5.

18. Garg AX, Suri RS, Barrowman N, et al. Long-term renal prognosis of diarrhea-associated hemolytic uremic syndrome: a systematic review, meta-analysis, and meta-regression. JAMA 2003;290(10):1360–70.

19. Levi M, van der Poll T. Disseminated intravascular coagulation: a review for the internist. Intern Emerg Med 2013;8(1):23–32.

20. McCoyd M, Gruener G, Foy P. Neurologic aspects of lymphoma and leukemias. Handb Clin Neurol 2014;120:1027–43.

21. DeAngelis LM. Neuro-oncology: primary CNS lymphoma treatment–the devil is in the details. Nat Rev Neurol 2015;11(6):314–5.

22. Raheja D, Specht C, Simmons Z. Paraproteinemic neuropathies. Muscle Nerve 2015;51(1):1–13.

23. Bayat E, Kelly JJ. Neurological complications in plasma cell dyscrasias. Handb Clin Neurol 2012;105:731–46.

24. Mauermann ML. Paraproteinemic neuropathies. Continuum (Minneap Minn) 2014;20(5 Peripheral Nervous System Disorders):1307–22.

25. Eurelings M, Notermans NC, Van de Donk NW, et al. Risk factors for hematological malignancy in polyneuropathy associated with monoclonal gammopathy. Muscle Nerve 2001;24(10):1295–302.

26. Ramchandren S, Lewis RA. An update on monoclonal gammopathy and neuropathy. Curr Neurol Neurosci Rep 2012;12(1):102–10.

27. Richardson PG, Xie W, Mitsiades C, et al. Single-agent bortezomib in previously untreated multiple myeloma: efficacy, characterization of peripheral neuropathy, and molecular correlations with response and neuropathy. J Clin Oncol 2009; 27(21):3518–25.

28. Richardson PG, Briemberg H, Jagannath S, et al. Frequency, characteristics, and reversibility of peripheral neuropathy during treatment of advanced multiple myeloma with bortezomib. J Clin Oncol 2006;24(19):3113–20.

29. Dispenzieri A, Kyle RA. Neurological aspects of multiple myeloma and related disorders. Best Pract Res Clin Haematol 2005;18(4):673–88.

30. Ropper AH, Gorson KC. Neuropathies associated with paraproteinemia. N Engl J Med 1998;338(22):1601–7.

31. Plasmati R, Pastorelli F, Cavo M, et al. Neuropathy in multiple myeloma treated with thalidomide: a prospective study. Neurology 2007;69(6):573–81.

32. Chaudhry V, Cornblath DR, Polydefkis M, et al. Characteristics of bortezomib- and thalidomide-induced peripheral neuropathy. J Peripher Nerv Syst 2008; 13(4):275–82.
33. Velasco R, Bruna J. Neurologic complications in multiple myeloma and plasma- cytoma. European Association of NeuroOncology Magazine 2012;2(2):71–7.
34. Dispenzieri A, Kyle RA. Multiple myeloma: clinical features and indications for therapy. Best Pract Res Clin Haematol 2005;18(4):553–68.
35. Talamo G, Farooq U, Zangari M, et al. Beyond the CRAB symptoms: a study of presenting clinical manifestations of multiple myeloma. Clin Lymphoma Myeloma Leuk 2010;10(6):464–8.
36. Saliou G, Kocheida el M, Lehmann P, et al. Percutaneous vertebroplasty for pain management in malignant fractures of the spine with epidural involvement. Radiology 2010;254(3):882–90.
37. Kapoor P, Paludo J, Vallumsetla N, et al. Waldenström macroglobulinemia: What a hematologist needs to know. Blood Rev 2015;29(5):301–19.
38. Marini A, Carulli G, Lari T, et al. Myelomatous meningitis evaluated by multiparam- eter flow cytometry: report of a case and review of the literature. J Clin Exp Hem- atop 2014;54(2):129–36.
39. Chamberlain MC, Glantz M. Myelomatous meningitis. Cancer 2008;112(7):1562–7.
40. Brum M, Antonio AS, Guerreiro R. Myelomatous meningitis: a rare neurological involvement in complete remission of multiple myeloma. J Neurol Sci 2014; 340(1–2):241–2.
41. Nieuwenhuizen L, Biesma DH. Central nervous system myelomatosis: review of the literature. Eur J Haematol 2008;80(1):1–9.

Imaging Manifestations of Neurologic Complications in Anemia

Ritesh Patel, MD[a], Shyam Sabat, MD[a], Sangam Kanekar, MD[a,b,*]

KEYWORDS

• Imaging • Neurologic complications • Anemia

KEY POINTS

• The hallmark signs and symptoms of anemia are directly related to a decrease in oxygen delivery to vital tissues and organs and include pallor, fatigue, lightheadedness, and shortness of breath. Neurologic complications are often nonspecific and can include poor concentration, irritability, faintness, tinnitus, and headache.

• If undiagnosed or untreated, depending on the cause, anemia can progress to cognitive dysfunction, psychosis, encephalopathy, myelopathy, peripheral neuropathy, as well as more focal syndromes, such as stroke, seizures, chorea, and/or transverse myelitis.

• Imaging can play a very important role in the early diagnosis and treatment of these neurologic and systemic complications associated with anemia, and hence, better outcome.

INTRODUCTION

Anemia, the most common disorder of the blood, affects more than 3 million Americans.[1] It is defined as a condition marked by a deficiency of red blood cells (RBCs) and/or hemoglobin diminishing the bloods ability to carry oxygen to vital organs leading to symptoms such as fatigue, lightheadedness, and shortness of breath. Anemia is divided into 3 main classes based on pathophysiology, including

1. Blood loss,
2. Increased destruction,
3. Impaired production of RBCs.

More commonly, anemia is classified by various causes and RBC parameters, including size/volume and hemoglobin content of the RBC. This morphologic

[a] Department of Radiology, Hershey Medical Center, The Pennsylvania State University, 500 University Drive, Hershey, PA 17033, USA; [b] Department of Neurology, Hershey Medical Center, The Pennsylvania State University, 500 University Drive, Hershey, PA 17033, USA
* Corresponding author. Department of Radiology, Hershey Medical Center, The Pennsylvania State University, 500 University Drive, Hershey, PA 17033.
E-mail address: skanekar@hmc.psu.edu

Hematol Oncol Clin N Am 30 (2016) 733–756
http://dx.doi.org/10.1016/j.hoc.2016.03.002   hemonc.theclinics.com
0889-8588/16/$ – see front matter © 2016 Elsevier Inc. All rights reserved.

classification is based on mean corpuscular volume (MCV) and on hemoglobin content of the RBC. The categories include normocytic (MCV between 80 and 100 fL), microcytic (MCV <80 fL), and macrocytic (MCV >100 fL), as well as normochromic (normal hemoglobin content) and hypochromic (low hemoglobin content).

The clinical manifestations of anemia vary markedly due to various causes, rate of progression, and severity. The hallmark signs and symptoms of anemia are directly related to a decrease in oxygen delivery to vital tissues and organs and include pallor, fatigue, lightheadedness, and shortness of breath. Neurologic complications are often nonspecific and can include poor concentration, irritability, faintness, tinnitus, and headache. If undiagnosed or untreated, depending on the cause, anemia can progress to cognitive dysfunction, psychosis, encephalopathy, myelopathy, peripheral neuropathy, as well as more focal syndromes, such as stroke, seizures, chorea, and/or transverse myelitis. Imaging can play a very important role in the early diagnosis and treatment of these neurologic and systemic complications associated with anemia, and hence, better outcome.

IMAGING MODALITIES

Anemia is a diagnosis made by routine blood workup. Type and associated cause are invariably diagnosed by clinical examination, blood smear, and bone marrow examination. Imaging is not a commonly used technique for evaluation of anemia. However, imaging plays an important role in the early diagnosis of the neurologic and systemic complications associated with anemia. Commonly used imaging techniques include plain radiography, ultrasonography, nuclear medicine, computed tomography (CT), and MRI.

Plain radiography is a fast and relatively inexpensive imaging technique for evaluation of bones, chest, and soft tissues. However, because of its low specificity and sensitivity, compared with the newer imaging techniques, it has lost its importance and application in the evaluation of the early disease process. Ultrasound is inexpensive, is easy to perform, and does not use ionizing radiation. It is predominately used to assess the intra-abdominal and soft organ abnormalities. Bone radionuclide scan is mainly used to assess bony abnormalities, such as metastasis and bone marrow abnormalities. It is very sensitive but lacks specificity to the abnormality. The advent of PET-CT and PET MR, which provide whole body evaluation, has provided a modality that is very useful in staging and assessing the response to various hematologic malignancies following therapy. CT remains the primary modality of choice in the evaluation of various neurologic disorders because of its easy availability and shorter scanning time. It is sensitive in diagnosing various acute neurologic complications, like intracranial hemorrhage, infarctions, and parenchymal and calvarial metastasis. However, it lacks sensitivity to detect posterior fossa lesions, leptomeningeal and dural abnormalities, or metabolic-related disorders. MRI remains the modality of choice for most brain and spine abnormalities because of its excellent soft tissue differentiation and multiplanar acquisition. It is very sensitive in diagnosing abnormalities ranging from neoplastic, metabolic, and inflammatory to infection. In respect to the hematologic disorders, it is very sensitive in diagnosing intracranial bleeds, infarctions, and leptomeningeal and dural abnormalities. It is also very sensitive in the diagnoses of bone marrow abnormalities.

IRON DEFICIENCY ANEMIA

Iron deficiency anemia (IDA) is the most common cause of anemia, often related to decreased dietary intake or an overall decrease in iron due to chronic bleeding (eg, gastrointestinal loss, menorrhagia), malabsorption disorders, or increased demand (eg, pregnancy).[2] Iron deficiency is a microcytic (MCV <80 fL), hypochromic (central pallor) anemia consistent with decreased iron, increased total iron binding capacity, and decreased ferritin. The workup for iron deficiency anemia involves identifying the source of the deficiency. Identifying the source of the deficiency often includes a through history, physical examination, complete blood count, blood smear, and stool and urine analysis. Rarely, imaging may be used, particularly to diagnose associated central nervous system (CNS) and musculoskeletal complications.

Neurologic symptoms are often nonspecific and include tiredness, fatigue, weakness, poor concentration, irritability, faintness, dizziness, tinnitus, and headache. These findings in an undiagnosed case of anemia are very challenging to link to a specific cause. The most common imaging finding seen in a patient with anemia is marrow reconversion. These findings are best appreciated on an MRI of the spine. Normally as the age advances, yellow marrow, which is predominately fat, replaces the appendicular as well as axial skeleton. Thus, a normal adult spine shows hyperintensity in the vertebral bodies on T1-weighted and fast-spin T2-weighted images (**Fig. 1**). In cases of marrow reconversion, diffuse hypointensity is seen throughout the axial skeleton due to red marrow (**Fig. 2**). These changes may be associated with diffuse dull back pain.

Various case reports have also shown an association of IDA with benign intracranial hypertension and cerebral venous sinus thrombosis.[2–4] Waxing and waning of the benign intracranial hypertension symptoms have been documented with recurrence and resolution of the iron deficiency anemia. On the background of carotid vessels atherosclerosis, iron deficiency anemia may cause focal neurologic signs. These changes are particularly seen in elderly patients with severe anemia. These symptoms may rapidly improve following blood transfusion and an increase in hemoglobin. Restless legs syndrome has also been shown to be strongly associated with IDA.[5]

Some patients may present with thrombocytosis due to repeated stimulation of the bone marrow from chronic anemia. This increase in the platelet mass may cause transient blockade of the intracranial vessels, giving rise to transient cerebral ischemic attacks (TIAs), amaurosis fugax, or cerebral infarction. Diffusion-weighted imaging– apparent diffusion coefficient images are very sensitive for the diagnosis of this tiny lacunar infarction in the supratentorial and infratentorial brain parenchyma. Profound anemia, if associated with thrombocytopenia (mostly in adults) and erythroblastopenia (in childhood), frequently presents with ocular symptoms. These ocular symptoms may include papilledema, cotton-wool exudates, flame-shaped hemorrhages, retinal edema, and very rarely, detachment.

Thalassemia

Thalassemia is an autosomal-recessive disorder that results in a microcytic, hypochromic anemia similar to that of iron deficiency anemia (**Fig. 3**). Normal adult hemoglobin consists of 98% hemoglobin A (HbA; 2 α-globin chains and 2 β-globin chains) and 2% HbA2 (2 α-chains and 2 δchains). In thalassemia, a genetic defect causes the patient to produce a deficient amount of either α- or β-globin, resulting in a quantitative problem of globin synthesis. Thalassemia is classified depending on the globin chain (αor β) that is reduced. The diagnosis of thalassemia can be confirmed via hemoglobin electrophoresis.

The clinical presentation of these patients widely depends on the severity of the disease. The ineffective erythropoiesis leads to anemia, hepatosplenomegaly, and extramedullary erythropoiesis with skeletal deformities. Skeletal abnormalities are often due to the expansion and invasion of erythroid bone marrow, which widen the marrow

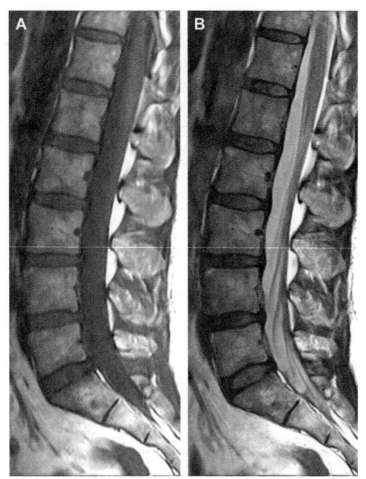

Fig. 1. Normal bone marrow appearance on MRI. Sagittal T1-weighted (T1W) (*A*), and T2-weighted (T2W) (*B*) images of the lumbar spine show normal hyperintensity in comparison with disc signal and slightly hypointense compared with subcutaneous fat on T1W and T2W image.

spaces, attenuate the cortex, and produce osteopenia/osteoporosis. These changes are typically seen in the spine, the skull, and the facial bones, as well as the ribs and the metaphyses of the long bones.

The spine shows diffuse marrow conversion, osteopenia, and a decrease in the subchondral bone thickness leading to multisegmental end-plate compression fractures. On imaging, vertebrae are biconcave or wedge shaped. As the disease progresses, compression fractures as well as paravertebral expansion of extramedullary masses become more prominent. These changes can progress to back pain, spinal asymmetry and scoliosis, cord compression from intraspinal collections of hematopoietic tissue, and intervertebral disc degeneration. Organs such as the liver, spleen, and kidneys are often enlarged due to extramedullary hematopoiesis.

Marrow hyperplasia widens the diploic space with thinning of the outer skull, reduction of trabeculae, granular osteopenia, and solitary or multiple circumscribed osteolytic areas. The classic "hair-on-end" appearance is due to a periosteal reaction that

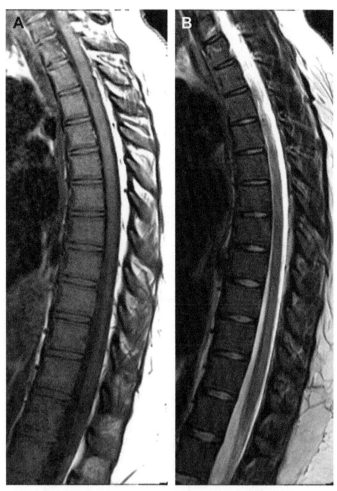

Fig. 2. IDA with marrow reconversion. Sagittal T1W (*A*) and T2W (*B*) images of the thoracic spine show diffusely T1 hypointense marrow signal throughout the vertebrae, consistent with red marrow reconversion.

manifests as perpendicular trabeculations interspersed with radiolucent marrow hyperplasia along the skull vault. The expansion of the facial bones inhibits the pneumatization of the paranasal sinuses leading to lateral displacement of the orbits and maxillary protrusion with ventral displacement, ultimately producing the characteristic "chipmunk facies" (**Fig. 4**).

Extramedullary hematopoiesis (EMH) is a compensatory process associated with chronic hemolytic anemia that occurs in the hematopoietic elements outside the bone marrow when the bone marrow is unable to maintain sufficient RBC production to suffice for the body's demand. It often occurs in patients with a myeloproliferative disorder or hemoglobinopathies such as sickle cell disease (SCD), thalassemia, or hereditary spherocytosis (HS). Common sites include the spleen, liver, and lymph nodes leading to organomegaly. EMH is commonly seen in the paraspinal region, which may extend into the spinal canal, leading to cord compression and myelopathic changes. These masses are isointense on both T1- and T2-weighted images. In addition,

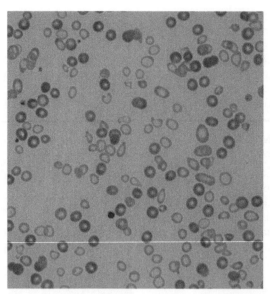

Fig. 3. Peripheral smear from a child with thalassemia. The child had hemoglobin of 7.5 g/dL, RBC of 5.9 × 106/μL, and an MCV of 47 fL, consistent with a diagnosis of thalassemia. Smear shows marked RBC microcytosis and hypochromia. The child had received an RBC transfusion before the smear was performed, accounting for the dual population of RBCs. Wright-Giemsa stain, original magnification ×100.

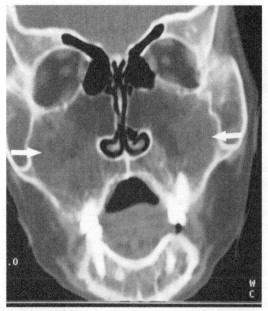

Fig. 4. Chipmunk facies in thalassemia. Coronal CT scan of the paranasal sinuses shows expansion of the facial bones with nonpneumatization of the bilateral maxillary sinuses (*arrows*) and ethmoid air cells, leading to mild lateral displacement of the orbits producing the characteristic "chipmunk facies."

vertebral bodies are found to have low- to intermediate-signal intensity due to the displacement of fatty marrow with hematopoietic marrow.[6]

Patients that are adequately treated with repeated transfusions have less medullary expansion but high serum iron levels. This iron overload gets deposited in the various organs of the body, including bone marrow. MRI in these patients shows low signal intensity of the axial, appendicular skeleton and other soft tissue organs on T2 and gradient echo sequence (**Fig. 5**).

VITAMIN DEFICIENCY ANEMIA
Vitamin B12 Deficiency

Vitamin B12 deficiency causes a characteristic megaloblastic anemia (MCV >100 fL) and an ineffective erythropoiesis. Pernicious anemia, or the absence or deficiency of intrinsic factor, is the most common cause of vitamin B12 deficiency.[7] Other causes include nutritional deficiency (vegans, elderly, alcoholics), malabsorption syndromes, type B atrophic gastritis, abnormality of the distal ileum (Crohn, resection, Whipple), colonization of small bowel with bacteria or intestinal parasite, and chronic infections,

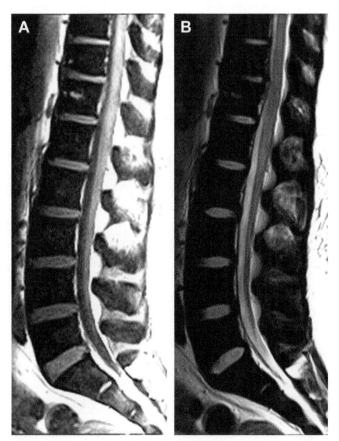

Fig. 5. Thalassemia with hemosiderosis. Sagittal T1W (A) and T2W (B) images of the lumbar spine show diffusely hypointense marrow signal related to iron overload from chronic transfusions.

such as human immunodeficiency virus (HIV), congenital syndromes (Imerslund-Gras-beck syndrome), and medications.

Vitamin B12 deficiency may take decades to develop. Patients may be asymptom-atic or present with a wide spectrum of hematologic and neuropsychiatric manifesta-tions. Vitamin B12 deficiency causes a typical pattern of degeneration of the white matter in the CNS that can be manifested clinically as encephalopathy, myelopathy, peripheral neuropathy, and optic neuropathy.

Subacute combined degeneration of the cord is associated with vitamin B12 defi-ciency, due to demyelination and axonal degeneration of the most heavily myelinated fibers, such as posterior and lateral columns of the cord. It is most commonly seen at the midthoracic level. Clinical presentations include paresthesia in the hands and feet, with progression to sensory loss, gait ataxia, and distal weakness, especially in the legs.

On MRI, linear T2 hyperintensity is seen on the posterior aspect of the cord, specif-ically on sagittal T2 images. On an axial plane, symmetric bilateral areas of T2 hyper-intensity are seen in the dorsal columns, giving an "inverted V sign" appearance (**Fig. 6**). The signal changes typically begin in the upper thoracic region, with ascending or descending progression. The lateral corticospinal tracts and sometimes lateral spinothalamic tract may also have similar signal intensity changes. Unfortu-nately, symptoms often precede months or years before any imaging abnormality is identified. Therefore, spinal cord abnormality on MRI is not very sensitive as an early test for subacute combined degeneration.[8,9]

Cerebral white matter parenchyma may also show focal or diffuse areas of demye-lination with little evidence of glial cell proliferation or axonal degeneration. These changes predominate in the corpus callosum and in the frontal and parietal white mat-ter. Clinically, they may present with signs and symptoms of encephalopathy. Symp-toms may include disorders of mood, mental slowing, poor memory, confusion,

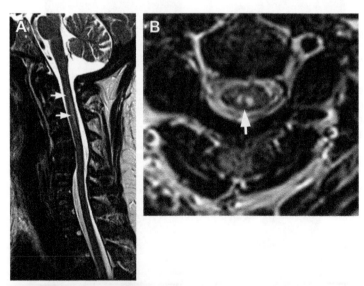

Fig. 6. (*A, B*) Megaloblastic anemia with subacute combined degeneration. Sagittal T2W (*A*) image of the cervical spine shows linear T2 hyperintensity (*arrows*) in the posterior aspect of the cervical cord. Axial T2W (*B*) image shows symmetric bilateral T2 hyperintensity in the dorsal columns, giving an "inverted V sign" appearance (*arrow*).

agitation, delusions, visual and auditory hallucinations, aggression, dysphasia, and in-continence. Fluid-attenuated inversion recovery (FLAIR) and T2-weighted images can demonstrate extensive areas of high-intensity signal in the periventricular white matter, often bilateral and symmetric. Infantile encephalopathy due to vitamin B12 deficiency may show MRI changes similar to many other metabolic disorders with bilateral and symmetric hyperintensity in the putamen, anterior thalamus, periaqueductal, and posterior parts of the brainstem.

Other neurologic presentations in vitamin B12 deficiency include peripheral neuropathy and optic neuropathy; these are diagnosed clinically and supplemented with evoked potentials studies. Imaging offers very limited information in the diagnosis of these conditions.

FOLATE DEFICIENCY

Like vitamin B12 deficiency, folate deficiency also gives a megaloblastic anemia (MCV >100 fL). Causes include malnutrition (eg, alcoholics), malabsorption, medications (eg, methotrexate, trimethoprim, phenytoin), and increased requirement (eg, pregnancy). Unlike vitamin B12 deficiency, folate deficiency results in increased homocysteine levels, but normal methionine levels and therefore results in minimal to no neurologic symptoms.

Kearns-Sayre Syndrome

Kearns-Sayre syndrome (KSS) is a condition caused by a defect in mitochondria due to a single, large deletion of mitochondrial DNA resulting in impaired oxidative phosphorylation and decreased cellular energy production. Because KSS is a multisystem disorder, it can result in various clinical features, including short stature, cardiac conduction defects, muscle weakness, anemia, renal abnormalities, diabetes, deafness, ataxia, and cognitive deficits. The choroid plexus, the main site of active folate transport to the CNS, is a target organ of KSS. It is suggested that the accumulation of mitochondrial DNA mutations in the choroid plexus leads to increased levels of protein in the cerebrospinal fluid (CSF; >100 mg/dL) and reduced levels of 5-methyltetrahydrofolate, resulting in a profound cerebral folate deficiency.

Diagnosis of KSS is made by history, physical examination, laboratory analysis (eg, CSF protein levels, serum creatine kinase, and folate levels), imaging, muscle biopsies, and genetic testing. Neuroimaging is often helpful in documenting the abnormality in the deep gray matter nuclei and cerebral white matter. CT or MRI shows cerebral, cerebellar, and brainstem atrophy. CT scan shows siderocalcific deposits in the basal ganglia and subcortical region. The characteristic MRI findings include high T2 signal intensity in subcortical cerebral white matter, brainstem, globus pallidus, or thalamus (**Fig. 7**). These areas may also show high signal on T1-weighted images.[10,11]

PAROXYSMAL NOCTURNAL HEMOGLOBINURIA

Paroxysmal nocturnal hemoglobinuria (PNH) is an acquired intravascular hemolytic disorder of a hematopoeitic stem cell caused by a mutation within the phosphatidyl inositol glycan-class A gene, resulting in increased sensitivity to complement-mediated erythrocyte lysis. A diagnosis of PNH can be confirmed by a positive Ham test (hemolysis acid test) and a positive sucrose hemolysis test.

Major clinical features include severe hemolysis, hemoglobinuria, and venous thrombosis. Most neurologic symptoms and complications in PNH are related to large vessel thrombosis. Thrombosis may be arterial or venous and may occur in cerebral or spinal cord vessels leading to hemorrhagic infarction. MRI is the method of choice for

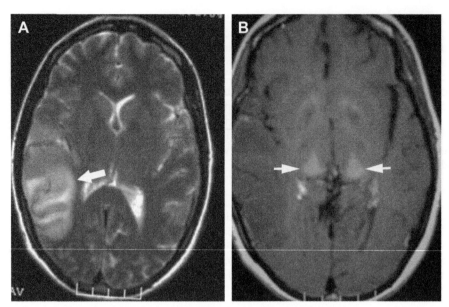

Fig. 7. KSS. Axial T2W (*A*) image of the brain shows subacute infarction (*arrow*) in the right parieto-occipital lobe. Axial T1W (*B*) image at the level of thalamus shows bilateral symmetric hyperintensity in the thalami (*arrows*) due to siderocalcific deposition.

assessing vascular patency and associated cerebral parenchymal abnormality. MR angiogram (MRA) and MR venogram will show the acute blockade of the thrombosed artery or nonvisualization of the venous sinuses (**Fig. 8**). In the acute crises of PNH, the patient may present with TIAs and subarachnoid hemorrhage.[12–14]

HEREDITARY SPHEROCYTOSIS

HS is the most common normocytic, hemolytic anemia due to a red cell membrane defect. It is most commonly caused by an alteration in the ankyrin gene and results in an unusual spherical shape of the RBCs. These abnormally shaped cells are sequestered by the spleen leading to jaundice, splenomegaly, reticulocytosis, and variable degrees of anemia. The diagnosis can be established by either an eosin-5-maleimide binding test, osmotic gradient ektacytometry, or osmotic fragility testing in conjunction with careful examination of peripheral blood smears.[15]

Long-standing, undetected HS can result in skeletal changes in the skull and vertebrae in the form of marrow hyperplasia, osteopenia, and coarsened trabeculations. The hair-on-end sign is a common feature found on radiographs. EMH associated with bone marrow reconversion has also been reported in HS. EMH can involve the posterior paravertebral mediastinum extending into the central canal and causing compression of the cord. On MRI, EMH masses are isointense lesions on T1- and T2-weighted images. Paramagnetic agents may cause an intermediate enhancement of the mass. The vertebral bodies have low-to-intermediate signal intensity because of the displacement of fatty marrow by hematopoietic marrow.[15]

APLASTIC ANEMIA

Aplastic anemia is characterized by diminished or absent hematopoietic precursors resulting in pancytopenia and a hypocellular bone marrow. Stem cell failure can be

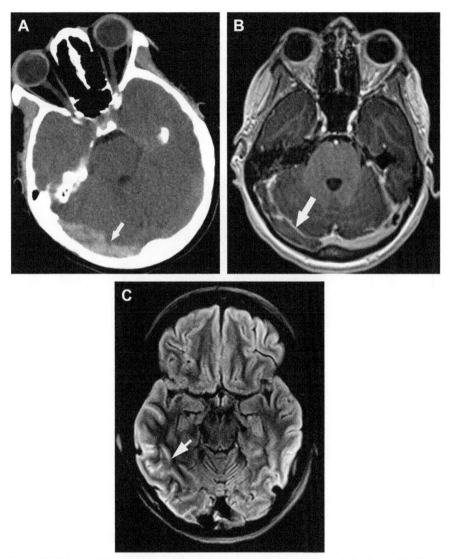

Fig. 8. PNH in an 11-year-old patient with seizures. Axial CT scan of the brain (*A*) shows expansion and hyperdensity (*arrow*) in the right lateral and sigmoid sinus. Axial contrast-enhanced T1W image (*B*) shows nonopacification (*arrow*) of the right lateral and sigmoid sinus compatible with sinus thrombosis. Axial FLAIR image (*C*) shows right temporo-occipital gyri hyperintensity (*arrow*) due to cerebral edema.

congenital (eg, Fanconi anemia) or acquired via ionizing radiation, medications (chloramphenicol, carbamazepine, phenytoin, sulfonamides), or viruses (parovirus B19, HIV). In most patients, the pathogenesis cannot be determined and is termed idiopathic.[16]

Aplastic anemia has a varied clinical course, which ranges from mild symptoms that necessitate little or no therapy to life-threatening pancytopenia that necessitates bone marrow transplantation and high-dose immunosuppression. Clinical presentation is due to anemia (fatigue and cardiac/pulmonary symptoms), neutropenia (recurrent infections), and thrombocytopenia (hemorrhages). Diagnosis is confirmed by bone marrow aspirate and trephine biopsy. The bone marrow biopsy will be hypocellular with a decrease in all elements. Bone marrow space will be predominately composed of fat cells and stroma.

MRI is useful in detecting the differences in fatty and active hematopoietic marrow. Because of the absence of cellular elements and abundant presence of fatty marrow in aplastic anemia, MR will show increased signal intensity on T1- and T2-weighted images (**Fig. 9**). Active hematopoietic cells may be seen as focal areas of low-signal

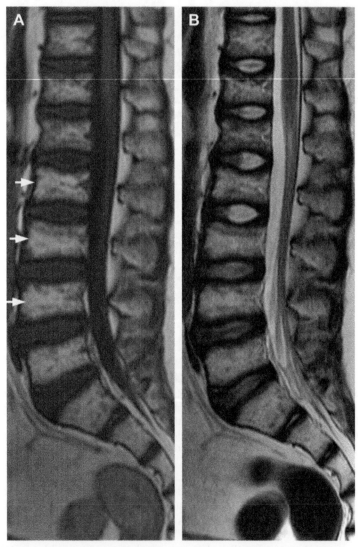

Fig. 9. Aplastic anemia. Sagittal T1W (*A*), and T2W (*B*) images of the lumbar spine show increased signal intensity (*arrows*) on T1W and T2W images due to the absence of cellular elements and abundant presence of fatty marrow in aplastic anemia.

interspersed on the background of high-signal intensity. This finding is nonspecific and may be seen in myelodysplastic disorders, lymphoma, myeloma, and metastases. MRI is also an effective method for evaluating bone marrow recovery in aplastic anemia after treatment. The MRI of the spine of a patient responding to therapy will initially be patchy and later present as diffuse hypointensity on T1-weighted images.

Thrombocytopenia, regardless of cause, is a risk factor for spontaneous intracranial hemorrhage. Development of spontaneous subdural hematomas and/or large intraparenchymal hemorrhages is a potential complication of aplastic anemia. Intracranial bleeds are seen in about 20% of patients with aplastic anemia.[17] A CT scan is usually the first imaging modality used to assess patients with suspected intracranial hemorrhages. An acute bleed is hyperdense relative to brain parenchyma on CT (**Fig. 10**). Subdural hematomas are interposed between the dura and arachnoid and are easily detected on CT scans. The appearance of subdural hematomas varies based on the age of the clot and therefore is divided into acute (1–3 days, hyperdensce on CT), subacute (4 days to 2 weeks, isodence on CT), and chronic (>2 weeks, hypodence on CT) (**Fig. 11**).

Fanconi Anemia

Fanconi anemia is a rare inherited blood disorder caused by genetic defects in various genes responsible for DNA repair. This disorder is characterized by pancytopenia, macrocytic anemia, congenital malformations, and an increased risk of acute myeloid leukemia as well as other tumors. Approximately 90% of people with Fanconi anemia have impaired bone marrow function that leads to aplastic anemia. These patients may also develop myelodysplastic anemia. Clinical symptoms include hypopigmentation, café-au-lait spots, malformed limbs, short stature, defects in the kidneys and

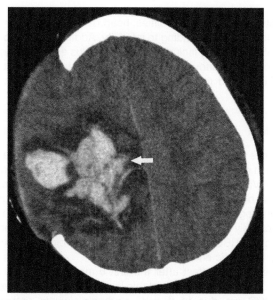

Fig. 10. Aplastic anemia. CT scan of the brain shows large intracranial bleed (*arrow*) in the right frontoparietal lobe in an aplastic anemia patient who presented with acute head and left-sided hemiplegia. Craniectomy was performed as a treatment for raised intracranial pressure.

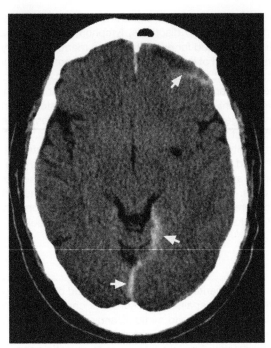

Fig. 11. Aplastic anemia with thrombocytopenia. CT scan of the brain shows acute subdural hematoma (*arrows*) along the tentorium and a subacute subdural hematoma in the left frontal lobe. Wright-Giemsa stain, original magnification ×100.

urinary tract, gastrointestinal abnormalities, heart defects, eye abnormalities, hearing loss, and reproductive defects leading to infertility. Additional symptoms include brain and spinal cord abnormalities, including hydrocephalus and microcephaly. Brain and spine may be involved by various primary or metastatic tumors. Most commonly seen is the leptomeningeal and parenchymal involvement from acute myeloid leukemia (**Fig. 12**).

SICKLE CELL ANEMIA

Sickle cell disease is an autosomal-recessive hereditary condition caused by a single nucleotide mutation of the β-globin gene that replaces the sixth amino acid, glutamic acid, with valine.[18] Valine is hydrophobic, which causes the hemoglobin to collapse on itself. The resultant, hemoglobin molecules, hemoglobin S, tend to clump together into long polymers, making the RBC elongated (sickle shaped) (**Fig. 13**), rigid, and unable to deform appropriately when passing though small vessels, resulting in vascular occlusion. The abnormal RBCs are also removed from the bloodstream at an increased rate, leading to a hemolytic anemia.

Clinical findings often manifest after the first 6 months, because babies are protected by elevated levels of fetal hemoglobin in the first 6 months. Neurologic complications in the SCD are due to 3 main pathophysiologic processes: increased destruction of the sickle cells leading to chronic anemia, clumping of the sickle cells leading to vaso-oclusion, and damage to the immune system leading to increased rate of infection.

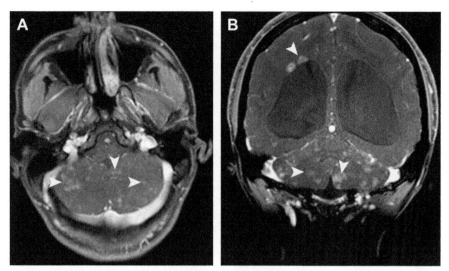

Fig. 12. Fanconi anemia. Contrast-enhanced axial (*A*) and coronal (*B*) T1W images show diffuse leptomeningeal metastasis (*arrowheads*) in the supratentorial and infratentorial brain parenchyma with moderate hydrocephalus.

Changes of chronic anemia cause marrow reconversion in the axial skeleton and expansion of the medullary space. Bone marrow expansion is manifested in the skull as a widening of diploic space with thinning of the inner and outer tables. Vertical hair-on-end striations are also seen due to prominence of trabeculae and new bone formation. Vaso-occlusion due to sickling leads to blood stasis and sequestration, which leads to ischemia and hypoxia in the bone. These infarcts are often the source of pain in acute bone crises. Infarcts are best appreciated on short time inversion recovery (STIR) and fat-saturated T2-weighted images, where they appear as hyperintense areas with irregular margins (**Fig. 14**). Another manifestation of infarction is H-shaped

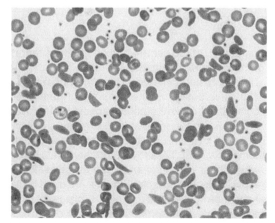

Fig. 13. Peripheral smear from a patient with SCD illustrates the spectrum of RBC findings, which include sickle cells, polychromatophilic RBCs, target cells, and Howell-Jolly bodies.

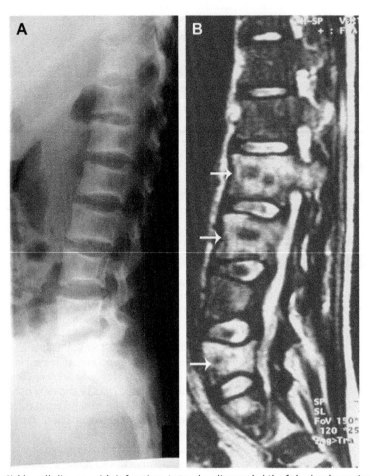

Fig. 14. Sickle cell disease with infarction. Lateral radiograph (*A*) of the lumbar spine shows "H-shaped" vertebral bodies, which are classic in SCD. Sagittal T2W (*B*) image of the lumbar spine shows abnormal heterogeneous T2 signal in the multiple lumbar vertebrae (*arrows*) consistent with infarcts.

vertebrae due to the infarction of the central portion of the vertebra from occlusion of the long branches of the vertebral nutrient artery.[19]

Osteomyelitis is commonly encountered in sickle cell patients due to functional asplenia, diminished opsonic activity of the serum, and poor antibody response to the polysaccharide component of the bacterial capsule. Osteomyelitis of long bones and vertebrae presents as fever, tenderness, and swelling and is clinically difficult to differentiate from infarction. MRI with contrast is the imaging method of choice for the diagnosis of osteomyelitis. MRI, T2, and STIR demonstrate increased signal intensity in the vertebrae with enhancing prespinal and paraspinal soft tissue. There may be an intraspinal or paraspinal abscess present (**Fig. 15**). Although MRI is very sensitive in identifying the signal changes in the bone and surrounding soft tissues, it lacks specificity in differentiating early infection from infarct.[20,21]

The incidence of neurologic manifestations in patients with SCD is seen in approximately 25%. These manifestations are mainly due to damage to the intima by sickled

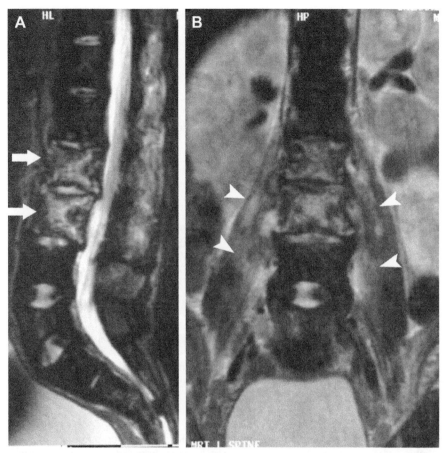

Fig. 15. Sickle cell disease with osteomyelitis. Sagittal T2W (*A*) image of the lumbar spine shows hyperintensity in the 2 contiguous vertebrae (L2 and L3) (*arrows*). Coronal T2W (*B*) image shows loculated hyperintense collections (*arrowheads*) within bilateral psoas muscles consistent with osteomyelitis with psoas abscess.

cells, leading to vascular stenosis and occlusion. Intimal damage may result from high-velocity blood flow, the shape of the sickle cells, adherence of RBCs to the endothelium, endothelial damage, intravascular sludge, intimal hyperplasia, or thrombosis. Vascular changes in SCD have 4 angiographic manifestations: proximal arterial occlusion/stenosis, distal branch occlusion secondary to thrombosis or embolism, moyamoya syndrome, and aneurysm.

Cerebrovascular involvement leading to brain infarction is one of the most severe and common complications of SCD, affecting 25% of patients with the disease (**Fig. 16**). Stenosis of the intracranial internal carotid artery (ICA), especially the distal portion, is more common than extracranial ICA stenosis. Intracranial velocities greater than 170 to 200 cm/s indicate significant risk for infarction and are shown to correlate with areas of MRI abnormality and vessel narrowing. Clinical signs and symptoms are mostly related to either cerebral ischemia or hemorrhage. Ischemic events with the classic scenario of alternating hemiparesis are seen early

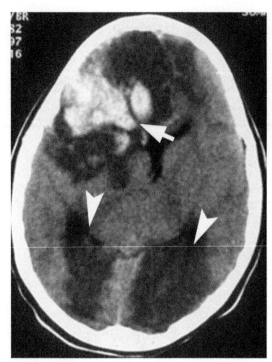

Fig. 16. Sickle cell disease with cerebral infarctions and bleed. Axial CT scan of the brain shows bilateral posterior cerebral artery territory infarctions (*arrowheads*) and acute intra-parenchymal bleed in the right frontal lobe (*arrow*).

in the course of vaso-occlusion. Ischemic stroke is more common in younger patients, whereas parenchymal hemorrhage is more frequent in older individuals. MRI of the brain may show multiple tiny dilated vessels in the region of deep gray matter nuclei with various small- and medium-sized areas of infarctions in the cerebral parenchyma. There may be scattered foci of microhemorrhages or macrohemorrhages.[19–21]

Occlusion or stenosis of the distal ICA leads to reduced cerebral blood flow and development of fine collateral vascular channels, usually from the thalamoperforate and lenticulostriate arteries. This process is named moyamoya, meaning puff of smoke in Japanese (**Fig. 17**). MRA or CT angiogram of head shows stenosis or occlusion of distal internal carotid arteries and/or proximal portions of the middle and/or anterior cerebral arteries combined with an abundance of dilated, thin-walled collateral branches of the circle of Willis. A fine network of vessels at the base of the brain is seen as a hazy, puff-of-smoke appearance, hence the name. As the middle and anterior cerebral arteries become affected, there is development of leptomeningeal, extracranial, transdural, and transosseous collaterals. Perfusion studies may show a severe decrease in the blood flow throughout the supratentorial white matter with an increase in the mean transit time.[22]

Endothelial damage of the vessel wall may lead to aneurysm formation. Aneurysms are multiple in the majority (57%) of patients with SCD and often originate from the vertebrobasilar system. Aneurysms may manifest as subarachnoid hemorrhage and rarely as intraparenchymal hemorrhage (**Fig. 18**).

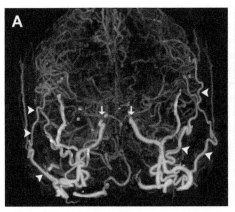
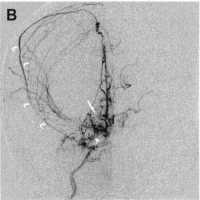

Fig. 17. SCD with moyamoya. Time-of-flight MRA head (*A*) shows severe stenosis of distal ICAs and proximal MCAs bilaterally (*arrows*) with extensive collaterals from external carotid artery (*arrowheads*), suggestive of moyamoya. Frontal view of the conventional angiogram of the head (*B*) shows severe narrowing of the right ICA (*arrowhead*) with multiple extracranial (*curved arrows*), transdural, and intracranial (*arrow*) collaterals. Please note multiple dilated collaterals from the lenticulostriate vessels "puff of smoke" (*arrow*).

GLUCOSE-6-PHOSPHATE DEHYDROGENASE DEFICIENCY

Glucose-6-phosphate dehydrogenase (G6PD) deficiency is an inherited, X-linked, metabolic disorder and the most common enzyme disorder in humans, affecting 400 million people worldwide.[23] It is most prevalent in people of Africa, Asian, and

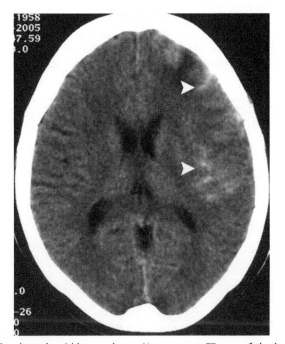

Fig. 18. SCD with subarachnoid hemorrhage. Noncontrast CT scan of the brain shows acute subarachnoid hemorrhage (*arrowheads*) in the left frontoparietal convexity.

Mediterranean descent. G6PD catalyzes the oxidation of glucose-6-phosphate and the reduction of NADP+ to NADPH in the pentose monophosphate shunt. NADPH is important in maintaining glutathione in its reduced form, which protects the RBC against oxidative stress. In a patient with G6PD deficiency, oxidative stress can lead to intravascular hemolysis and therefore anemia.

Neurologic symptoms are mostly related to the bilirubin encephalopathy resulting from increasing levels of unconjugated bilirubin levels from hemolysis. Kernicterus is more likely to occur in premature infants of less than 32 weeks gestation than in term neonates. Signs and symptoms include jaundice, lethargy, weakness, seizures, spasticity, and choreoathetosis. Unconjugated bilirubin is highly lipid soluble; it enters the brain and binds to neurons, resulting in neuronal necrosis. Toxic effects of bilirubin are most concentrated in the striatum, globus pallidus, hippocampus, substantia nigra, brainstem nuclei, and the dentate nucleus of cerebellum. MRI of the brain shows changes of necrosis in these regions, mainly in the deep gray matter nuclei (**Fig. 19**).

PYRUVATE KINASE DEFICIENCY

Pyruvate kinase deficiency is an enzymatic defect of the erythrocyte that clinically manifests as hemolytic anemia. Pyruvate kinase is a mitochondrial enzyme that is required for the conversion of pyruvate to acetyl-CoA. Similar to G6PD deficiency, pyruvate kinase deficiency results in growth delay, hyperbilirubinemia, jaundice, and splenomegaly.[24]

Laboratory findings consist of normochromic, normocytic anemia with reticulocytosis, elevated blood lactate and pyruvate levels, as well as a normal lactate-to-pyruvate ratio. The diagnosis can be confirmed with an enzyme assay or a DNA analysis with polymer chain reaction. Imaging studies are useful in demonstrating findings of marrow expansion in severe anemia.

Interestingly, the neurologic presentation of PDHA1 deficiency is variable and differs between male and female patients. Imaging features in male patients include subependymal cysts and agenesis of corpus callous. In female patients, brain anomalies include absence or hypoplasia of the corpus callosum thin cerebral mantle and

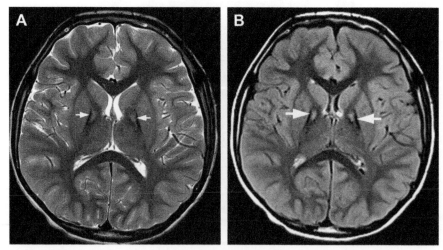

Fig. 19. G6PD deficiency. Axial T2 (*A*) and FLAIR (*B*) images show bilateral symmetrical hyperintensity in the globus pallidi (*arrows*) due to neuronal necrosis from kernicterus.

enlargement of the ventricles. Brain imaging reveals asymmetric enlargement of the lateral and third ventricles, often sparing the fourth ventricle. Intraventricular septations are also present as well as prominent paucity of cerebral white matter volume and a small pons. An incomplete corpus callosum, specifically missing the posterior body and splenium, can be seen on sagittal T1 and axial T2 images. The recognition of these MRI patterns should prompt further investigation for molecular testing for PDHA1 mutations/pyruvate kinase deficiency.

SECONDARY CAUSES OF ANEMIA

Secondary anemia is defined as anemia that does not result from a hematologic disease process. Secondary anemia could be due to various causes and may vary widely from mild to severe anemia. Common causes of the secondary anemia include chronic infection, liver or renal disease, metabolic disorders, and underlying neoplasm with penetration of malignant cells in bone marrow. It is important to diagnose and treat the underlying cause in cases of secondary anemia.[25]

Myeloma

Multiple myeloma is the most primary malignant bone neoplasm in adults characterized by neoplastic proliferation of plasma cells producing a monoclonal immunoglobulin that infiltrate hematopoietic locations. This plasma cell proliferation in the bone marrow leads to anemia as well as a decrease in the precursors of the other blood cells. Anemia seen with myeloma is a normocytic, normochromic anemia and is related to bone marrow replacement or kidney damage.

Imaging, in the setting of multiple myeloma, serves many roles, including diagnosing, assessing pathologic complications, and assessing disease progression. MRI is more sensitive in detecting multiple lesions and allows for great visualization of infiltration and replacement of the bone marrow. Multiple myeloma shows 2 common radiological appearances:

1. Numerous, well-circumscribed lytic bone lesions
2. Generalized osteopenia or marrow replacement, with or without vertebral compression fractures (**Fig. 20**).

For detailed imaging appearances of multiple myeloma, please refer to (see Amos B, Kanekar S, Agarwal A: Imaging of Multiple Myeloma, in this issue).

Systemic Lupus Erythematosus

Systemic lupus erythematosus (SLE) is a chronic autoimmune and inflammatory disease that results in tissue damage in multiple organs by autoantibodies and immune complexes. The diagnosis of SLE is based on a combination of clinical and laboratory findings. Hematologic abnormalities are common in SLE and include anemia, leukopenia, thrombocytopenia, and antiphospholipid syndrome. Anemia is found in almost half of SLE patients and is thought to be due to multifactorial mechanisms including inflammation, erythropoietin deficiency, renal insufficiency, blood loss, dietary insufficiency, medications, hemolysis, infection, hypersplenism, myelodysplasia, and/or aplastic anemia. As a result, in the setting of anemia in an SLE patient, one must identify the underlying cause to treat the patient appropriately.

The neurologic manifestations of SLE are highly diverse, and the cause is often not entirely understood. SLE can affect the central, peripheral, and autonomic nervous system and produce symptoms such as cognitive dysfunction, psychosis,

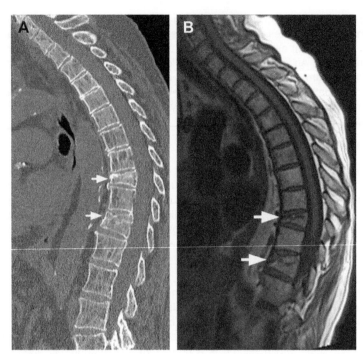

Fig. 20. Multiple myeloma. Sagittal reconstructed (*A*) image from the CT scan of the thora-columbar spine shows diffuse osteopenia. There are compression deformities of the T7 and T9 (*arrows*). Sagittal T1W (*B*) image of the thoracic spine shows diffuse hypointense marrow signal throughout the vertebrae, consistent with red marrow reconversion. Again seen are chronic compression deformities (*arrows*) of the T7 and T9.

depression, headache, confusion, as well as more focal syndromes, such as stroke, seizures, chorea, and/or transverse myelitis. SLE can also lead to CNS vasculitis.

Evaluation of CNS complications in SLE requires a brain MRI, MRA, and a spinal tap. Principal findings include mild prominence of convexity sulci and widespread confluent T2 hyperintensities in the white matter due to chronic hypoperfusion. MRA may show associated changes of vasculitis. Unfortunately, in a large group of patients with SLE, no MRI abnormalities are usually found, even with the presence of clinical signs and symptoms for active disease.

Myelodysplastic Syndrome

Myelodysplastic syndrome (MDS) is characterized by ineffective hematopoiesis with bone marrow dysplasia. MDS is further divided into primary or secondary. Primary MDS is characterized by a lack of causal factors and associated with genetic predis-position and somatic mutations. Secondary MDS, also recognized as treatment-related MDS, is associated with previous anticancer treatment and is observed in patients after chemotherapy or radiation therapy. The final diagnosis of MDS involves a bone marrow aspiration and biopsy. The major causes of death in MDS are the development of leukemia and hemorrhage or infection related to the pancytopenia.

Imaging is mostly used to diagnose marrow changes in the spine and for any intra-cranial hemorrhage or infarctions. Because MRI is sensitive in the assessment of bone marrow, it allows the detection and evaluation of infiltrations of neoplastic cells in the spine. T1-weighted images show focal or diffuse hypointensities, with corresponding hyperintensity on T2-weighted images.

REFERENCES

1. Anemia. American Society of Hematology. 2016. Available at: http://www. hematology.org/Patients/Anemia/. Accessed May 15, 2016.
2. Mollan SP, Ball AK, Sinclair AJ, et al. Idiopathic intracranial hypertension associated with iron deficiency anemia: a lesson for management. Eur Neurol 2009; 62(2):105–8.
3. Kinoshita Y, Taniura S, Shishido H, et al. Cerebral venous sinus thrombosis associated with iron deficiency: two case reports. Neurol Med Chir (Tokyo) 2006; 46(12):589–93.
4. Beri S, Khan A, Hussain N, et al. Severe anemia causing cerebral venous sinus thrombosis in an infant. J Pediatr Neurosci 2012;7(1):30–2.
5. Allen RP, Earley CJ. The role of iron in restless legs syndrome. Mov Disord 2007; 22(Suppl 18):S440–8.
6. Chourmouzi D, Pistevou-Gompaki K, Plataniotis G, et al. MRI findings of extramedullary haemopoiesis. Eur Radiol 2001;11(9):1803–6.
7. Sen A, Chandrasekhar K. Spinal MR imaging in vitamin B12 deficiency: case series; differential diagnosis of symmetrical posterior spinal cord lesions. Ann Indian Acad Neurol 2013;16(2):255–8.
8. Sethi N, Robilotti E, Sadan Y. Neurological manifestations of vitamin B-12 deficiency. Internet J Nutr Wellness 2004;2(1).
9. Locatelli E, Laureno R, Ballard P, et al. MRI in vitamin B12 deficiency myelopathy. Can J Neurol Sci 1999;26(1):60–3.
10. Serrano M, García-Silva MT, Martin-Hernandez E, et al. Kearns-Sayre syndrome: cerebral folate deficiency, MRI findings and new cerebrospinal fluid biochemical features. Mitochondrion 2010;10(5):429–32.
11. Chu BC, Terae S, Takahashi C, et al. MRI of the brain in the Kearns-Sayre syndrome: report of four cases and a review. Neuroradiology 1999;41(10):759–64.
12. Verswijvel G, Vanbeckevoort D, Maes B, et al. Paroxysmal nocturnal haemoglobinuria. MRI of renal cortical haemosiderosis in two patients, including one renal transplant. Nephrol Dial Transplant 1999;14:1586–9.
13. Kim S, Han MC, Lee JS, et al. Paroxysmal nocturnal hemoglobinuria. Acta Radiol 1991;32(4):315–6.
14. Mathieu D, Rahmouni A, Villeneuve P, et al. Impact of magnetic resonance imaging on the diagnosis of abdominal complications of paroxysmal nocturnal hemoglobinuria. Blood 1995;85(11):3283–8.
15. Gogia P, Goel R, Nayar S. Extramedullary paraspinal hematopoiesis in hereditary spherocytosis. Ann Thorac Med 2008;3(2):64–6.
16. Young NS, Calado RT, Scheinberg P. Current concepts in the pathophysiology and treatment of aplastic anemia. Blood 2006;108(8):2509–19.
17. Menger R, Dossani R, Thakur J, et al. Extra-axial hematoma and trimethoprim-sulfamethoxazole induced aplastic anemia: the role of hematological diseases in subdural and epidural hemorrhage. Case Rep Hematol 2015;2015:374951.
18. Ejindu VC, Hine AL, Mashayekhi M, et al. Musculoskeletal manifestations of sickle cell disease. Radiographics 2007;27(4):1005–21.
19. Thust SC, Burke C, Siddiqui A. Neuroimaging findings in sickle cell disease. Br J Radiol 2014;87(1040):20130699.

20. Madani G, Papadopoulou AM, Holloway B, et al. The radiological manifestations of sickle cell disease. Clin Radiol 2007;62(6):528–38.

21. Agha M, Fathy A, Sallam M. Sickle cell anemia: imaging from head to toe. The Egyptian Journal of Radiology and Nuclear Medicine 2013;44(3):547–61.

22. Tarasów E, Kułakowska A, Łukasiewicz A, et al. Moyamoya disease: diagnostic imaging. Pol J Radiol 2011;76(1):73–9.

23. Cappellini M, Fiorelli G. Glucose-6-phosphate dehydrogenase deficiency. Lancet 2008;371(9606):64–74.

24. Mew N, Loewenstein J, Kadom N, et al. MRI features of 4 female patients with pyruvate dehydrogenase E1 alpha deficiency. Pediatr Neurol 2011;45(1):57–9.

25. Davis SL, Littlewood TJ. The investigation and treatment of secondary anaemia. Blood Rev 2012;26(2):65–71.

Central Nervous System Complications of Hemorrhagic and Coagulation Disorders

Irina Filatova, MD[a], Lindsay L. Stratchko, DO[a],
Sangam Kanekar, MD[a,b,*]

KEYWORDS

• Hemorrhagic and coagulation disorders • Neurologic complications • MRI • CT

KEY POINTS

• Hematologic disorders can affect the central nervous system in a variety of ways, producing wide range of neurologic disturbances.
• It is important to identify these complications as early as possible for early intervention and better outcome.
• Cross-sectional imaging, mainly CT and MRI, plays an important role in identifying brain abnormalities and thus helps the clinician in deciding the appropriate course of action and treatment.

INTRODUCTION

Hematologic disorders can affect the central nervous system (CNS) in a variety of ways, producing a wide range of neurologic disturbances. It is important to identify these complications as early as possible for early intervention and better outcome. If untreated some of these complications may have irreversible deficit to fatal outcome. Today cross-sectional imaging, mainly computed tomography (CT) and MRI, plays an important role in identifying brain abnormalities and thus helps the clinician in deciding the appropriate course of action and treatment. This article reviews the basics of hemostasis including the coagulation cascade and the application of basic laboratory evaluation of hematologic function. The standard classification of the hematologic disorders is used to categorize the clotting and bleeding diatheses. The imaging features of various neurologic disorders associated with these clotting and bleeding diatheses are then discussed in detail.

[a] Department of Radiology, Hershey Medical Center, The Pennsylvania State University, 500 University Drive, Hershey, PA 17033, USA; [b] Department of Neurology, Hershey Medical Center, The Pennsylvania State University, 500 University Drive, Hershey, PA 17033, USA
* Corresponding author. Department of Radiology, Hershey Medical Center, The Pennsylvania State University, 500 University Drive, Hershey, PA 17033.
E-mail address: skanekar@hmc.psu.edu

Hematol Oncol Clin N Am 30 (2016) 757–777
http://dx.doi.org/10.1016/j.hoc.2016.03.003   hemonc.theclinics.com
0889-8588/16/$ – see front matter © 2016 Elsevier Inc. All rights reserved.

COAGULATION CASCADE

Normal hemostasis is an elaborate, multifactorial process involving the interaction of multiple elements to produce two main physiologic effects: the maintenance of liquidity of blood and prevention of bleeding after vessel damage. Normal platelet function maintains hemostasis in an undamaged vessel. Active hemostasis, or formation of fibrin in blood vessels, depends on progression through three main processes: (1) vascular, (2) platelet, and (3) coagulation stages of clot formation.[1] The vessel and vascular endothelium play an important primary role in the initiation of clotting. Vascular constriction at the time of injury can be the sole mechanism of preventing minor bleeding. In addition, vascular endothelium damage exposes blood to collagen, fibrinogen, and von Willebrand factor (vWF), which stimulates platelet adhesion. Conversely, intact endothelium is responsible for inhibition of hemostasis through prostacyclin and nitrogen oxide, which inhibit platelet aggregation.[1]

Platelet aggregation contributes to the next phase of hemostasis by binding circulating vWF and collagen released from injured endothelium to its surface receptors. After aggregation and activation, platelets undergo morphologic change forming a plug that releases substances, such as calcium, serotonin, and ADP, which promote further coagulation. Many additional factors, which play a role in coagulation, are released from dense granules secreted by aggregating platelets. These factors include platelet factor 3; β-thromboglobulin; platelet-derived growth factor; thrombospondin; factor V; and plasma proteins, such as fibrinogen and IgG.[1]

The final stage of the clotting process is the coagulation cascade, where a series of coagulation factors become sequentially activated to produce a fibrin clot (**Fig. 1**). There are two coagulation pathways, which culminate into a final common pathway. The liver produces factors involved in these pathways, therefore liver disease

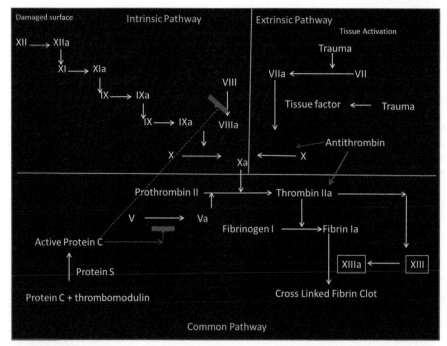

Fig. 1. Clotting cascade.

predisposes to dysfunction of the coagulation cascade. The intrinsic coagulation pathway begins with the activation of factor XII and conversion into factor XIIa; this activates the conversion of factor XI to XIa. Factor XIa activates the conversion of factor IX to IXa, which ultimately leads to the conversion of factor X to factor Xa, which is the initial step of the common pathway. The shorter, extrinsic pathway begins with the simultaneous activation of factor VII to VIIa and activation of factor III (tissue thromboplastin). Both of these factors cause the conversion of factor X to Xa. The activation of the common pathway begins with factor Xa, which activates the conversion of thrombin to prothrombin I. Prothrombin I in turn activates the conversion factor XIII to XIIIa. At the same time, thrombin activates polymerization of fibrinogen to fibrin polymers, which are converted to a fibrin meshwork making up the clot by the action of factor XIIIa.

LABORATORY EVALUATION

The disturbance of these pathways, and alteration in production or function of coagulation factors, are responsible for producing the spectrum of clotting and bleeding disorders. Several basic laboratory tests help in their distinction:

- Bleeding time: an older test, now mostly replaced by quantitative tests that measure platelet function under conditions of high sheer stress. Bleeding time test was used in the past to assess in vivo response to vascular injury by measuring a standard time for an induced skin puncture to stop bleeding.
- Platelet count: a test to quantify platelet availability by counting the number of platelets by an electronic counter in an anticoagulated blood sample. The count is then confirmed by visual inspection of a comparative blood smear. Disorders of platelet number, such as thrombocytopenia, are diagnosed by this method.
- Prothrombin time (PT): a test of the extrinsic and common coagulation pathways. After addition of calcium ion and tissue thromboplastin to a sample of plasma, time to coagulation is assessed. Prolonged coagulation time points to deficiency or dysfunction of factors V, VII, X, prothrombin, or fibrinogen.
- Partial thromboplastin time (PTT): similar to PT, this test evaluates the function of the intrinsic coagulation pathway. Clotting time of plasma is assessed after the addition of calcium ion with kaolin and cephalin. The function and amount of available factors V, VII, IX, X, XI, XII, prothrombin, or fibrinogen may be assessed.

In addition, various other tests may be performed to diagnose or classify the underlying pathology. Some of these tests may include peripheral smear, bone marrow biopsy, and organ biopsy. Discussion of these investigations is beyond the scope of this article.

CLASSIFICATION

This article is organized under two main headings: hemorrhagic and coagulation disorders. Hemorrhagic disorders may be caused by a disorder of one or more factors that participate in hemostasis. Most hemorrhagic syndromes are related to blood vessel disorders (vasculopathies), platelet number (thrombocytopenias) and function disorders (thrombocytopathies), or coagulopathies **Table 1**. Coagulopathies are caused by the absolute absence or decrease of the synthesis of certain coagulation factors, or the production of abnormal coagulation factor molecules or increased destruction during intravascular coagulation, or by the presence of inhibitors. This deficiency may be inherited or, more frequently, may result from organ disorders participating in the formation of coagulation factors.

Table 1
Classification and causes of common hemorrhagic and coagulation disorders

Vasculopathies (functional abnormalities of vascular wall)	Hereditary	Hereditary hemorrhagic telangiectasia Hereditary disorders of connective tissue (eg, Ehlers-Danlos syndrome)
	Secondary	Infections Chemical factors or drugs Disorders of metabolism (vitamin C or substance P deficiency) Pathologic changes of vascular wall (atherosclerosis) Connective tissue diseases
	Allergy: allergic purpura	Henoch-Schönlein purpura, purpura simplex, senile purpura, mechanic purpura, paraproteinemia
Platelet disorders	Thrombocytopenia	See **Table 2**
	Thrombocytosis	Primary: essential thrombocythemia Secondary: infections, injury, postsplenectomy chronic myelocytic leukemia, myeloproliferative disorders (polycythemia vera)
	Functional abnormalities of platelets	Congenital: thrombasthenia, giant platelet syndrome Acquired: drugs, uremia, liver diseases, and dysproteinemias
Coagulation disorders caused by coagulation factor deficiencies	Congenital	Hemophilia A (factor VIII deficiency) Hemophilia B (factor IX deficiency) Factor XI deficiency (hemophiliac), hypothrombinogenemia, hypofibrinogenemia Von Willebrand disease Hereditary thrombophilia: antithrombin deficiency, protein C deficiency, protein S deficiency, factor V Leiden (RQ506Q), prothrombin G:A 20210 mutation
	Acquired	Vitamin K deficiency Severe liver diseases Drugs (dicumarol) Disseminated intravascular coagulation
Hyperfibrinolysis	Primary	Congenital deficiency of α_2-antiplasmin, clinical use of urokinase, liver diseases, liberation of tissue plasminogen activator into the circulation
	Secondary	Disseminated intravascular coagulation

INCREASED VESSEL FRAGILITY

Functional abnormality in the vessel wall may cause either macrohemorrhages or microhemorrhages in the various organs of the body. These hemorrhages are predominately seen as small dermal and mucous membrane petechia or purpura. It is not uncommon for these disorders to present with neurologic deficit caused by intracranial hemorrhage or infarction. They may be hereditary, such as hereditary hemorrhagic telangiectasia (HHT) or Ehlers-Danlos syndrome (EDS), a heritable disorder of connective tissue. Alternatively they may be secondary to infections, chemical factors, drugs, disorders of metabolism (vitamin C or substance P deficiency), pathologic changes of vascular wall (atherosclerosis), or connective tissue diseases. Vessel wall abnormality may also be seen with allergic conditions, such as purpura and Henoch-Schönlein purpura. These disorders usually have a normal bleeding time, platelet count, PT, and PTT.

Hereditary Causes

Hereditary hemorrhagic telangiectasia

HHT, also referred to as Osler-Weber-Rendu disease, is an autosomal-dominant disorder characterized by multiple arteriovenous malformations (AVMs). As a result the disorder presents with dilated, tortuous blood vessels with thin vessel walls that rupture and bleed easily. The diagnosis is usually not suspected until adolescence or later when patients present with frequent epistaxis secondary to rupture of small AVMs near the skin surfaces and mucous membranes.[2]

HHT can present at any age, including infancy. CNS presentations in HHT may be caused by strokes usually secondary to pulmonary AVM/arteriovenous fistula (AVF), brain AVM with bleed, or subarachnoid hemorrhage from saccular aneurysm. In the brain parenchymal capillary telangiectasias are relatively rare compared with AVM. Disorder is thought to be caused by abnormal transforming growth factor-β signal transduction, which affects the vasculogenesis, angiogenesis, and endothelial cell properties. Diagnosis is often made by documenting multiple pulmonary AVM or cerebral AVM in a patient with recurrent epistaxis. There are several genes responsible for the disorder and diagnosis is made by clinical presentation followed by genetic testing including a search for pathologic variants of genes involved in the transforming growth factor-β/bone morphogenetic proteins (BMP) signaling cascade.[2]

On an unenhanced CT of the brain AVM appears as isodense serpentine vessels, which shows intense uniform enhancement of vascular channels and nidus on contrast-enhancement scans.[3] MRI evaluation shows cerebral AVMs as a tangle of vessels with flow voids and possible hemorrhages on T1- and T2-weighted images. T2-weighted sequences may also show edema, mass effect, and gliosis surrounding the AVMs (**Fig. 2**).[3] Additional large AVMs occur in the liver and lungs where they also present with bleeding or shunting complications. Treatment is based on symptoms, and in the brain, cerebral AVMs are treated surgically, embolized, or are treated with stereotactic radiosurgery. In diagnosed or suspected cases of HHT, screening for presence and evolution of cerebral AVMs is recommended with MRI in childhood (usually at the time of diagnosis) and again after puberty.[2]

Ehlers-Danlos syndrome

Vessel wall fragility producing microvascular bleeds may be seen because of impaired formation of collagen that is needed for vessel wall support. Such disorders include EDS, scurvy, and Cushing syndrome.

EDS is a heritable connective tissue disorder characterized by skin hyperextensibility, fragile and soft skin, delayed wound healing with formation of atrophic scars, easy bruising, and generalized joint hypermobility. Fifty percent of patients with classic EDS harbor mutations in the COL5A1 and the COL5A2 gene, encoding the 1- and the 2-chain of type V collagen, respectively.[4]

The diagnosis of EDS is established by clinical examination and family history. Cardiac lesions are common and include mitral and tricuspid valve prolapse, septal defects, and dilatation of the aortic root and pulmonary arteries.[5] The most important and frequent cerebrovascular complications are carotid-cavernous fistulas and arterial dissections.[6,7] Extracranial and intracranial aneurysms have also been reported. The internal carotid artery (ICA) is the most common site of aneurysm formation,

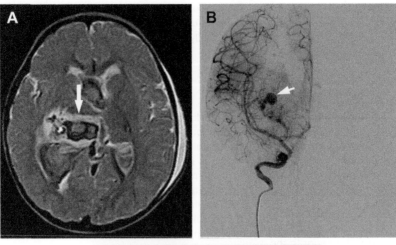

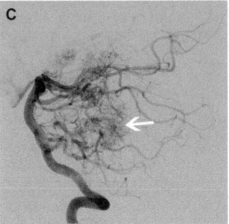

Fig. 2. Hereditary hemorrhagic telangiectasia. (*A*) Axial T2-weighted image at the level of the basal ganglia shows large hypointense bleed epicentered over the right thalamus (*arrow*). (*B*) Anteroposterior view of the cerebral angiogram shows an arteriovenous malformation with aneurysm (*arrow*) arising from thalamic perforator artery. (*C*) Lateral view of the cerebral angiogram with selective right vertebral injection shows large arteriovenous malformation (*arrow*) in the posterior fossa for the same patient.

typically in the cavernous sinus. Rupture of various systemic and cerebral vessels leads to frequent bleeding and subarachnoid hemorrhage (**Fig. 3**). Conventional angiography and angioplasty have a high rate of complications and therefore noninvasive techniques, such as MR angiography, are the primary investigation of choice in patients with EDS.[8] Surgery is difficult in these patients because the friable arteries are difficult to suture.

Secondary Causes of Vessel Wall Abnormality

Many secondary or acquired conditions, such as infections, chemical or drugs, disorders of metabolism (vitamin C or substance P deficiency), atherosclerosis, or connective tissue diseases, may affect vessel wall leading to weakness in the vessel wall and predisposing them to bleed.

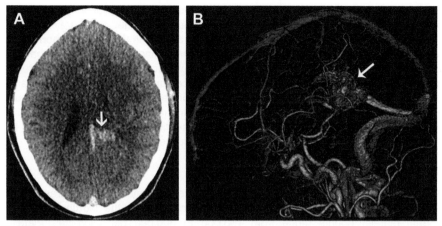

Fig. 3. Ehlers-Danlos syndrome with AVM. Axial CT of the brain (*A*) demonstrates acute hemorrhage (*arrow*) superior to the splenium of the corpus callosum. Three-dimensional reconstructed images of the CTangiography brain (*B*) shows a large AVM (*arrow*) posterior to the splenium supplied by the posterior cerebral artery and distal branches of anterior cerebral artery.

Septicemia, including meningococcemia and infective endocarditis (**Fig. 4**), results in microbial damage to the brain microvasculature, effectively producing a type of vasculitis. This vessel wall damage can be caused by organisms directly infecting the vessel wall or damage to blood vessels as they traverse purulent exudate in cisterns and along the cerebritis bed. Secondary vessel damage can be caused by postinfectious inflammatory toxins, such as immunoglobulin, complement,

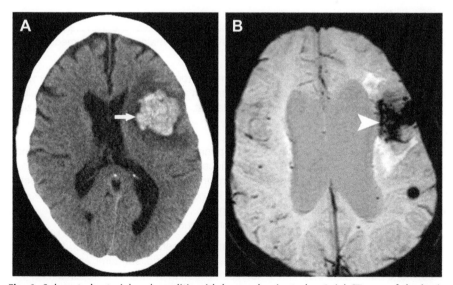

Fig. 4. Subacute bacterial endocarditis with hemorrhagic stroke. Axial CT scan of the brain (*A*) shows acute hemorrhage in the left frontal lobe (*arrow*). Axial gradient echo (GRE) image of the brain (*B*) shows hypointense signal intensity (*arrowhead*) in the same area caused by hemosiderin deposition.

lipoprotein, viral antigen or immune complex deposition, cold agglutinin formation, or vascular endothelial cell proliferation leading to vessel damage.

The proximal middle cerebral artery (MCA) and arteries in the posterior perforated substance are most often involved. MRI may show meningeal inflammatory changes as hyperintense signal in the basal cisterns and subarachnoid space on fluid attenuation inversion recovery images with thick enhancement on the postcontrast scans. Diffusion-weighted imaging may show changes of cerebritis, and associated acute brain infarction, whereas susceptibility-weighted imaging may show microhemorrhages from small vessel fragility. Hemorrhages in septicemia may also be caused by disseminated intravascular coagulation (DIC), discussed later.

PLATELET DISORDERS

Platelets play a critical role in hemostasis because they form temporary plugs that quickly stop bleeding and promote key reactions in the clotting cascade. Normal platelet counts range from 150,000 to 300,000 per microliter. Platelet counts lower than 100,000 per microliter are considered thrombocytopenia and spontaneous bleeding may occur when platelet counts fall below 20,000 per microliter. Both PT and PTT remain normal in thrombocytopenic bleeding, whereas the bleeding time is prolonged. Platelet abnormalities may be classified into three major groups:

1. Thrombocytopenia
2. Thrombocytosis
    a. Primary: essential thrombocythemia
    b. Secondary: infections, injury, postsplenectomy chronic myelocytic leukemia, other myeloproliferative disorders (eg, polycythemia vera)
3. Functional abnormalities of platelets
    a. Congenital: thrombasthenia, giant platelet syndrome (Bernard-Soulier syndrome)
    b. Acquired: because of drugs, uremia, liver diseases, and dysproteinemias

Thrombocytopenia

Decreased platelets counts could be caused by four major causes or mechanisms **Table 2**:

1. Decreased production of platelets (thrombocytopenia), which is most commonly seen with aplastic anemia, marrow infiltration by carcinoma, leukemia, myelofibrosis, infection, drugs that act on platelet production (eg, alcohol, thiazide diuretics)
2. Decreased platelet survival, such as:
    a. Immunologic (idiopathic thrombocytopenic purpura, systemic lupus erythematosus (SLE), posttransfusion, drug-induced thrombocytopenia)
    b. Nonimmunologic (DIC; thrombotic microangiopathies, such as thrombotic thrombocytopenic purpura [TTP] and hemolytic-uremic syndrome [HUS])
3. Sequestration of platelets (hypersplenism)
4. Platelet dilutional effects related to massive transfusions

Regardless of the underlying cause, thrombocytopenia less than 20 × 109/L may cause spontaneous hemorrhage. In the CNS, subarachnoid, subdural, and intracranial hemorrhage constitutes the most serious complication of thrombocytopenia (**Fig. 5**).[9]

Decreased production of platelets

Lymphoproliferative and myeloproliferative disorders diffusely involve the bone marrow. The abnormal proliferation and accumulation of pathologic cells within the

Table 2
Causes of thrombocytopenia

Decreased production of platelets	Generalized diseases of bone marrow Aplastic anemia: congenital and acquired Marrow infiltration: leukemia, disseminated cancer Selective impairment of platelet production Drug-induced: alcohol, thiazides, cytotoxic drugs Infections: measles, human immunodeficiency virus Ineffective megakaryopoiesis Megaloblastic anemia Myelodysplastic syndromes Effects of irradiation, drugs
Decreased platelet survival	Immunologic: idiopathic thrombocytopenic purpura, systemic lupus erythematosus Isoimmune: posttransfusion and neonatal Drug-associated: quinidine, heparin, sulfa compounds Infections: infectious mononucleosis, human immunodeficiency virus infection, cytomegalovirus Nonimmunologic: nonimmunologic destruction Disseminated intravascular coagulation Thrombotic thrombocytopenic purpura Giant hemangiomas Microangiopathic hemolytic anemias
Sequestration	Hypersplenism
Platelet dilutional	Massive transfusions

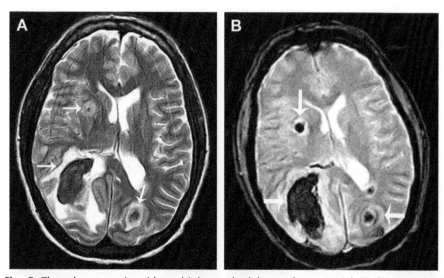

Fig. 5. Thrombocytopenia with multiple cerebral hemorrhages. Axial T2 (*A*) and axial gradient echo (GRE) (*B*) images show multiple areas of acute hemorrhage (*arrows*) with surrounding edema. Largest bleed is seen in the right occipital region with severe mass effect on the posterior horn of the right lateral ventricle.

bone marrow suppresses the normal marrow elements, resulting in anemia, leukopenia, and thrombocytopenia, which in turn may predispose to infection, and bleeding. Axial and appendicular skeleton may show diffuse osteopenia with marrow reconversion.

CNS involvement in leukemia is frequent and is a poor prognostic sign.[9] The CNS involvement in leukemia is caused by infiltration of leukemic cells, hemorrhage, infection, drug-radiation-induced neurotoxicity, or impaired circulation caused by leukostasis. The risk of cerebral hemorrhage is shown to be greater in leukemia than in uncomplicated idiopathic TTP, because of other associated hemostatic defects. It may occur during relapse and typically presents concomitantly with thrombocytopenia. Decreased platelet counts in leukemic states may be from DIC, which may occur because of the release of thromboplastins by leukemic cells, impaired platelet production, or chemotoxicity.[9] For example, DIC is a prominent feature of promyelocytic leukemia. The risk of DIC-related hemorrhage in leukemia is especially high during induction chemotherapy because of the release of thromboplastin from a large number of destroyed leukocytes. Cerebral white matter is most commonly involved with hemorrhage, but hemorrhage may happen anywhere in the brain (**Fig. 6**).

Leukemia may also cause thrombosis with hemorrhage from hyperviscosity due to hypercellularity of the disease state. Neurologic symptoms of hyperviscosity include visual and auditory disturbances, ataxia, impaired consciousness, lethargy, coma, transient ischemic attack, and stroke (**Fig. 7**).[9] Blood viscosity is increased in all types of leukemia; however, myelocytic leukemia causes symptoms at much lower cell counts than lymphocytic leukemia, likely because of the larger size of myelogenous leukemic cells.

Aplastic anemia is caused by a failure of the stem cells, characterized by decreased or absent hematopoietic precursors in the bone marrow. This results in pancytopenia in the peripheral blood. Aplastic anemia may be hereditary or acquired and may cause

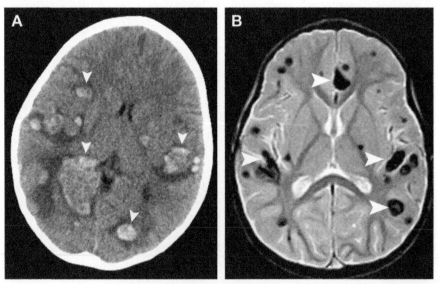

Fig. 6. Acute leukemia with blastic crisis. Axial head CT (*A*) and axial GRE (*B*) images of the brain show multiple areas of hemorrhages (*arrowheads*) involving bilateral cerebral parenchyma.

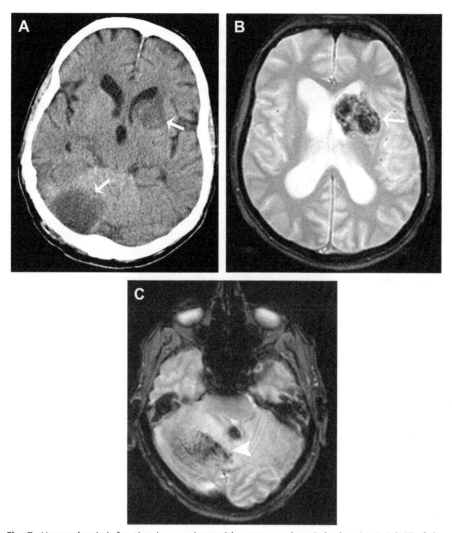

Fig. 7. Hemorrhagic infarction in a patient with acute myelocytic leukemia. Axial CT of the brain (*A*) shows hypodensity in the left caudate head and right cerebellar hypodensity (*arrows*) suggestive of infarction. Axial GRE images of the brain (*B*) and (*C*) at the level of deep gray matter nuclei (*arrow in B*) and posterior fossa (*arrow in C*) show areas of dark signal intensity in the infarcted areas caused by hemorrhage.

insult to the bone marrow. Unfortunately, in the more than 50% of the cases pathogenesis cannot be determined. In aplastic anemia, bleeding becomes a much greater problem when infection supervenes, presumably because of the superimposed hemostatic defect or intravascular coagulation. Because of associated thrombocytopenia, intraparenchymal, subarachnoid, and subdural hemorrhage may be seen.

Decreased platelet survival
Severe spontaneous thrombocytopenic hemorrhages are more likely to occur in disorders of platelet survival (idiopathic TTP, HUS).

Thrombocytopenic purpura TTP is a chronic or acute condition where platelets are destroyed through the formation of antiplatelet autoantibodies. Antibodies may be formed in response to exposure (eg, viral pathogens); however, the etiologic factor is often unknown (idiopathic TTP). The acute condition usually affects young children exposed to pathogens, most occurring following an acute febrile illness. Some have also been documented to occur after vaccination with measles-mumps-rubella, pneumococcus, *Haemophilus influenzae* B, hepatitis B virus, and varicella-zoster virus.[10] The acute illness is usually self-limited. The chronic condition usually affects adult women in their third and fourth decades. The disorder is characterized by formation of antibodies against the platelet membrane glycoproteins (usually IIb-IIIa and Ib-IX). The platelets are targeted, tagged, and subsequently removed by the functional spleen through a process termed opsonization. The characteristic signs of the disorder are bleeding at the skin and mucosal surfaces with relatively minor trauma. Additionally there may be melena, hematuria, and menorrhagia. Neurologic symptoms and complications largely depend on severity of the thrombocytopenia. The more common neurologic manifestations include headache, organic brain syndromes, coma, paresis, aphasia, dysarthria, syncope, vertigo, ataxia, visual symptoms, paresthesias, seizures, and cranial nerve palsies. Visual pathway and ocular changes are commonly affected resulting in homonymous field defects, exudative retinal detachment, retinal and choroidal hemorrhages, papilledema, anisocoria, and diplopia. Most of these symptoms are transient and fluctuating. On imaging the CNS most commonly manifests with subarachnoid and intracranial hemorrhage.[9]

Thrombotic microangiopathies Thrombotic microangiopathy is a clinical syndrome associated with the pentad of fever, thrombocytopenia, microangiopathic hemolytic anemia, transient neurologic deficits, and renal failure. Two most commonly encountered clinical syndromes associated with this microangiopathy include TTP and HUS.

HUS is a microangiopathy that typically affects children exposed to *Escherichia coli* 0157:H7 shiga-like toxin or *Shigella* toxin. Other less frequent causes include sporadic and familial HUS. The toxin, which is absorbed in the gastrointestinal mucosa, damages endothelium causing platelet activation and aggregation.[9] Patients often present with bloody diarrhea that may progress to irreversible renal damage because of damage of glomerular endothelium.

The CNS is involved in approximately 30% of children. The most common neurologic presentation includes generalized seizures, which may occur secondary to intracranial hemorrhages, which is associated with high mortality and long-term neurologic sequelae.[11] Other neurologic symptoms include behavioral changes, diplopia, dizziness, irritability, obtundation, coma, decerebrate posturing, cerebellar ataxia, hemiparesis, hemianopia, cortical blindness, cranial nerve palsies, vitreous hemorrhages, and retinal infarction.

MRI findings in microangiopathic conditions (TTP and HUS) include single or multifocal cortical and subcortical or gyral hyperintensities on T2-weighted images. In addition MRI may show features of infarction or hemorrhage.[12] Neurologic complications in HUS specifically include axonal neuropathy and small areas of infarctions in the basal ganglia; however, prognosis is favorable even with these findings (**Fig. 8**).[13] In the acute presentation, reversible posterior leukoencephalopathy has also been described, which on imaging shows bilateral symmetric hyperintensities in the juxtacortical and cortical areas of cerebral parenchyma on T2/ fluid attenuation inversion recovery images (**Fig. 9**).[13] A hemorrhagic component within these lesions is often associated with residual deficit. Long-term neurologic

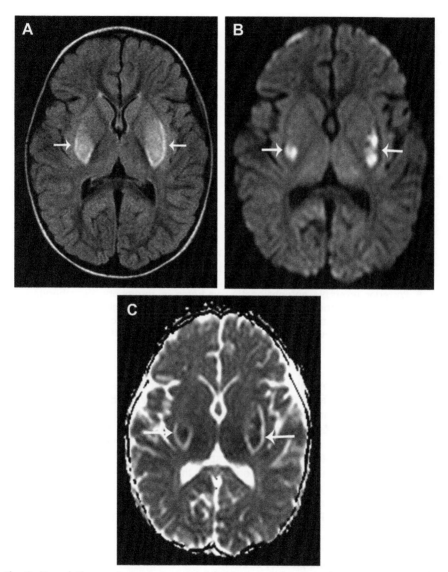

Fig. 8. Hemolytic uremic syndrome. Axial fluid attenuation inversion recovery image (*A*) shows bilateral symmetric hyperintensities in the posterior aspect of the putamen bilaterally (*arrows*). Axial diffusion-weighted image (*B*) and apparent diffusion coefficient image (*C*) show restricted diffusion in these areas (*arrows*).

complications are mostly seen because of residual hypertension and chronic renal failure.

Drug-induced immune thrombocytopenias Drug-induced immune thrombocytopenias may be seen with various drugs but are more frequently seen with quinine, quinidine, gold salts, phenytoin, valproic acid, carbamazepine, sulfonamides, certain cephalosporins, and heparin. These drugs may act as a hapten, binding to platelets

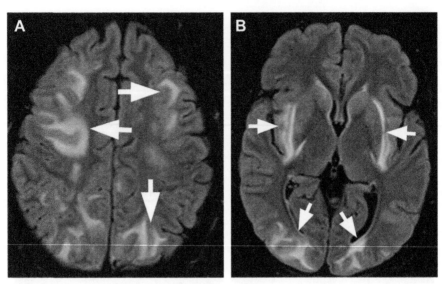

Fig. 9. Posterior reversible encephalopathy syndrome in thrombotic thrombocytopenic purpura. Axial fluid attenuation inversion recovery images at the level of cerebral convexity (*A*) and deep gray matter nuclei (*B*) show multiple cortical and subcortical hyperintensities in the frontoparietal lobes (*arrows in A*) and in the bilateral occipital lobes and external capsules (*arrows in B*).

and resulting in complement fixation leading to intravascular lysis or removal by the reticuloendothelial system. Clinically two types of heparin-induced thrombocytopenia (HIT) are encountered that largely vary in severity. Type I HIT is seen within first 1 to 3 days of heparin therapy and is characterized by a mild to moderate reduction in platelet counts (rarely less than $100 \times 10^9/L$). Platelet count may normalize despite continued heparin therapy. Type II HIT is more severe and is immunologically mediated. Platelet counts in this type can drop below 100 to $150 \times 10^9/L$. Neurologic complications, which include ischemic cerebrovascular events, cerebral venous thromboses, and a transient confusional state, are seen mainly with type II HIT. Massive intracranial hemorrhage is seen only in severe thrombocytopenia.

Platelet sequestration and platelet dilution
Platelet sequestration is related to conditions of hypersplenism and platelet dilutional effects are related to massive transfusions. Both conditions may affect the CNS by decreasing the number of platelets, causing thrombocytopenic bleeds.

Platelet dysfunction, or qualitative defect, may also be responsible for abnormal bleeding, despite normal platelet counts. These disorders are either congenital or acquired. Fortunately congenital qualitative defects are much rarer compared with quantitative and acquired platelet dysfunction. Most congenital platelet dysfunctions are seen with syndromes, such as Bernard-Soulier syndrome, Wiskott-Aldrich syndrome, and Glanzmann thrombocytopenia. Acquired platelet dysfunctions result from use of drugs, such as aspirin, nonsteroidal anti-inflammatory drugs, and ticlopidine, and renal or liver dysfunction.[9] Main dysfunction is seen in the platelet adhesion, aggregation, secretion, and procoagulant activity or a combination of abnormalities of number and function.

Bernard-Soulier syndrome is a disorder of platelet adhesion caused by an inherited deficiency of the platelet membrane glycoprotein complex Ib-IX, which is essential for normal platelet adhesion to subendothelial matrix. Glanzmann thrombasthenia is an autosomal-recessive disorder where platelets lack glycoprotein IIb/IIIa, and therefore fail to aggregate in response to ADP, collagen, epinephrine, or thrombin. This prevents the clot retraction and significantly prolongs bleeding time. Several drugs (mainly nonsteroidal anti-inflammatory drugs) in addition to chronic conditions, such as organ failure, may lead to platelet dysfunction. For example, aspirin is an irreversible inhibitor of the enzyme cyclooxygenase, which is required for the synthesis of thromboxane A_2 and prostaglandins. The later plays an important role in platelet aggregation.

COAGULATION DISORDERS CAUSED BY COAGULATION FACTOR DEFICIENCIES

Coagulation is heavily dependent on the availability and function of the clotting factors involved in forming the fibrin clot. A deficiency or dysfunction of any clotting factors (except factor XII) can lead to hemorrhagic disorders. The difference in bleeding from factor deficiency and platelet deficiency is the lack of small bleeds, such as petechia and ecchymosis, and, rather, the prevalence of larger bleeds, such as hemarthrosis, hematomas, and prolonged bleeding.

Coagulation factor deficiencies may be classified into two groups: hereditary and acquired. Hereditary clotting factor deficiencies typically involve a single factor. The most common hereditary factor deficiencies include hemophilia A (factor VIII deficiency), hemophilia B (factor IX deficiency), factor XI deficiency (formerly hemophilia C), hypothrombinogenemia, hypofibrinogenemia, von Willebrand disease, and hereditary thrombophilia (antithrombin deficiency, protein C and S deficiencies, factor V Leiden [RQ506Q], prothrombin G:A 20210 mutation). Acquired disease is mostly caused by the systemic processes, which causes deficiency of single or multiple clotting factors. Common causes include vitamin K deficiency, severe liver disease, drugs (dicumarol), and DIC.

Hemophilia A (Factor VIII Deficiency) and Hemophilia B (Factor IX Deficiency)

Hemophilia involves the reduction of factor VIII (hemophilia A) or deficiency of factor IX (hemophilia B), which serve as factors in activation of the common final pathway. Hemophilia A and B are X-linked recessive disorders and occur in males and in homozygous females. Hemophilia A is the most common hereditary disease associated with serious bleeding.

Clinically these two diseases are nearly indistinguishable and both prolong PTT, but do not affect PT and bleeding time. Spontaneous hemorrhages and massive hemorrhages after trauma, particularly hemarthrosis, are characteristic for this disease when the factor level is less than 1%.

Intracranial bleeds are the leading cause of mortality with rates of bleeding from 2.2% to 13.8%.[9] The most common cause of intracranial hemorrhage in a young patient with hemophilia is trauma, whereas in the older population it is hypertension (**Fig. 10**). Bleeding may occur anywhere including subdural (most common with delayed onset of symptoms, 4 ± 2.2 days), subarachnoid, cerebral hemispheres, cerebellar hemispheres, and the brainstem. Subdural and subarachnoid bleeds carry a better prognosis than parenchymal hemorrhages.[9] Increased risk of seizures and rebleeding are more commonly associated with intracerebral hemorrhages. Other CNS complications in patients with hemophilia include hemiparesis, aphasia, hemianopia, ataxia, and mental retardation.

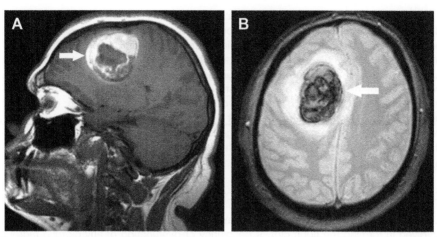

Fig. 10. Intraparenchymal hemorrhage in a patient with hemophilia. Sagittal T1-weighted (A) and axial T2 GRE (B) images show a large hemorrhage in the frontal lobe (arrow) with surrounding edema and mass effect.

Imaging appearance of hemophilia differs depending on presence of an acute event or sequel of chronic disease. Acute events are mostly caused by acute intracranial or spinal canal bleed. CT remains the imaging modality of choice in the acute presentation. An acute bleed is hyperdense on CT and may be seen in any compartment of the intracranial cavity, intraparenchymal, subarachnoid, subdural, and extradural (**Fig. 11**). Imaging findings of sequela of chronic hemophilia are generally related to prior hemorrhage or nonhemorrhagic events, such as infarctions. These findings are better appreciated on MRI, which show posthemorrhagic findings in approximately

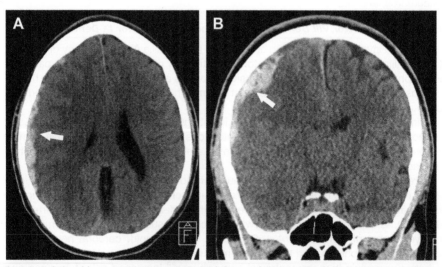

Fig. 11. Subdural hematoma in a patient with hemophilia. Axial (A) and coronal (B) CT scan of the brain shows acute right frontoparietal subdural hematomas (arrow) with effacement of the underlying convexity sulci and mild mass effect on ipsilateral lateral ventricle and mild leftward midline shift.

20% of subjects and nonhemorrhagic findings in about 11% of subjects.[9] Hemorrhagic findings include focal atrophy with either focal or diffuse superficial siderosis. Nonhemorrhagic findings include generalized cerebral atrophy with multifocal hyperintensities in the cerebral white matter on T2 weighted images.

Bleeding may occur in the spinal canal and around peripheral nerves, which may cause radiculopathy or more severe paraparesis, quadriparesis, and various peripheral nerve palsies. Small epidural hemorrhages, with mild clinical symptoms, may recover completely with intensive factor VIII replacement therapy alone. Large hematomas with severe cord compression require surgical decompression with intensive coverage of factor VIII replacement.

Von Willebrand Factor

Von Willebrand disease is one of the most common inherited disorders of bleeding in humans with an estimated frequency of 1%. It is characterized by deficiency or malfunction of vWF, which is a carrier for factor VIII and is also required for normal platelet adhesion. The bleeding complications caused by von Willebrand disease are relatively mild. Neurologic complications are rare; however, serious intracranial hemorrhages are seen as a complication of deficiency of vWF following trauma (**Fig. 12**). Because vWF is a carrier for factor VIII, patients with such hemorrhages require immediate factor VIII replacement therapy to prevent further bleeds.[9] Additionally, because deficiency of vWF is a type of hypercoagulable state, dural venous sinus thrombosis may occur.[14]

Hereditary Thrombophilia

Hereditary thrombophilias are caused by a defect or deficiency in the natural anticoagulant mechanisms predisposing to the development of venous thrombosis. Deficiencies of various anticoagulants, such as antithrombin, protein C and S deficiencies, factor V Leiden, the G20210A prothrombin gene mutation, and MTHFR C677T mutation (resulting in hyperhomocysteinemia), have been found to

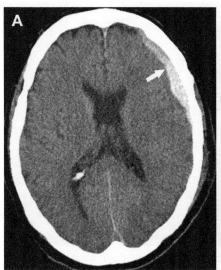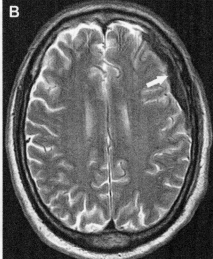

Fig. 12. Intracranial hemorrhage in a patient with von Willebrand disease. Axial CT scan (*A*) of the brain shows left frontal acute subdural hematoma (*arrow*). Axial T2-weighted image (*B*) of the brain shows hypointense subdural hematoma causing mild effacement of the convexity sulci.

predispose patients to thrombosis, including systemic or intracranial venous thrombo-embolism. Genetic or acquired predisposing factors are identified in 80% of patients who develop cerebral venous sinus thrombosis. In the cerebral venous system, throm-bosis is predominately seen in the superior sagittal and transverse sinuses (**Fig. 13**).

Antithrombin deficiency
Antithrombin belongs to the serine protease inhibitor, and as the name suggest it is an inhibitor of thrombin formation. It also inhibits other activated serine proteases of the coagulation cascade, including factors IXa, Xa, XIa, XIIa, and kallikrein. Antithrombin deficiency may be inherited (defect on chromosome 1 band q23.1–23.9) or acquired because of sepsis, renal or liver failure, pregnancy, bone transplant, or drug related. Hereditary antithrombin deficiency affects around 1 in 2000 to 5000 of the population. Inherited or acquired deficiency of antithrombin may be associated with cerebral venous thrombosis.

Protein C and S deficiency
Protein C and S are a vitamin K–dependent glycoproteins synthesized in the liver. Protein C circulates in the blood as an inactive zymogen. When bound to thrombomo-dulin, an endothelial cell surface protein, it is converted into an active protease by the action of thrombin. Protein C and protein S proteolyses factors Va and VIIIa, thereby reducing thrombin formation and promoting fibrinolysis. Protein C deficiency is inherited in an autosomal-dominant fashion. Prevalence of protein C deficiency is thought to be 1 in 30,000. Sagittal sinus and cerebral venous thromboses are reported in association with deficiency of protein C and S.

Factor V Leiden (RQ506Q)
Hypercoagulable states also results from factor V Leiden disease (RQ506Q). This dis-ease results from a point mutation in factor V at Arg 506, where protein C cleaves and

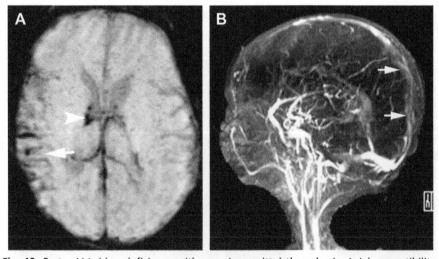

Fig. 13. Factor V Leiden deficiency with superior sagittal thrombosis. Axial susceptibility-weighted image of the brain (*A*) shows focal hypointensity in the genu of the right internal capsule (hemorrhage) (*arrowhead*). There is low signal intensity seen over the right parietal convexity suggestive of subarachnoid hemorrhage (*arrow*). Sagittal reformatted image from MR venogram (*B*) shows thrombosis of the superior sagittal sinus (*arrows*).

inactivates Va procoagulant. This results in poor downregulation of blood coagulation and hypercoagulability. This is one of the most common procoaguable states, with prevalence in white persons of 2% to 10%.[9] Venous thromboembolism can occur at any site, with most common intracranial complications of cerebral venous thrombosis. Infarcts from thrombi are the leading cause of morbidity. Although the risk of thrombosis in factor V Leiden disease is mild to moderate, the prevalence of the disease in the population increases the risk for thrombosis compared with all other factor deficiencies combined.[9]

DISSEMINATED INTRAVASCULAR COAGULATION

The fibrinolytic pathway removes a clot through the function of plasmin. Plasminogen, the inactive from of plasmin, is activated by fibrin among other activators. Activated plasmin degrades fibrinogen and factors V, VIII, and vWF, which activates clot-degrading pathways.[15]

When fibrinolysis is excessive or deficient, hemostasis is disrupted. Primary hyperfibrinolytic disorders cause bleeding by increased activation of fibrinolytic enzymes. These are rare disorders, such as congenital deficiency of α_2-antiplasmin.[15] More common disorders, such as liver disease, promote excessive fibrin breakdown by increased endothelial release and decreased hepatic clearance of tissue plasminogen activator, and decreased synthesis of α_2-antiplasmin and plasminogen activator inhibitor.[16]

DIC can be an acute, subacute, or chronic thrombohemorrhagic disorder, which may be considered as secondary hyperfibrinolysis. It is difficult to distinguish DIC from primary hyperfibrinolysis clinically; however, primary hyperfibrinolysis (especially when caused by liver cirrhosis) is characterized specifically by elevated factor VIII, stable platelet count, and absence of the multiorgan failure, which is often associated with DIC.[16]

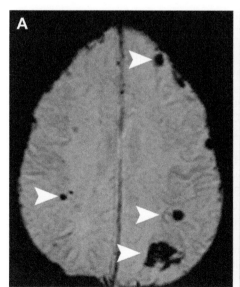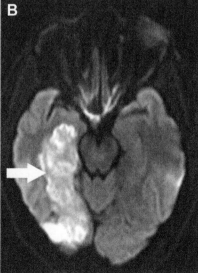

Fig. 14. Disseminated intravascular coagulation. Axial susceptibility-weighted image (A) of the brain shows multiple areas of signal drop outs (arrowheads) suggestive of multiple intraparenchymal bleeds. Axial diffusion-weighted image (B) through the brain shows large area of restricted diffusion consistent with acute infarction in the right posterior cerebral artery (PCA) territory (arrow).

In DIC, overactive fibrinolysis occurs from a myriad of causes, which lead to activation of the coagulation cascades and impairment of inhibitory mechanisms of clotting. Some of the major contributory causes include release of tissue thrombotic substances as a result of obstetric complications, infections (gram-negative sepsis, meningecoccus, aspergillus, histoplasma, and so forth), neoplasms (especially from certain adenocarcinomas, which directly activate factor X), and extensive endothelial injury from burns, trauma, surgery, vasculitides, aortic aneurysms, and giant hemangiomas. Acute promyelocytic leukemia is also among the known causes of DIC, because these cancers release thrombotic substances, including tissue factors, proteolytic enzymes, and mucin. Patients with cancer more often present with chronic DIC, which at least initially predominates with thrombotic, rather than hemorrhagic, complications.

CNS complications of DIC are characteristic with hemorrhagic and ischemic components. Massive cerebral, intraventricular, and subarachnoid hemorrhages may occur. Thrombi are found in multiple cerebral vessels with surrounding hemorrhages (**Fig. 14**).

SUMMARY

Hematologic disorders cause a variety of CNS complications ranging from thrombotic to hemorrhagic. Deficiencies of clotting factors may lead to hemorrhages or infarcts caused by thrombosis. Platelet deficiencies or dysfunction may also lead to several hemorrhagic complications. Vessel wall malformation may cause aneurysmal dilations and wall fragility may cause spontaneous rupture, leading to catastrophic hemorrhagic events in the brain. It is useful for the clinician to be aware of the appearance of these multiple complications of hematologic disorders because some may significantly contribute to the morbidity and mortality of the patient.

REFERENCES

1. Baklaja R. Hemostasis and hemorrhagic disorders. Fermentation-Biotecc GmbH Rudolf-Huch-Str. Bad Harzburg (Germany); 2008.
2. McDonald J, Pyeritz R. Hereditary hemorrhagic telangiectasia. In: Pagon R, Adam MP, Ardinger HH, et al, editors. Genereviews [Internet]. Seattle (WA): University of Washington; 2000. p. 1993–2015 [Updated 2014 July 24].
3. Jaskolka J, Wu L, Chan RP, et al. Imaging of hereditary hemorrhagic telangiectasia. Am J Roentgenol 2004;183(2):307–14.
4. Malfait F, Wenstrup RJ, De Paepe A. Clinical and genetic aspects of Ehlers-Danlos syndrome, classic type. Genet Med 2010;12(10):597–605.
5. Leier CV, Call TD, Fulkerson PK, et al. The spectrum of cardiac defects in the Ehlers-Danlos syndrome types I and III. Ann Intern Med 1980;92:171–8.
6. Mathew T, Sinha S, Taly AB, et al. Neurological manifestations of Ehlers–Danlos syndrome. Neurol India 2005;53(3):339–41.
7. North KN, Whiteman DA, Pepin MG, et al. Cerebrovascular complications in Ehlers-Danlos syndrome type IV. Ann Neurol 1995;38(6):960–4.
8. Roach ES. Ehlers-Danlos syndrome. In: Caplan LR, editor. Uncommon causes of stroke. 2nd edition. Cambridge: Cambridge University Press; 2008. p. 139–44.
9. Davies-Jones GAB, Sussman JD. Neurological manifestations of hematological disorders. Neurol Gen Med. In: Aminoff MJ, editor. Neurology and General Medicine (Fourth Edition). Churchill Livingstone;2008. p. 227–263.
10. Cines DB, Bussel JB, Liebman HA, et al. The ITP syndrome: pathogenic and clinical diversity. Blood 2009;113(26):6511–21.
11. Eriksson KJ, Boyd SG, Tasker RC. Acute neurology and neurophysiology of haemolytic-uraemic syndrome. Arch Dis Child 2001;84:434.

12. Zheng XL, Sadler JE. Pathogenesis of thrombotic microangiopathies. Annu Rev Pathol 2008;3:249–77.
13. Steinborn M, Leiz S, Rudisser K, et al. CT and MRI in haemolytic uraemic syndrome with central nervous system involvement: distribution of lesions and prognostic value of imaging findings. Pediatr Radiol 2004;34:805.
14. Teksam M, Moharir M, Deveber G, et al. Frequency and topographic distribution of brain lesions in pediatric cerebral venous thrombosis. AJNR Am J Neuroradiol 2008;29(10):1961–5.
15. Carpenter SL, Mathew P. α2-Antiplasmin and its deficiency: fibrinolysis out of balance. Haemophilia 2008;14:1250–4.
16. Nair GB, Lajin M, Muslimani A. A Cirrhotic patient with spontaneous hematoma due to primary hyperfibrinolysis. Clin Adv Hematol Oncol 2011;9(3):249–52.

Neurologic and Head and Neck Manifestations of Sickle Cell Disease

Andrew Steven, MD[a],*, Prashant Raghavan, MD[a],
Tanya J. Rath, MD[b], Dheeraj Gandhi, MD[a]

KEYWORDS

- Sickle cell disease • Sickle cell anemia • Sickle cell • Moyamoya • Stroke

KEY POINTS

- Clinical symptoms of sickle cell disease (SCD) occur primarily as a result of hemolytic anemia, vasocclusion, infection, or a combination thereof.
- Hemorrhagic and ischemic stroke is the leading cause of death and a major cause of morbidity in SCD patients.
- SCD results in diffuse gray and white matter abnormalities, which may account for accelerated neurocognitive deficits even in patients without focal lesions on conventional MRI.
- SCD-associated vasculopathy may result in vascular narrowing or aneurysm formation. Chronic progressive occlusion of the internal carotid artery with prominent lenticulostriate collaterals produces the stereotypical "moyamoya" angiographic pattern.
- Although less well-known, many patients suffer from head and neck manifestations of SCD, which may affect the inner ears, orbits, sinuses, lymphoid tissue, and bone.

BACKGROUND

Sickle cell disease (SCD) is an autosomal-recessive inherited disorder characterized by an abnormal oxygen-carrying hemoglobin molecule that results in deformed red blood cells (RBC). This widely studied entity was the first disease where the exact genetic and molecular defect was identified, attributable to a single nucleotide mutation of the β-globin gene located on the short arm of chromosome 11. The disease requires 2 defective genes for full disease penetrance and most patients are homozygotic HbS carriers. Although the term SCD refers to a somewhat varied population with clinically important compound heterozygous variants, including sickle D, sickle C, and sickle B thalassemia.[1]

Disclosure: The authors have nothing to disclose.
[a] Department of Diagnostic Radiology, University of Maryland Medical System, 22 S Greene St., Baltimore, MD 21201, USA; [b] Department of Radiology, University of Pittsburgh Medical Center, 200 Lothrop Street, Suite 200 East Wing, Pittsburgh, PA 15213, USA
* Corresponding author.
E-mail address: asteven@umm.edu

SCD is common, with approximately 300,000 children born annually with the disease, predominating in sub-Saharan African and among African descendants around the world. The Centers for Disease Control and Prevention estimates that 90,000 to 100,000 Americans suffer from the disease. Despite recent advances in treatment, the high morbidity and mortality rates of SCD remain a major public health concern resulting in an average of 75,000 hospitalizations and US health care costs approaching $475 million annually.[2]

Low oxygen tension results in polymerization of the abnormal hemoglobin tetramer, which becomes relative insoluble when deoxygenated. Aggregates form long chains, disrupting the microstructural and macrostructural appearance of the cell. The normally plastic biconcave erythrocytes morph into crescentic or sickle-shaped cells that are more friable and easily hemolyzed. Preceding events may include infection, trauma, and other stressful conditions that may promote intracellular hypoxia and acidosis.

Acute and chronic clinical manifestations of SCD primarily occur as a result of hemolysis and vasoocclusion. Changes in membrane structure and function, loss of normal plasticity, disorganized cell volume control, increased sheer stress, and increased endothelial adherence are all thought to contribute to these phenomena. A typical RBC from a sickle cell patient has a life span on the order of just 10 to 20 days in comparison with the normal 90 to 120 days. Chronic anemia results in profound stresses on both the hematopoietic and cardiovascular systems.

After RBC sickling, vasoocclusion occurs through a cascade of events including endothelial adhesion and damage, arterial narrowing, and aggregation, ultimately leading to ischemia and/or infarction. Ischemic events may occur throughout the body, resulting in repeated acutely painful episodes known as crises. Hemolysis and vasoocclusion result in end organ damage affecting virtually every organ system to some degree. This review focuses on the central nervous system and the less recognized head and neck manifestations of the disease.

VASCULAR DISEASE

SCD vasculopathy results in large vessel arterial stenosis and occlusion with the distal internal carotid arteries, proximal anterior cerebral arteries, and middle cerebral arteries (MCA) most commonly affected (**Fig. 1**). Pathologic studies describe smooth muscle hyperplasia and intraluminal thrombus rather than inflammation or atherosclerosis as the underlying pathophysiology. This process occurs slowly over time as evidenced by extensive collateral vessel formation, particularly the lenticulostriate vessels coursing through the basal ganglia. The angiographic appearance of stenosis with an extensive network of ill-defined collateral vessels was likened to "a puff of smoke" by the original Japanese angiographers who coined the term "moyamoya" (**Fig. 2**). This moyamoya pattern has been described in several other disease entities including neurofibromatosis and postradiation vasculopathy.

Blood supply is tenuous, even in the setting of collateral vessel formation with regional perfusion abnormalities. These collateral vessels exhibit stress-related changes, including thinned walls and microaneurysm formation, predisposing them to both hemorrhage and thrombosis.[3]

In addition to stenosis, SCD may result in arterial dilatation. Reported rates of aneurysm formation in SCD patients appear much higher than that of the general population (>1% in children and 10% in adults), with a high prevalence of patients with multiple aneurysms. Chronic high-flow states, changes in circulatory patterns,

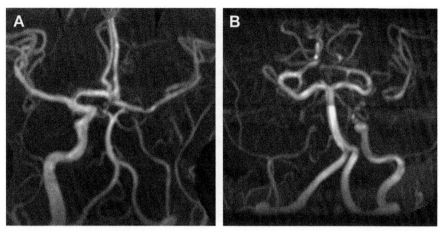

Fig. 1. Three-dimensional maximum intensity projection images of time-of-flight MR angiography from 2 different patients with narrowing of the internal carotid artery (ICA). (*A*) shows severe narrowing of the left ICA, which is essentially occluded in its supraclinoid segment. (*B*) shows bilateral ICA stenosis with minimal signal in the supraclinoid ICAs, both anterior cerebral arteries and the right middle cerebral arteries.

and underlying vessel wall damage all likely contribute to the increased rates of aneurysms. Nonsaccular arterial enlargement (or ectasia) has also been described in the setting of SCD, most commonly affecting the basilar artery, but also seen within the anterior circulation as well[4] (**Fig. 3**).

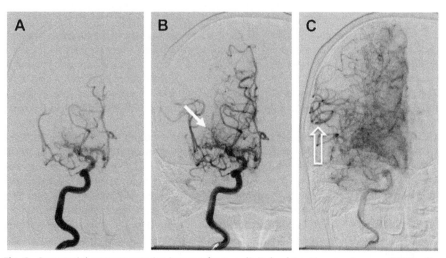

Fig. 2. Sequential anteroposterior images from a digital subtraction angiogram (DSA) after right internal carotid artery (ICA) injection in a patient with chronic ICA stenosis. (*A*) Severe narrowing of the supraclinoid ICA with absence of the M1 segment of the middle cerebral arteries (MCA). (*B*) A prominent ill-defined network of collateral vessels in the expected region of the MCA (*arrow*) consistent with moyamoya phenomenon, with normal filling of the anterior cerebral arteries. (*C*) Delayed filling of distal MCA branches (*open arrow*) through lenticulostriate and pial collaterals.

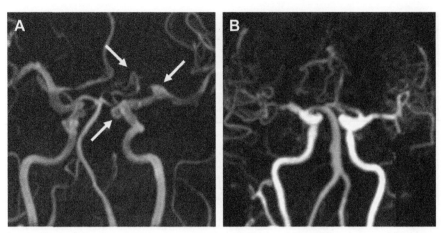

Fig. 3. Three-dimensional maximum intensity projection images from time-of-flight MR angiography showing vascular dilatation in 2 different patients. Patient in (*A*) has multiple intracranial aneurysms (*arrows*), which are arising from the left internal carotid artery (ICA), left middle cerebral arteries and distal left posterior cerebral artery. Patient in (*B*) exhibits fusiform enlargement, or ectasia, of the basilar artery and both supraclinoid ICAs.

Transcranial Doppler ultrasonography may be used to assess the blood flow within internal carotid arteries and MCA.[5] The velocity of flowing blood is inversely proportional to arterial diameter; therefore, stenosis may be identified by localizing areas of increased velocity and high-resistance waveforms. Absent waveforms suggest complete occlusion. Although there are significant limitations related to specificity and anatomic accuracy, the technique is helpful in identifying patients with stenoses and those at risk for stroke.

Computed tomography (CT) and MR angiography are excellent noninvasive imaging techniques to identify areas of vascular narrowing.[6] Each technique has its own strengths and limitations; however, both focus on evaluation of flowing blood within the arterial lumen. CT angiography offers improved spatial resolution and is less susceptible to artifact. However, MR angiography is generally recommended in patients who are expected to undergo repeated examinations and routine follow-up to minimize radiation exposure.

Although dedicated evaluation of the vasculature is not included in a typical MRI of the brain, subtle findings may indicate the presence of stenosis and collateral formation, even in the absence of ischemic changes. Loss of the normal internal carotid arterial flow voids with punctate basal ganglia flow voids on T2-weighted images are highly suspicious. Tiny foci of postcontrast enhancement within the basal ganglia or an ill-defined enhancing structure replacing the normal MCA in the Sylvain fissure indicates collateral vessel formation (**Fig. 4**). The "ivy sign" refers to leptomeningeal enhancement in the cerebral sulci indicating engorged pial collateral vessels.[7]

Aneurysms should be readily identifiable on CT or MR angiography as focal saccular outpouchings. These tend to occur at predictable locations—vascular branch points including the anterior communication artery, posterior communicating artery, and middle cerebral artery bifurcation. However, the typical search pattern should be expanded to avoid missing aneurysm in atypical locations, especially including the posterior circulation.

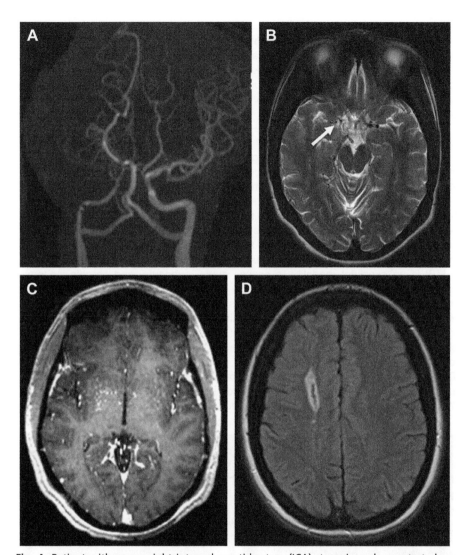

Fig. 4. Patient with severe right internal carotid artery (ICA) stenosis as demonstrated on 3-dimensional maximum intensity projection images of time-of-flight MR angiography (*A*). Corresponding T2-weighted image (*B*) shows absent right middle cerebral artery flow void, which is replaced by an ill-defined network of collaterals (*arrow*). These collaterals manifest as punctate foci of enhancement in the basal ganglia on postcontrast T1-weighted images (*C*). Axial fluid-attenuated inversion recovery image (*D*) shows chronic ischemic changes in the right centrum semiovale, corresponding to a deep ICA watershed distribution.

NEUROLOGIC COMPLICATIONS
Infarction

Stroke is a major complication associated with SCD, and the leading cause of death in both children and adults with the disease. CDC estimates a 300-fold increased likelihood of stroke for children with SCD, with an age-adjusted incidence is 0.61 to 0.76 per 100 patient-years. Cerebral infarction affects approximately

30% of all individuals with SCD.[2] Normal brain function requires a continuous supply of oxygen to maintain aerobic metabolism.[8] Ischemic infarctions occur as a result of both occlusive disease and hemodynamic factors, including a reduction in arterial oxygen concentration. Clinically, a stroke is manifested as an acute onset focal neurologic deficit lasting for more than 24 hours. Symptoms vary with the site and size of the lesion, but may include motor or sensory deficits, vision or hearing loss, or disruption of language function.

CT serves as the initial study of choice for acutely symptomatic stroke patients owing to its widespread availability and speed of imaging. It accurately distinguishes hemorrhagic from ischemic lesions, facilitating triage and time-sensitive treatments such as intravenous or intraarterial thrombolytics. Classic CT findings in a large vessel acute ischemic infarction include decreased attenuation with loss of gray–white differentiation conforming to a specific vascular distribution. CT findings of ischemic stroke may take hours to develop, so a normal appearing scan does not exclude the diagnosis. The presence of a hyperattenuating vessel, the so-called hyperdense MCA sign, is another finding that may indicate a thrombus in a vessel. Mass effect from infarction develops in the first few days and wanes in the subacute to chronic phases (**Fig. 5**).

MRI is an excellent modality to assess acute, subacute, and chronic ischemic changes. After a screening CT examination, diffusion-weighted imaging has become the standard of care for MR evaluation of stroke in the last few decades. Cytotoxic edema from infarction restricts the free diffusivity of water molecules resulting in increased diffusion-weighted imaging signal and decreased signal on apparent diffusion coefficient maps. In contradistinction to CT, diffusion-weighted imaging may identify infarcted brain tissue in a matter of minutes (**Fig. 6**). Signal changes on T2-weighted images and fluid-attenuated inversion recovery develop in the first 6 to 12 hours, and commonly persist. Gliosis and encephalomalacia from chronic infarcts manifest as focal volume loss with increased signal on T2-weighted images (**Fig. 7**).

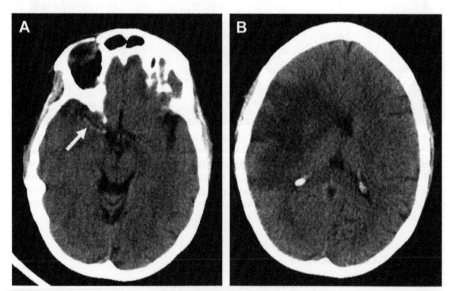

Fig. 5. Axial noncontrast computed tomography images in a patient with an acute middle cerebral artery (MCA) infarct. Thrombus within the vessel manifests as a classic "hyperdense MCA" (*arrow*) in (*A*). (*B*) A large wedge-shaped area of hypoattenuation with swelling and loss of gray-white differentiation throughout the affected territory.

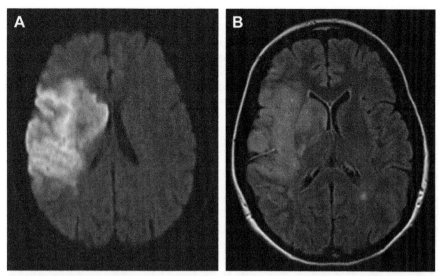

Fig. 6. Diffusion-weighted (*A*) and fluid-attenuated inversion recovery (FLAIR; *B*) images demonstrate the appearance of an acute right middle cerebral arteries infarct on MRI. There is restricted diffusion and FLAIR hyperintensity throughout the vascular territory with modest mass effect.

In addition to large vascular distribution infarcts, SCD patients may present with small vessel "lacunar-type" infarcts or a watershed pattern of disease. Lacunar infarcts associated with thrombosis of small perforating vessels tend to be more centrally located in the brain. Watershed infarcts occur at the border zone between

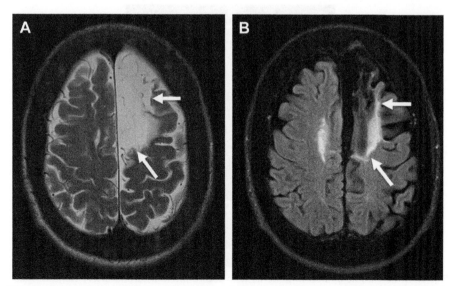

Fig. 7. Chronic left anterior cerebral artery infarct on axial T2-weighted (*A*) and fluid-attenuated inversion recovery (*B*) images. Gliosis and encephalomalacia are manifested as increased signal with focal volume loss (*arrows*). Relatively subtle chronic ischemic changes are also found in the paramedian right frontal subcortical white matter.

large arterial territories, that is, between the middle cerebral artery and posterior cerebral artery distributions[9] (**Fig. 8**).

CT and MR perfusion imaging allows for assessment of regional blood flow.[10,11]
These emerging techniques has been explored as a methodology for assessing sickle
cell and moyamoya patients with encouraging early results (**Fig. 9**). There is increased
incidence of right–left asymmetry when compared with general populations. This
promising technique may ultimately prove useful in identifying patients at high risk
for stroke and stratify those patients that may benefit from intervention.

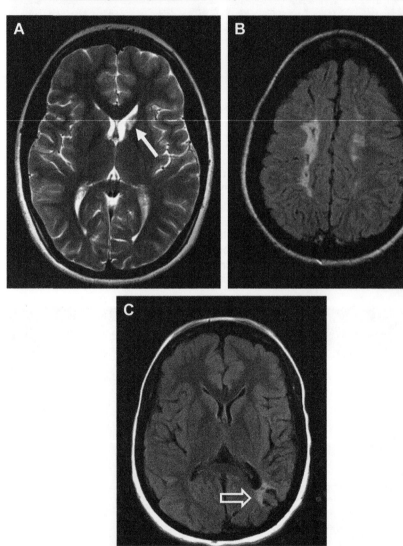

Fig. 8. Three chronic infarcts in patients with severe internal carotid artery stenosis. Axial
T2-wieghted image (*A*) demonstrates a remote lacunar infarct in the left caudate head
(*arrow*). Axial fluid-attenuated inversion recovery (FLAIR) image (*B*) shows bilateral deep white
matter watershed ischemic changes. Left parietal infarct (*open arrow*) on axial FLAIR image (*C*)
corresponds to the middle cerebral arteries-posterior cerebral artery watershed territory.

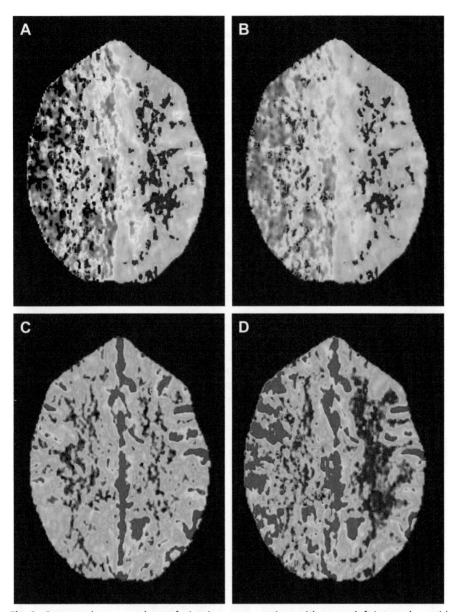

Fig. 9. Computed tomography perfusion images on patient with severe left internal carotid artery stenosis demonstrates increased mean transit time (*A*) and time to peak (*B*) throughout the entire left cerebral hemisphere. However, there was no infarction, because collateral vessels maintain cerebral blood flow (*C*) and cerebral blood volume (*D*).

Hemorrhage

Approximately one-third of all strokes in SCD are hemorrhagic, and these insults carry much higher mortality rates. Risk factors include low steady-state hemoglobin and high leukocyte count. There is significant overlap in the clinical presentation of acute intracranial hemorrhage and ischemic stroke, and both may present with focal neurologic deficits such as paresis or language difficulty. However, intracranial hemorrhage is more often associated with headache, seizures, alterations in consciousness, and signs of increased intracranial pressure. An initial noncontrast head CT is critical to distinguishing hemorrhagic from ischemic strokes in SCD patients who present with acute neurologic symptoms.

Intraparenchymal hematomas tend to be round or ovoid, well-circumscribed lesions with only modest surrounding edema (**Fig. 10**). Acute hematomas are hyperdense on CT relative to the adjacent brain parenchyma. Hematomas decrease in size and radiodensity as they evolve through the subacute phase, although the associated edema may initially increase. A chronic hematoma manifests as a low attenuation, slitlike cavity or focal volume loss.

MRI is helpful in identifying and characterizing intracranial hemorrhage. Historically T2*-weighted or gradient echo images have been used to identify hemorrhagic foci on MRI. These sequences are extremely sensitive to magnetic field inhomogenity caused by blood products. Susceptibility weighted imaging is a more recently developed MR sequence used for detection of blood product that increases sensitivity for microhemorrhage.[12] These sequences detect inhomogeneity in the magnetic field that may be induced by paramagnetic substances found in certain blood products, manifesting as foci of signal void or "blooming artifact." A diffuse pattern of microhemorrhage has been described in the SCD patients resulting from cerebral fat embolism syndrome[13] (**Fig. 11**).

In addition to intraparenchymal hemorrhage, SCD patients are prone to subarachnoid and intraventricular hemorrhage (**Fig. 12**). This may occur from rupture of the abnormal dilated collateral vessels formed in the setting of moyamoya or rupture of saccular aneurysms. Aneurysmal subarachnoid hemorrhage manifests as increased CT attenuation in and around the basal cisterns extending to overlying fissures and cerebral sulci. The blood may distribute diffusely, although tends to center around the

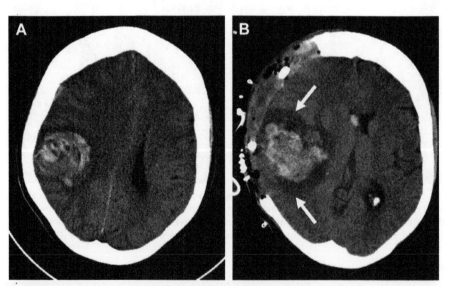

Fig. 10. Axial noncontrast CT images (*A, B*) on 2 different patients with large intraparenchymal hemorrhages. Acute blood products are hyperdense compared with the brain. Patient in (*B*) has considerable surrounding edema (*arrows*) and mass effect, requiring a decompressive craniectomy.

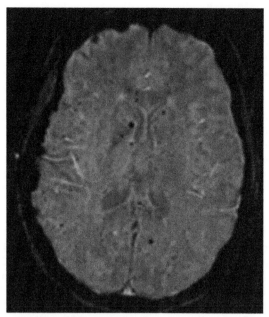

Fig. 11. Axial susceptibility weighted imaging image of a patient with cerebral fat embolism syndrome demonstrating numerous scattered foci of microhemorrhage manifesting as punctate foci of susceptibility artifact (signal void).

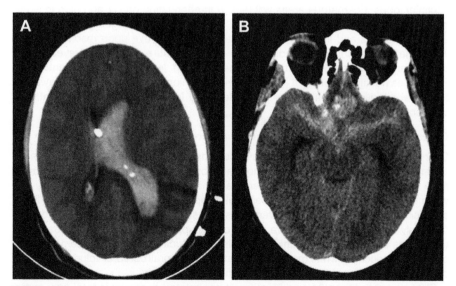

Fig. 12. Axial noncontrast CT images from 2 different patients with intracranial hemorrhage. (*A*) Intraventricular hemorrhage with a large cast of blood filling the left lateral ventricle. (*B*) Subarachnoid hemorrhage centered in the anterior interhemispheric fissure, suprasellar cistern, and bilateral Sylvian fissures from an anterior communicating artery aneurysm rupture.

site of rupture. MRI offers a sensitive, although nonspecific, assessment for detection of intraventricular or subarachnoid hemorrhage and may identify even small amounts of blood imperceptible on CT.

Subarachnoid and intraventricular hemorrhages are often associated with hydrocephalus. This may occur acutely from direct obstruction of the ventricles and their outlet foramina or in a delayed fashion as breakdown of RBCs disrupts the resorption of cerebrospinal fluid at the level of the arachnoid granulations. Hydrocephalus appears as enlargement of the ventricular system without corresponding enlargement of the sulci. Distention of the temporal tips and rounding of the front horns are helpful features to differentiate from cerebral volume loss.

Nontraumatic epidural hematomas may occur in the setting of calvarial infarcts.[14] These lesions have a characteristic biconvex or lentiform configuration as blood accumulates between the closely adherent dura mater and periosteum in a high-pressure fashion.

Posterior Reversible Leukoencephalopathy Syndrome

Numerous reports describe posterior reversible leukoencephalopathy syndrome (PRES) occurring in the setting of SCD. The exact etiology of PRES is not entirely understood, but is thought to be related to loss of autoregulation of the cerebral vasculature.[15,16] Most commonly associated with neurotoxic medications, hypertension, and eclampsia, the pattern has been described in a wide variety of inflammatory conditions. Factors that may predispose SCD patients to PRES include chronic high cardiac output states, elevated blood pressure, endothelial damage with abnormal cerebral vasculature, repeated infection and sepsis, and blood transfusions.

Characteristic findings include patchy but fairly symmetric areas of vasogenic edema centered in the subcortical white matter of both cerebral hemispheres. There is typical posterior predominance with preferential involvement of the parietal and occipital lobes. Edematous areas will be low in attenuation on CT and high in signal on fluid-attenuated inversion recovery and T2-weighted MR images (**Fig. 13**).

The symptoms and imaging appearance typically improve upon resolution of the insult, that is, discontinuing medication or blood pressure control. However, severe cases can progress to infarction and hemorrhage leading to permanent injury. PRES does not always present in characteristic fashion and atypical cases may affect the basal ganglia, cerebellum, or brain stem and lesions may have asymmetric or unilateral distributions.

Generalized Cerebral Volume Loss and Leukoencephalopathy

Changes in neurocognitive function have been described in SCD patients, even in the absence of localized ischemic or hemorrhagic brain lesions.[17] Several recent studies have been performed to assess generalized changes in both brain morphology and volume. Historical assessment of cerebral atrophy relied on a qualitative analysis, assessing for enlargement of the ventricles and sulci greater than expected for age, obviously limited by the subjective nature of this approach. Recent advances in MRI techniques allow for a quantitative analysis, and studies have clearly demonstrated distinct differences in white matter, gray matter, and overall cerebral volumes between children with SCD and the general population.

Chen and colleagues[18] found "significant age-related decrease in total gray matter volume in children with sickle cell disease." This decrease was widely spatially distributed throughout both cerebral hemispheres, although somewhat patchy. Kirk and colleagues[19] also found decreased overall gray matter volume, with different regions

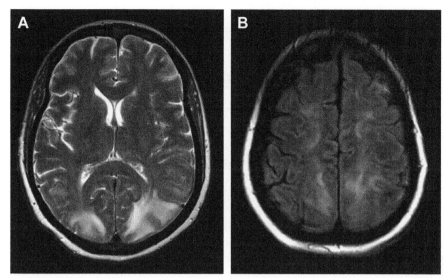

Fig. 13. Bilateral symmetric subcortical and cortical edema manifesting as increased signal on T2-weighted (A) and fluid-attenuated inversion recovery (B) images. This pattern of edema is highly consistent with posterior reversible leukoencephalopathy syndrome in the appropriate clinical scenario.

of cortical thinning. The largest regions were the precuneus and posterior cingulate gyrus.

Diffusion tensor imaging studies demonstrate changes in white matter in patients with no or minimal apparent anatomic or signal changes on traditional MR pulse sequences.[20] Investigators found increased diffusivity and decreased anisotropy throughout the white matter of SCD patients, including major white matter bundles such as the corpus callosum. Although certainly not a specific finding, this does suggest a generalized leukoencphalopathy.

HEAD AND NECK COMPLICATIONS
Inner Ears

There is a known association of SCD and sensorineural hearing loss with estimated prevalence rates as high as 60%.[21] Extent of hearing loss ranges from mild to profound, and may be unilateral or bilateral. The highly vascular cochlea and organ of Corti are susceptible to ischemic changes, and even brief periods of ischemia may be damaging as minimal collateral vessels exist. Deficits are often permanent; however, there are reports of hearing recovery after resolution of a crisis.

Imaging of these patients is often negative. However, several reports exist of spontaneous, nontraumatic labyrinthine hemorrhage in SCD patients who experience a sudden onset of sensorineural hearing loss. Imaging findings for labyrinthine hemorrhage may be subtle, and dedicated thin-section imaging of the inner ears using a small field of view is helpful. Increased fluid-attenuated inversion recovery signal and postcontrast enhancement is typical for any inflammatory process of the inner ear, but increased intrinsic T1-weighted signal is fairly specific for hemorrhage, because subacute blood products result in marked T1 shortening[22] (**Fig. 14**).

Labyrinthitis ossificans occurs as a result of pathologic bone formation within the otic capsule as a reparative response to an inflammatory process such as infection

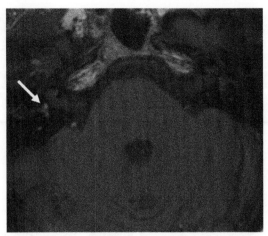

Fig. 14. Axial T1-weighted MRI through the inner ears demonstrates increased signal intensity in the right vestibule (*arrow*) and semicircular canals consistent with hemolabyrinth.

or vascular insult, both of which occur with increased frequency in SCD patients.[23] The resultant characteristic findings on CT include increased density within or frank osseous lesions encroaching on the membranous labyrinth (**Fig. 15**). Imaging findings may be apparent earlier on MRI as low signal fibroosseous material replaces the normal high signal endolymph on T2-weighted imaging.

Orbits

Vasoocclusive events can have a profound effect on the globe and optic apparatus with devastating visual effects. Optic disc and retinal abnormalities are diagnosed typically on funduscopic examination without imaging. However, macroscopic

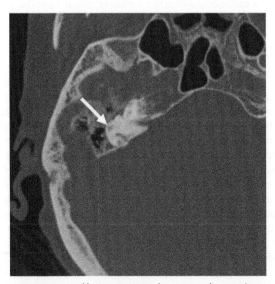

Fig. 15. Axial noncontrast temporal bone computed tomography scan in a patient with labyrinthitis ossificans. Bone deposition results in increased density throughout the inner ear (*arrow*).

changes, including retinal detachment, vitreous hemorrhage, cataracts, or phthisi bulbi, may be readily identifiable with orbit imaging.

Orbital crises and orbital bone infarction are relatively uncommon but fairly unique manifestations of SCD. Rapidly progressive pain and swelling occur during a crisis with resultant proptosis and visual changes[24] (**Fig. 16**). Bone changes can be identified on MRI as heterogenous increased signal on T2-weighted or short T1 inversion recovery images or increased uptake on nuclear medicine bone scintigraphy. Intraorbital or periorbital soft swelling occurs, manifesting as ill-defined stranding. Subperiosteal hematomas may further complicate the matter and may require surgical evacuation (**Fig. 17**). Differentiation from orbital cellulitis may be difficult, because there is significant clinical and radiographic overlap between these entities, and antibiotic coverage is often given presumptively.

Lymphoid Tissue

Children with SCD have increased lymphoid tissue in the head and neck region relative to the general population.[25] This is manifested by prominence of the adenoids and palatine tonsils, as well as the retropharyngeal and deep cervical lymph nodes (**Fig. 18**). This is postulated to occur as a compensatory response for functional asplenia. Resultant narrowing of the upper airway results in increased rates of sleep-disordered breathing. This obstructive sleep apnea may play an important role in the previously described neurocognitive dysfunction seen in SCD patients.[26] Direct imaging and quantitative assessment of the lymphoid tissue is rarely performed; however, the findings of lymphoidal hypertrophy are frequently identifiable on routine imaging of the brain, spine, or neck (see **Fig. 18**).

Bone

Chronic anemia has a profound effect on the hematopoietic system, and as such bony changes are the most commonly described clinical and imaging manifestation of SCD. Elevated erythropoietin levels induce red marrow hyperplasia.[27,28] Expansion of the diploic space with trabecular thinning and osteoporosis may be seen throughout the calvarium and skull base on CT scan. A significant decrease in T1-weighted signal of the marrow cavity is typical on MRI[29] (**Fig. 19**).

Focal disruption of the trabecular architecture from acute bone infarcts has been described on CT scan; however, this subtle finding is difficult to detect. Chronic

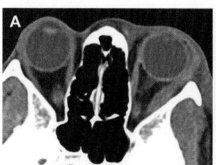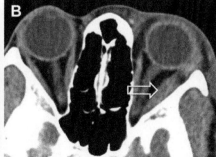

Fig. 16. Two axial images from a contrast enhanced computed tomography scan in a patient with acute orbital crisis. Note the periorbital soft tissue swelling in (*A*) with thickening and stranding along the lateral rectus muscle (*open arrow*) in (*B*). (*Courtesy of* T. York, MD, Baltimore, MD.)

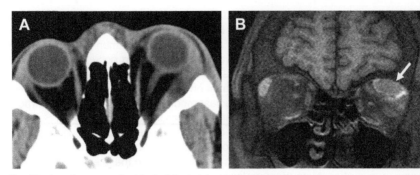

Fig. 17. Another case of orbital crisis. Axial noncontrast computed tomography scan (*A*) demonstrates left-sided proptosis, with periorbital soft tissue and thickening of the lateral rectus muscle. Coronal T1-fat saturated MRI (*B*) demonstrates an associated subperiosteal hematoma in the roof of the left orbit (*arrow*). (*Courtesy of* J. Matsumoto, MD, Charlottesville, VA.)

infarctions may induce well-defined geographic areas of sclerosis. MRI offers a much more sensitive evaluation for acute bone marrow edema, which manifests as high signal on T2-weighted and short T1 inversion recovery sequences, with possible adjacent subperiosteal blood or fluid. Avascular necrosis may follow infarction. When involving the mandibular condyle, this can lead to advanced degenerative and temporomandibular joint disorders (**Fig. 20**).

Damage to the spleen and functional asplenia also leaves patients at greater risk for infection. This immune deficiency results in a particular susceptibility to infection from encapsulated bacteria, because necrotic bone is a suitable environment for infection. The facial bones, especially the mandible, are at prone to osteomyelitis (**Fig. 21**). Differentiating bone infection from infarction is difficult with imaging alone. Fluid collections communicating with the bone marrow through cortical defects is particularly concerning for infection.

Although rare in the head and neck, extramedullary hematopoiesis has been described, most commonly in the paranasal sinuses. When severe, there may be

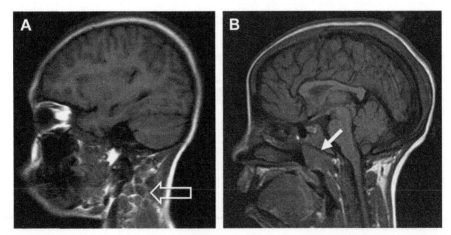

Fig. 18. Sagittal T1-weight MRIs in 2 different sickle cell patients. Off-midline image (*A*) shows numerous prominent upper cervical lymph nodes (*open arrow*). Adenoidal hypertrophy (*arrow*) in (*B*) results in narrowing of the nasopharyngeal airway.

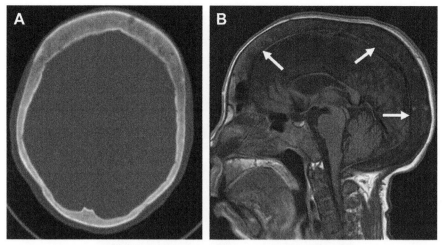

Fig. 19. Axial noncontrast computed tomography scan on bone windows (A) exhibits marked expansion of the bony calvarium. Sagittal T1-weighted MRI in a different patient (B) also shows an expanded calvarium (*arrows*). Note the heterogeneity and diffusely decreased signal intensity throughout all of the visualized osseous structures.

associated nasal obstruction. Pneumatization of the paranasal sinuses is typically delayed, and the sinuses may be relatively underpneumatized compared with normal populations (**Fig. 22**).

MANAGEMENT AND TREATMENT

The focus of management in SCD populations involves preventative treatments and supportive care for acute crises.[30,31] Infection prevention includes daily penicillin prophylaxis and immunizations.

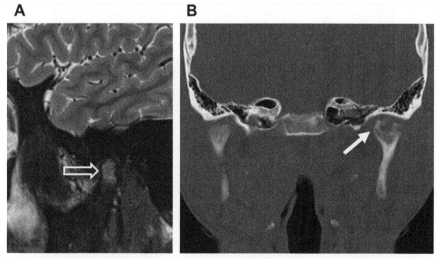

Fig. 20. Sagittal short T1 inversion recovery image (A) shows edema in the left mandibular condyle (*open arrow*) from an acute bone infarct. Coronal computed tomography image (B) shows chronic degenerative changes with avascular necrosis (*arrow*). (*Courtesy of* E. Zan, MD, Baltimore, MD)

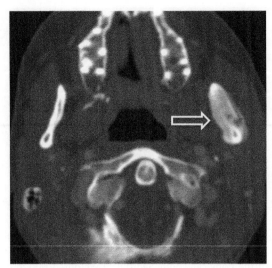

Fig. 21. Chronic osteomyelitis of the left mandibular ramus results in marked thickening and sclerosis (*open arrow*) on this axial computed tomography image.

Expert panel supports annual transcranial Doppler ultrasonography screening for SCD patients from age 2 through at least 16 as well regular ophthalmologic evaluation. More costly neuroimaging, such as CT and MRI, should be reserved for symptomatic patients or those with abnormalities identified on screening studies.

Patients with SCD should be managed according to standard guidelines including controlling risk factors and using antiplatelet agents in those with prior stroke, transient ischemic attack, or symptomatic stenoses. Disease-modifying treatments

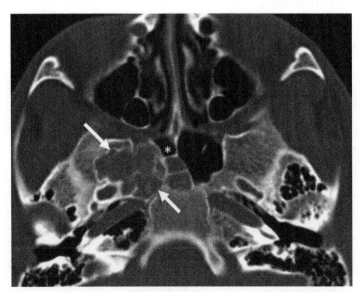

Fig. 22. Axial noncontrast computed tomography image of the skull base shows arrested pneumatization of the sphenoid sinus. The sinus (*asterisk*) is diminutive in size, replaced by a heterogenous osteosclerotic lesion (*arrows*).

such us hydroxyurea and long-term transfusion have shown significant results. Unfortunately, these treatments seem to be underused, because continuity of care in SCD patients is often lacking. Revascularization procedures, both direct and indirect, should be considered for advanced occlusive disease.

SUMMARY

SCD is a common chronic condition characterized by hemolysis and vasoocclusive episodes. Damage to the cerebral vasculature can cause thrombosis, stenosis, dilatation, and rupture. Resulting infarction and hemorrhage are major causes of mortality and mortality in this devastating disease.

Head and neck manifestations are less commonly discussed, but are a significant component of the disease. Bony changes and lymphoid enlargement are characteristic. Orbital and inner ear crises may induce significant visual and hearing impairments.

ACKNOWLEDGMENTS

Special thanks to Brigitte Pocta, MLA, for assistance in the preparation of this article.

REFERENCES

1. Bunn HF. Pathogenesis and treatment of sickle cell disease. N Engl J Med 1997; 337:762–9.
2. Centers for Disease Control and Prevention. Sickle cell disease. Available at: www.cdc.gov/ncbddd/sicklecell/index.html. Accessed November 1, 2015.
3. Scott RM, Smith ER. Moyamoya disease and moyamoya syndrome. N Engl J Med 2009;360(12):1226–37.
4. Diggs LW, Brookoff D. Multiple cerebral aneurysms in patients with sickle cell disease. South Med J 1993;86(4):377–9.
5. Adams RJ, McKie VC, Hsu L, et al. Prevention of a first stroke by transfusions in children with sickle cell anemia and abnormal results on transcranial Doppler ultrasonography. N Engl J Med 1998;339(1):5–11.
6. Krejza J, Chen R, Romanowicz G, et al. Sickle cell disease and transcranial Doppler imaging: inter-hemispheric differences in blood flow Doppler parameters. Stroke 2011;42(1):81–6.
7. Maeda M, Tsuchida C. "Ivy sign" on fluid-attenuated inversion-recovery images in childhood moyamoya disease. AJNR Am J Neuroradiol 1999; 20(10):1836–8.
8. Debaun MR, Derdeyn CP, McKinstry RC 3rd. Etiology of strokes in children with sickle cell anemia. Ment Retard Dev Disabil Res Rev 2006;12(3):192–9.
9. Mangla R, Kolar B, Almast J, et al. Border zone infarcts: pathophysiologic and imaging characteristics. Radiographics 2011;31(5):1201–14.
10. Noguchi T, Kawashima M, Nishihara M, et al. Arterial spin-labeling MR imaging in Moyamoya disease compared with clinical assessments and other MR imaging findings. Eur J Radiol 2013;82(12):e840–7.
11. Gevers S, Nederveen AJ, Fijnvandraat K, et al. Arterial spin labeling measurement of cerebral perfusion in children with sickle cell disease. J Magn Reson Imaging 2012;35(4):779–87.
12. Winchell AM, Taylor BA, Song R, et al. Evaluation of SWI in children with sickle cell disease. AJNR Am J Neuroradiol 2014;35(5):1016–21.

13. Gibbs WN, Opatowsky MJ, Burton EC. AIRP best cases in radiologic-pathologic correlation: cerebral fat embolism syndrome in sickle cell beta-thalassemia. Radiographics 2012;32(5):1301–6.
14. Resar LM, Oliva MM, Casella JF. Skull infarction and epidural hematomas in a patient with sickle cell anemia. J Pediatr Hematol Oncol 1996;18(4):413–5.
15. Henderson JN, Noetzel MJ, McKinstry RC, et al. Reversible posterior leukoencephalopathy syndrome and silent cerebral infarcts are associated with severe acute chest syndrome in children with sickle cell disease. Blood 2003;101(2):415–9.
16. Bartynski WS. Posterior reversible encephalopathy syndrome, part 1: fundamental imaging and clinical features. AJNR Am J Neuroradiol 2008;29(6):1036–42.
17. Steen RG, Reddick WE, Glass JO, et al. Evidence of cranial artery ectasia in sickle cell disease patients with ectasia of the basilar artery. Stroke 1998;7(5):330–8.
18. Chen R, Pawlak MA, Flynn TB, et al. Brain morphometry and intelligence quotient measurements in children with sickle cell disease. J Dev Behav Pediatr 2009; 30(6):509–17.
19. Kirk GR, Haynes MR, Palasis S, et al. Regionally specific cortical thinning in children with sickle cell disease. Cereb Cortex 2009;19(7):1549–56.
20. Balci A, Karazincir S, Beyoglu Y, et al. Quantitative brain diffusion-tensor MRI findings in patients with sickle cell disease. AJR Am J Roentgenol 2012;198(5): 1167–74.
21. Al Okbi MH, Alkindi S, Al Abri RK, et al. Sensorineural hearing loss in sickle cell disease–a prospective study from Oman. Laryngoscope 2011;121(2):392–6.
22. Liu BP, Saito N, Wang JJ, et al. Labyrinthitis ossificans in a child with sickle cell disease: CT and MRI findings. Pediatr Radiol 2009;39(9):999–1001.
23. Saito N, Nadgir RN, Flower EN, et al. Clinical and radiologic manifestations of sickle cell disease in the head and neck. Radiographics 2010;30(4):1021–34.
24. Ganesh A, William RR, Mitra S, et al. Orbital involvement in sickle cell disease: a report of five cases and review literature. Eye (Lond) 2001;15(Pt 6):774–80.
25. Strauss T, Sin S, Marcus CL, et al. Upper airway lymphoid tissue size in children with sickle cell disease. Chest 2012;142(1):94–100.
26. Rosen CL, Debaun MR, Strunk RC, et al. Obstructive sleep apnea and sickle cell anemia. Pediatrics 2014;134(2):273–81.
27. Yildirim T, Agildere AM, Oguzkurt L, et al. MRI evaluation of cranial bone marrow signal intensity and thickness in chronic anemia. Eur J Radiol 2005;53(1):125–30.
28. Elias EJ, Liao JH, Jara H, et al. Quantitative MRI analysis of craniofacial bone marrow in patients with sickle cell disease. AJNR Am J Neuroradiol 2013;34(3):622–7.
29. Loevner LA, Tobey JD, Yousem DM, et al. MR imaging characteristics of cranial bone marrow in adult patients with underlying systemic disorders compared with healthy control subjects. AJNR Am J Neuroradiol 2002;23(2):248–54.
30. Dobson SR, Holden KR, Nietert PJ, et al. Moyamoya syndrome in childhood sickle cell disease: a predictive factor for recurrent cerebrovascular events. Blood 2002;99(9):3144–50.
31. Yawn BP, Buchanan GR, Afenyi-Annan AN, et al. Management of sickle cell disease: summary of the 2014 evidence-based report by expert panel members. JAMA 2014;312(10):1033–48.

Neuroimaging in Central Nervous System Lymphoma

Seyed Ali Nabavizadeh, MD[a], Arastoo Vossough, MD[b],
Mehrdad Hajmomenian, MD[b], Reza Assadsangabi, MD[b],
Suyash Mohan, MD, PDCC[a],*

KEYWORDS

- Lymphoma • Central nervous system • MRI • CT

KEY POINTS

- Most cases of primary central nervous system lymphoma (PCNSL) are of the B-cell type (90% are diffuse large B-cell lymphoma) and a small subset are of T-cell lineage.
- PCNSLs are highly cellular lesions with tightly compacted cells, which translate into high density on computed tomography scan, low signal on T2-weighted imaging, and restricted diffusion on diffusion-weighted imaging.
- A variety of intracranial pathologic conditions can mimic PCNSL, such as high-grade gliomas, toxoplasmosis, subacute infarction, and tumefactive demyelinating lesions.

INTRODUCTION

Primary central nervous system lymphoma (PCNSL) is a rare aggressive high-grade type of extranodal lymphoma.[1] In PCNSL, the lymphoma is restricted to brain parenchyma, meninges, spinal cord, or eyes, without evidence of disease outside the central nervous system (CNS) at the time of initial diagnosis.[1,2] Most cases of PCNSL are of the B-cell type (90% are diffuse large B-cell lymphoma), and a small subset are of T-cell lineage.[3] PCNSL is more frequently seen in immunocompromised patients but it can occur in the immunocompetent population. The incidence of PCNSL has shown a growing trend from 3.3% before 1978 to 6.6% to 15.4% of all primary brain tumors in the early 1990s, due to increased prevalence of human immunodeficiency virus (HIV) infection and use of immunosuppressive drugs for transplantation.[1] However, subsequently, the incidence of PCNSL declined secondary to the introduction of highly active antiretroviral therapy (HAART).[4,5]

The mean age of diagnosis for PCNSL is 60 years old and it is more common in women.[6] Patients with acquired immunodeficiency syndrome (AIDS) are generally

[a] Department of Radiology, Division of Neuroradiology, Perelman School of Medicine at University of Pennsylvania, 3400 Spruce Street, Philadelphia, PA 19014, USA; [b] Department of Radiology, Children's Hospital of Philadelphia, Perelman School of Medicine at the University of Pennsylvania, 3401 Civic Center Boulevard, Philadelphia, PA 19104, USA
* Corresponding author.
E-mail address: Suyash.Mohan@uphs.upenn.edu

Hematol Oncol Clin N Am 30 (2016) 799–821
http://dx.doi.org/10.1016/j.hoc.2016.03.005
0889-8588/16/$ – see front matter © 2016 Elsevier Inc. All rights reserved.
hemonc.theclinics.com

diagnosed at a younger age than those without this disease.[7] A smaller peak is also observed in the first decade of life due to pediatric AIDS.[1]

Clinically, PCNSL may mimic other intracranial pathologies on imaging such as encephalitis, demyelination, and stroke. Personality changes, cerebellar signs, headache, seizure, and motor dysfunction may occur. Constitutional symptoms may also be present[1] but they are more common in T-cell lymphoma.[8] Early diagnosis and treatment can sometimes reduce the irreversible deficits of this disease.

In addition to primary lymphoma, the CNS can be secondarily involved by systemic lymphoma in 10% to 15% of patients,[9] with a tendency to occur early at a median lag of 5 to 12 months after the primary diagnosis of non-Hodgkin lymphoma (NHL).[10] The systemic lymphoma is almost always aggressive NHL and patients with systemic Hodgkin disease are at very low risk of CNS involvement.[10]

IMAGING FINDINGS
Secondary Central Nervous System Lymphoma

CNS involvement by systemic lymphoma presents as leptomeningeal disease in two-thirds and as parenchymal disease in one-third of patients.[10] Approximately half of the patients with secondary CNS lymphoma have progressive systemic lymphoma. Most of the remaining patients with apparently isolated CNS involvement will develop systemic disease within months.[10,11] In addition, systemic lymphoma of the face (nasal cavity and paranasal sinus) can spread to the orbit and CNS via extra-ocular muscle involvement and direct perineural spread of neoplasm.[12]

Contrast-enhanced MRI is the imaging modality of choice and can detect enhancement along the pial surface of the brain and spinal cord, subependymal ventricular system, and cranial or spinal nerve roots.[10] It is more sensitive compared with contrast-enhanced computed tomography (CT).[13] Leptomeningeal disease can also invade the brain parenchyma and cause superficial cerebral lesions. Communicating hydrocephalus is frequently observed in patients with leptomeningeal disease.[10]

Parenchymal CNS involvement in systemic lymphoma can present as single or multiple parenchymal masses (**Figs. 1** and **2**) and may accompany leptomeningeal disease.[14,15] In a study of 18 subjects with parenchymal lymphoma, Senocak and colleagues[16] demonstrated that homogenous nodular enhancement and supratentorial white matter involvement were present in all subjects with secondary lymphoma, with a butterfly pattern and infiltrative or perivenular enhancement in half of the subjects, with no significant distinctive radiologic characteristics between primary and secondary lymphoma of the brain parenchyma.

Primary Central Nervous System Lymphoma

General features

The most common presentation of PCNSL is a single intracranial mass.[17] However, multiple masses are also quite common, and are seen in 20% to 40% of immunocompetent cases and 50% of the immunocompromised patients.[17–19] The classic location of PCNSL is supratentorial in up to 70% of cases and has a predilection to involve the periventricular white matter. Basal ganglia are involved in 13% to 20% of patients.[17–20] Involvement of the corpus callosum and extension to the other side of the brain can mimic the butterfly glioma appearance of glioblastoma multiforme (GBM).[21] Superficial locations are also sometimes seen.[10] Less commonly, lymphoma may involve other CNS structures (**Fig. 3**) such as the hypothalamus, brainstem, cerebellum pituitary talk, and spinal cord.[3,21]

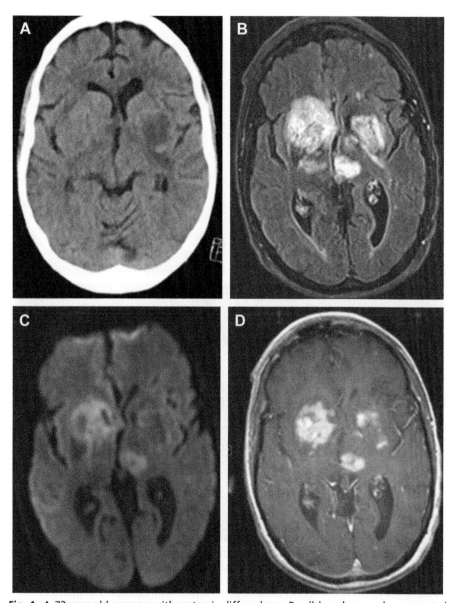

Fig. 1. A 72-year-old woman with systemic diffuse large B-cell lymphoma who presented with change in mental status. CT scan (*A*) demonstrated multiple hyperdense lesions in bilateral basal ganglia and thalami, which correspond to enhancing masses with restricted diffusion on MRI (*B–D*) consistent with secondary CNS involvement.

Primary dural lymphoma is a rare subtype of PCNSL, which is usually a low-grade marginal zone lymphoma[22,23] that primarily arises from the dura mater and may mimic meningioma and other dural based lesions.[24] It can be single or multiple and, although it has a predilection for cerebral convexities, it may involve other dural structures.[22–24] Primary leptomeningeal lymphoma, which has a better prognosis, is a rare subset of PSCNSL with estimated incidence of 7% of all PCNSLs.[25] In a study of 48 subjects

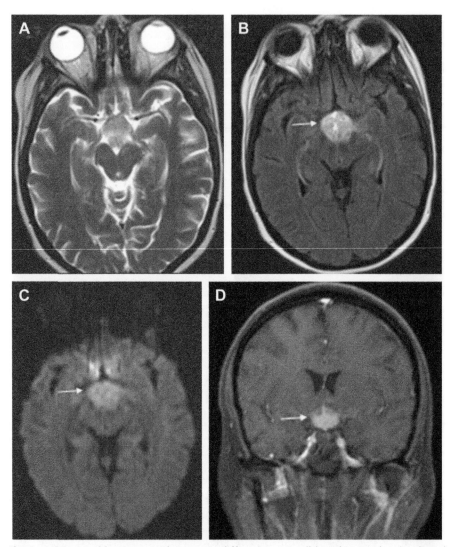

Fig. 2. A 23-year-old woman with systemic diffuse large B-cell lymphoma who developed memory loss, confusion, and mood changes during the course of treatment. MRI of the brain (*A–D, white arrows*) demonstrates an enhancing mass with restricted diffusion involving the optic chiasm and hypothalamus consistent with secondary lymphoma.

with primary leptomeningeal lymphoma, 62% had B-cell lymphoma, 19% T-cell, and 19% unclassified.[25] These patients usually present with multifocal symptoms. Imaging demonstrates leptomeningeal enhancement and CSF analysis is the mainstay of diagnosis[25] (**Fig. 4**).

Ocular lymphoma can be a secondary extension of PCNSL and has been reported in up to 25% of patients or, very rarely, PCNSL is restricted to the eye. Ocular lymphoma can be diagnosed by slit lamp examination or cytologic examination of vitreal aspirate. On dedicated orbital imaging (with application of fat-saturation sequences), ocular lymphoma can be detected as a nodular enhancing mass.[26] However, sensitivity is not high and a negative study does not exclude intraocular lymphoma.[26]

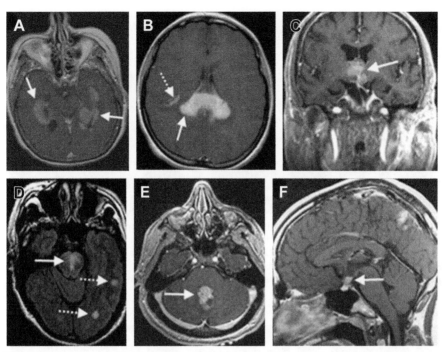

Fig. 3. Spectrum of various locations of CNS lymphoma in the brain. (*A*) Periventricular (*arrows*). (*B*) Corpus callosum (*arrow*) involvement mimicking a butterfly glioma, and a nearby linear branching parenchymal lymphomatous lesion (*dashed arrow*) mimicking a developmental venous anomaly. (*C*) Involvement of hypothalamus (*arrow*). (*D*) A 52-year-old man with new dysarthria, right facial weakness, right-sided weakness, and ataxia. FLAIR hyperintense lesion seen in pontomesencephalic junction (*arrow*) with other parenchymal lesions (*dashed arrows*). (*E*) Cerebellar lesion adjacent and protruding into the fourth ventricle (*arrow*). (*F*) Another patient presenting with diabetes insipidus. Thickening and enhancement of the pituitary stalk (*arrow*).

Conventional imaging

One of the histopathologic features of PCNSL is high cellularity with tightly compacted cells and high nuclear to cytoplasmic ratio, which translates into some important imaging characteristics of PCNSL, such as high density on CT scan, low signal on T2-weighted imaging, and restricted diffusion on diffusion-weighted imaging (DWI).[1,2,6–10] One of the important considerations in imaging of patients with PCNSL is the effect of steroids, which can cause apoptosis and necrosis in the mass, and can change the pattern of enhancement, metabolic activity, and also histopathologic findings.[27]

On CT scanning, PCNSL usually present as a hyperdense mass (**Fig. 5**) with contrast enhancement.[28,29] This is an important diagnostic feature of PCNSL; however, less commonly it may also be isodense or hypodense, which may be misdiagnosed as infarction, demyelination, or encephalomalacia.[19]

On MRI, PCNSLs are usually characterized by their periventricular locations, well-defined margin, moderate or marked edema, and intense and homogeneous nodular enhancement (**Fig. 6**). On T2-weighted images, PCNSL shows short T2 relaxation times in most instances and thus appears isointense to hypointense in relation to gray matter, which is not common for most intracranial lesions.[17,18] This feature is

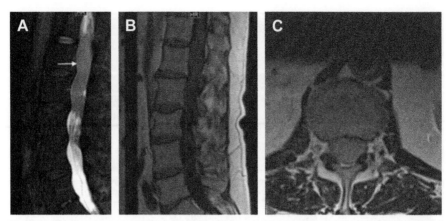

Fig. 4. A 62-year-old man with marginal B-cell lymphoma of the spleen who presented with lower extremity weakness and incontinence. MRI of the lumbar spine demonstrates complete filling of the spinal canal by a T1/T2 isointense soft tissue mass (*A, B, arrow*) completely enveloping and compressing the conus and proximal cauda equina (*C*), consistent with leptomeningeal involvement by lymphoma. Biopsy of the mass confirmed the diagnosis.

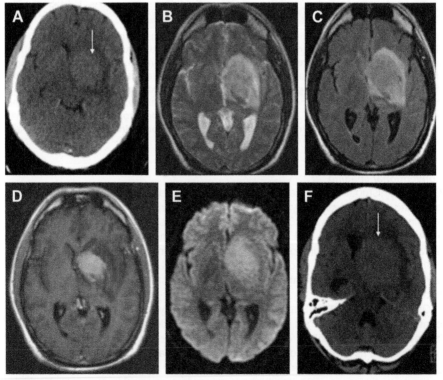

Fig. 5. Initial brain CT scan in 48-year-old HIV-positive patient demonstrates a hyperdense mass in left basal ganglia (*A, arrow*). MRI from the same day (*B–E*) demonstrated a T2 isointense, enhancing mass with restricted diffusion. Subsequent CT scan after 9 days (*F*) demonstrates marked enlargement of the mass (*arrow*) which was proven to be PCNSL.

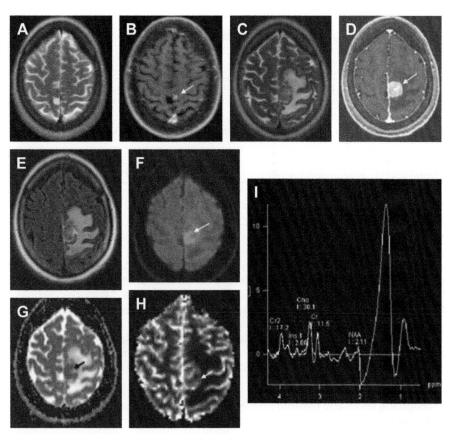

Fig. 6. Initial brain MRI in 59-year-old woman with sudden loss of consciousness demonstrated a subcentimeter left parafalcine enhancing lesion (*A, B, arrow*). Follow-up MRI after 5 weeks demonstrated marked enlargement of the enhancing mass, which is hypointense on T2 (*C, D, arrow*), with surrounding edema on FLAIR (*E*) and demonstrates restricted diffusion (*F, G, arrows*). DSC perfusion (*H, arrow*) demonstrates only mild elevation of cerebral blood volume. Magnetic resonance spectroscopy (*I*) of the mass demonstrates elevation of Cho/Cr ratio and prominent lipid/lactate peak. The mass was resected and histopathology was PCNSL.

due to compact cells and a high nuclear-to-cytoplasmic ratio. A long T2 relaxation time is uncommon for PCNSL and is correlated to the degree of necrosis.[30] On the other hand, similar to many other lesions in the brain, PCNSL is hypointense to gray matter on T1-weighted imaging. Perilesional edema is usually present and is typically vasogenic in nature.[8,17] However, cytotoxic edema has been reported in angiotropic large cell lymphoma (intravascular lymphomatosis) due to infiltration and cerebral infarction caused by vessel occlusion.[31]

PCNSL typically enhances avidly and homogeneously in immunocompetent patients (**Table 1**). Ring enhancement is seen in only 0% to 13% of immunocompetent cases.[10] The pattern of enhancement is more variable in immunocompromised patients. Ring enhancement is the dominant pattern due to central necrosis and occurs in up to 75% of the patients. Homogeneous enhancement is less common in this group. Leptomeningeal enhancement has been reported in 16% to 41% of

Table 1
Typical imaging appearances of central nervous system lymphoma in immunocompetent versus immunocompromised patients

	Immunocompetent	Immunocompromised
Location	White matter (central hemispheric or periventricular), superficial, corpus callosum	Gray matter (basal ganglion or other deep gray matter nuclei)
Number of lesions	Single, less likely multiple (20%–40%)	Single or multiple
Hemorrhage	Rare	Uncommon
Enhancement	Solid (ring in 0%–13%)	Ring (up to 75%)

PCNSL at initial diagnosis.[32] Rarely, PCNSL can present as T2 hyperintense lesions without contrast enhancement.[17,33] Nonenhancing PCNSLs have been shown to be low-grade, less aggressive, lesions with a better prognosis in a few studies.[34,35] Lymphomatosis cerebri is a rare entity characterized by diffuse supratentorial and infratentorial white matter T2 hyperintensity without contrast enhancement, which can mimic gliomatosis cerebri. Previously reported cases were in immune competent patients and the presenting symptoms can be nonspecific and include personality changes, cognitive deficit, and gait ataxia.[33,36]

Calcification is rare at the time of presentation in PCNSL.[37] However, it may develop after chemotherapy or radiotherapy. Similarly, hemorrhage is rare in PCNSL (**Fig. 7**)[17,28] and is associated with VEGF immunoreactivity.[38]

Pattern of recurrence

Although the survival of patients with PCNSL has improved because as of multimodality treatment approaches, recurrence will eventually occur in most patients.[39,40] One of the features of PCNSL relapse is that, unlike primary gliomas such as glioblastoma, recurrence usually does not occur at the site of initial tumor presentation (**Fig. 8**). In a study of 16 immunocompetent subjects with PCNSL relapse, local recurrence at the site of the initial tumor presentation was found only in 25% of subjects, and subjects frequently presented with bilateral or contralateral recurrence.[41]

Intravascular lymphomatosis

Intravascular lymphomatosis is a rare type of diffuse large B-cell lymphoma that is characterized by proliferation of the B-cells in the vascular lumen with no or minimal parenchymal involvement. It usually affects the CNS or skin, although any organ can be involved.[42] If the CNS is involved, patients can present with a variety of symptoms, including focal sensory or motor deficits, generalized weakness, altered sensorium, rapidly progressive dementia, seizures, hemiparesis, dysarthria, ataxia, vertigo, and transient visual loss.[43–46] It can mimic entities such as stroke, encephalomyelitis, Guillain-Barré syndrome, vasculitis, or demyelination. Diagnosis is often delayed and is based on findings on biopsy.[42]

Imaging usually demonstrates multifocal areas of hypodensity on CT and increased signal on T2-weighted images without enhancement (**Fig. 9**), although enhancement can be seen in a subset of cases and can have gyriform, speckled, ring-like, or homogeneous patterns.[47–49] Due to intravascular nature of the disease, some patients can present with infarcts, which can be detected on diffusion weighted imaging.[50]

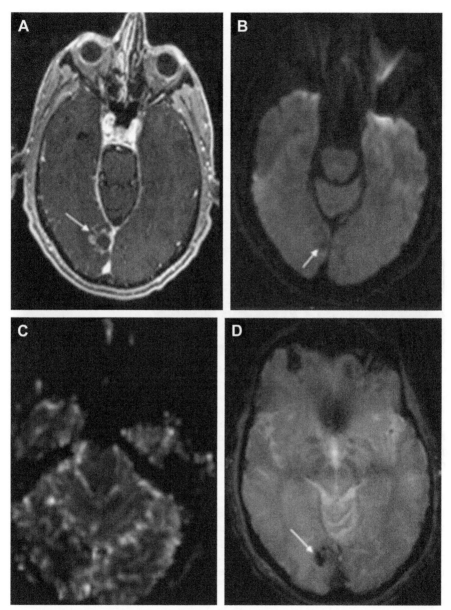

Fig. 7. Atypical imaging appearance of PCNSL. MRI in a 73-year-old patient with visual disturbance shows a superficial rim enhancing lesion in right occipital region (*A, arrow*). DWI trace image shows no clear diffusion restriction (*B, arrow*). No elevation in DSC perfusion rCBV maps (*C*). There is susceptibility effect on T2* images consistent with presence of hemorrhage and/or calcification (*D, arrow*), which are not common in untreated CNS lymphoma.

T-cell lymphoma

T-cell lymphomas are rare in both adults and children, comprising only 2% to 8% of PCNSL cases.[51–55] A review of 45 subjects with T-cell lymphoma revealed that the presentation and outcome seem similar to that of B-cell PCNSL.[56] Compared with

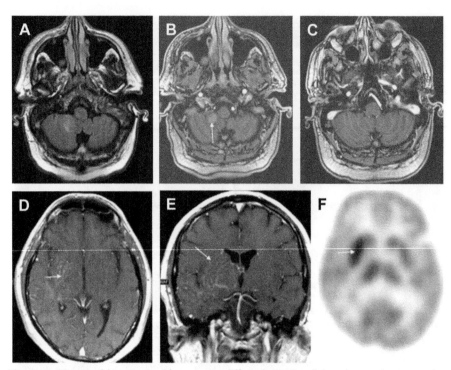

Fig. 8. A 56-year-old patient with systemic diffuse large B-cell lymphoma demonstrating distant recurrence. Initial MRI demonstrates an 11 mm superficial lesion in the right cerebellum consistent with secondary CNS lymphoma (*A, B, arrow*). Follow-up MRI after 3 months of treatment with high-dose methotrexate and Rituxan demonstrates resolution of the lesion (*C*). Another follow-up MRI, 7 months after the second MRI demonstrates interval development of predominantly perivascular enhancement centered in the right thalamus and basal ganglia consistent with CNS recurrence (*D, E, arrow*). FDG-PET demonstrates asymmetric increased FDG uptake involving the right thalamus and lentiform nucleus (*F, arrow*).

PCNSL of B-cell origin, there is less available literature with regard to imaging findings in subjects with T-cell PCNSL. Brain parenchymal involvement can be with solitary or multiple homogenously enhancing masses with a supratentorial predilection.[57,58] Some studies also report a predilection for a subcortical location, relatively high incidence of cortical or intratumoral hemorrhage (**Fig. 10**), and necrosis.[58] They showed lower relative cerebral blood volume (rCBV) ratios compared with high-grade glioma,[58] a finding shared by PCNSL of B-cell origin.[59,60]

Adult T-cell lymphoma-leukemia (ATLL)[61] is a T-cell neoplasm, associated with infection by the retrovirus human T-lymphotropic virus type 1. In patients with ATLL, secondary CNS involvement occurs in up to 25% of cases. The typical findings on imaging studies are multiple parenchymal lesions, with or without enhancement, involvement of the deep grey nuclei, and leptomeningeal disease.[61]

Advanced Imaging

With conventional imaging techniques, a wide range of differentials are often considered for an intraparenchymal mass, covering typical and atypical imaging presentation of various brain diseases. Recently, advanced imaging techniques have been used in

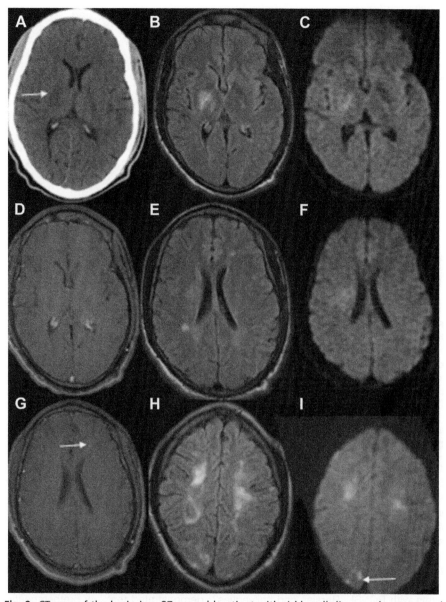

Fig. 9. CT scan of the brain in a 27-year-old patient with sickle cell disease who presented with dizziness demonstrated a hypodense lesion in right nucleocapsular region (*A, arrow*). Initial MRI (*B–D*) demonstrated T2 hyperintense lesions in right nucleocapsular region and right thalamus with mild restricted diffusion without enhancement. Additional small T2 hyperintense lesions with faint enhancement were noted in left frontal lobe (*E–G, arrow*). These lesions were presumed to be secondary to sickle vasculopathy or demyelination; however, the patient deteriorated clinically and developed multiple additional lesions on subsequent MRIs. An MRI 15 months later demonstrates multiple T2 hyperintense lesions in bilateral centrum semiovale and right parietal cortex with restricted diffusion (*H, I, arrow*). Cortical biopsy demonstrated intravascular B-cell lymphoma.

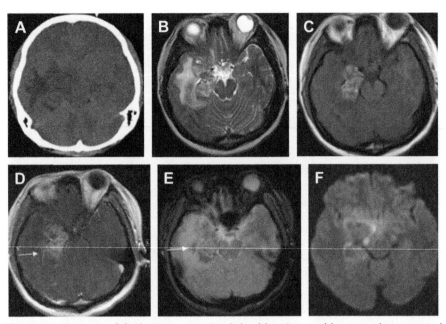

Fig. 10. Axial CT scan of the brain in a previously healthy 19-year-old woman demonstrated heterogeneous ill-defined area in the right medial temporal lobe (*A*). Brain MRI (*B*) performed on the same day demonstrates abnormal signal intensity (*B*) with gyriform areas of T1-hyperintensity and peripheral enhancement following contrast administration (*C, D, arrow*). T2* gradient echo images demonstrate foci of susceptibility, consistent with blood products (*E, arrow*). There was only mild peripheral restricted diffusion (*F*). The imaging findings were favoring herpes encephalitis; however, biopsy demonstrated T-cell PCNSL.

an effort to narrow the differential diagnosis and potentially change diagnostic and therapeutic decisions.

Diffusion-weighted imaging

DWI measures diffusion of water molecules in biological tissue. PCNSL commonly shows restricted diffusion due to high cellularity, appearing hyperintense on DWI trace images and hypointense on apparent diffusion coefficient (ADC) maps (**Fig. 11**).[10] Although cellular portions of GBM and cellular metastases may also show reduced diffusion, mean ADC values are usually lower in lymphoma.[62–65] ADC values are also higher in toxoplasmosis.[66] However, the overlap between the 2 groups is significant and makes the discrimination difficult except in the extreme ranges of ADC values.[67] In addition to added diagnostic value, ADC values have been shown to have prognostic value in patients with PCNSL. Barajas and colleagues[68] demonstrated that low pretherapeutic ADC tumor measurements within contrast-enhancing regions were predictive of shorter progression-free survival and overall survival. In addition, they demonstrated that serial ADC measurements can act as a biomarker for treatment response because patients with significant change in ADC values had a prolonged progression-free survival.[68] Diffusion tensor imaging (DTI) is a more advanced version of diffusion imaging, requiring image acquisition in at least 6 directions, which enables better assessment of alteration in the white matter and subsequent generation of fractional anisotropy (FA) maps. Multiple DTI metrics, including FA, have been extensively studied in intracranial masses, including PCNSL. Multiple studies have shown that FA values are lower in PCNSL compared with GBM.[69]

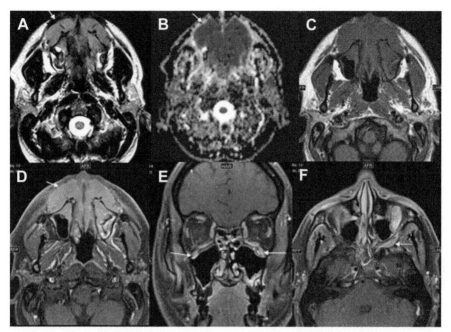

Fig. 11. A 42-year-old man with tooth and palate pain demonstrates a large mass centered at the level of the bilateral hard palate and alveolar ridge, with submucosal extraosseous extension at the level of the upper lip. The mass is isointense to hypointense on T2 (A, arrow), demonstrates marked restricted diffusion (B, arrow) with homogenous contrast enhancement (C and D, arrow). Coronal and axial T1-weighted images demonstrate perineural extension along bilateral infraorbital nerves (D, E, arrows) and left pterygopalatine fossa (F, arrow).

Perfusion and permeability imaging

PCNSL is seen as an avascular mass on angiography and this finding correlates with pathologic studies which report none to minimal neovascularization in PCNSL.[70] In the past 20 years, to go beyond the qualitative assessment of tumor vascularity on contrast-enhanced images, various imaging techniques have been used to quantitatively measure various parameters in tumor vasculature. Perfusion MRI techniques can be divided into 2 general categories: (1) those that use exogenous tracer, which is typically a gadolinium-based contrast agent, and (2) those that use an endogenous tracer such as blood, as in arterial spin labeling (ASL) and which primarily measures cerebral blood flow (CBF). Contrast-based perfusion methods can be further divided into 2 categories; T2*-weighted dynamic susceptibility weighted contrast-enhanced (DSC) MRI, and T1-weighted steady-state dynamic contrast-enhanced (DCE) MRI. Using DSC MRI, the primary output parameter in brain tumor imaging is CBV, which is often normalized to normal brain tissue as rCBV. Yamashita and colleagues[54] compared 19 subjects with PCNSL and 37 with GBM using ASL, and demonstrated that absolute and relative CBF (rCBF) were significantly higher in GBMs compared with PCNSLs. Similar results have been obtained using values from DSC perfusion studies (see **Fig. 6**).[60,71,72] There are also case series demonstrating that rCBV are higher in PCNSL compared with toxoplasmosis.[73–75] DCE MRI methods can be used for assessment of permeability of vessels, which have been shown to be significantly higher in PCNSL in comparison to GBM.[76] Schramm and colleagues[51] showed that CT perfusion can rather reliably differentiate high-grade gliomas and lymphomas based on quantitative measurements of CBV and volume transfer constant (k^{trans}). In their study, PCNSL displayed significantly increased mean k^{trans} values compared with the unaffected cerebral parenchyma (P = .0078) but no elevation of CBV compared with the marked elevation of CBV values in high-grade gliomas.[51]

Magnetic resonance spectroscopy

Magnetic resonance spectroscopy (MRS) provides in vivo measurement of different metabolic peaks that can provide diagnostic information in various brain diseases. On MRS, the most common features of PCNSL include extremely high lipid and macromolecule resonance but also high choline (Cho) and lactate, low N-acetyl aspartate (NAA) and creatine (Cr) and high Cho/Cr ratio (see **Fig. 6**).[10] Very high levels of lipid have been used for differentiation of PCNSL from GBM, in which the lipid peak is not as prominent as PCNSL.[77,78] In toxoplasmosis, lipid and lactate level are also high, which leads to overlap with PCNSL.[79] However, a study by Chang and colleagues[80] found that proton MRS alone helped correctly diagnose 94% of the brain lesions, without overlap between toxoplasmosis and lymphoma in 26 men with 35 AIDS-related brain lesions.

Susceptibility-weighted imaging

Blood and calcification produce intratumoral susceptibility signals that are depicted on susceptibility-weighted imaging (SWI) sequences as hypointense areas. Presence of microscopic bleeds is very characteristic of GBM on pathologic testing. Hemorrhage is much less common in PCNSL, although Lee and colleagues[81] reported blood product in as high as 18% of PCNSL cases. SWI can be used as an adjunct imaging measure to differentiate GBM from PCNSL.[62,82] In a study of 28 subjects with solid glioblastoma without necrosis and 19 immunocompetent subjects with PCNSL, Kickingereder and colleagues[62] found that presence of intratumoral susceptibility signals was significantly lower in subjects with PCNSL (32%) than in those with glioblastoma (82%). They also showed that a multiparametric approach using mean ADC, mean rCBV, and presence of intratumoral susceptibility signal will correctly predict histologic results in 95% of subjects with PCNSL and 96% of subjects with solid glioblastoma.

Nuclear radiology imaging

PCNSL can be assessed by nuclear imaging studies. Two tracers are more commonly used for PET of brain tumors: ^{18}F-fluorodeoxyglucose (FDG) PET and ^{11}C-methionine PET.[10] Because PCNSL has high cellular density with a high metabolic rate, it demonstrates high FDG uptake. However, it should be noted that normal FDG uptake is high in the basal ganglia, thalami and gray matter, which are also common locations for PCNSL. Therefore, FDG uptake by lymphoma in these areas can occasionally be masked by the high background uptake of these normal brain tissues. FDG-PET can be used for differentiating PCNSL and toxoplasmosis because decreased FDG is seen in toxoplasmosis in contrast to the high uptake observed in PCNSL.[83] In addition, FDG activity has been shown to be higher when compared with high-grade gliomas and brain metastasis.[84–86] Because methionine uptake is low in normal brain tissue, ^{11}C-methionine PET does not have the potential drawback of FDG-PET scans in normal high uptake areas, such as the basal ganglia.[10] Both of these tracers can be used to monitor the response of the tumor to radiotherapy and chemotherapy before the therapeutic effects are detectable on MRI.[87,88]

Different radioisotopes can be used for assessment of PCNSL by single-photon emission CT (SPECT). In contrast to toxoplasmosis, PCNSL has an avid uptake for thallium-201 (TL) and can be used as a tool for differentiation between the 2 entities.[89]

TL-SPECT has not been helpful in differentiation of GBM and PCNSL.[90] PCNSL also shows significantly higher uptake of N-isopropyl-123I-p-iodoamphetamine (I-IMP),[91] especially on delayed images after 24 hours in comparison with GBM.[92,93] Another radiotracer that is occasionally used to differentiate PCNSL from other intracranial lesions is 99Tc(m)-sestamibi (**Fig. 12**).[94] In a study of 17 AIDS subjects with intracranial enhancing lesions on either CT or MRI, Naddaf and colleagues,[94] found that sestamibi had higher specificity and equal sensitivity when compared with TL-201 scans.

LYMPHOMA MIMICS

Several disorders can mimic the imaging appearance of central nervous system lymphoma. The use of conventional and advanced imaging modalities can often help in distinguishing CNS lymphoma from these disorders (**Table 2**) but, occasionally, can be very challenging, requiring histopathologic confirmation. Preoperative differentiation of CNS lymphoma and its mimickers is important from a clinical standpoint because it will change surgical planning. Lymphoma itself, as opposed to GBM, will not require extensive resection and often a small biopsy is adequate for guiding management. Therefore, accurate preoperative evaluation of PCNSL has an important utility in the clinical decision-making process. Descriptions of the main mimickers of lymphoma follow.

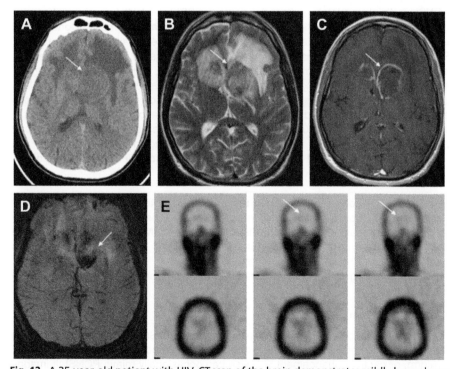

Fig. 12. A 25-year-old patient with HIV. CT scan of the brain demonstrates mildly hyperdense masses in bilateral basal ganglia (*A, arrow*). MRI brain demonstrates rim-enhancing masses with areas of internal blood products (*B–D, arrow*). Brain Tc-99m sestamibi scan demonstrates mild uptake in the area of abnormality on MRI more prominent in the right frontal periventricular region (*E, arrows*) favoring lymphoma versus toxoplasmosis. Subsequent biopsy demonstrated PCNSL.

Table 2
Imaging differentiation of central nervous system lymphoma from its 2 common mimickers: glioblastoma and toxoplasmosis

	Lymphoma vs GBM	Lymphoma vs Toxoplasmosis
DWI	Hyperintense vs hypointense	Hyperintense vs hypointense
ADC	Hypointense vs hyperintense	Hypointense vs hyperintense
MRS	Higher lipid vs lower lipid	Inconclusive literature
CT Perfusion	Low CBV vs high CBV	No study
DSC-MRI perfusion	Low rCBV vs high rCBV	No study
ASL-MRI perfusion	Low rCBF vs high rCBF	No study
SWI	No ITSS vs with ITSS	No study
FDG-PET	Higher SUV_{max} vs lower SUV_{max}	High uptake vs low uptake
11C-MET-PET	No study	No study
TI-SPECT	Not informative	High uptake vs low uptake
I-IMP-SPECT	High uptake vs low uptake	No study

Abbreviations: ITSS, intratumoral susceptibility signals; MET, ^{11}C-methionine.

High-Grade Glioma

PCNSL and high-grade gliomas, and in particular GBM, are both important differential diagnoses in an older patient presenting with an intra-axial mass. Conventional sequences are helpful in differentiating the very classic presentations of these tumors. PCSNL often has solid enhancement, whereas GBM has an irregular and often rim enhancement due to a central necrotic portion. However, there is sometimes considerable overlap in the imaging appearance of these neoplasms. For example, the less common forms of PCNSL with rim enhancement or atypical forms of GBM with solid enhancement would be hard to differentiate (**Fig. 13**). Location-wise, both lesions may involve the corpus callosum. In these circumstances, use of more advanced sequences such as ADC maps, MRS, perfusion imaging, SWI, FDG-PET, and I-IMP-SPECT can be useful tools in the preoperative assessment of these tumors.

Toxoplasmosis

PCNSL is the second most common mass lesion after toxoplasmosis in AIDS patients (**Fig. 14**). Sometimes, a CNS mass in an HIV-positive patient is presumed to be toxoplasmosis and empirical therapy is initiated. MRI is repeated and, if no changes are seen in the mass, or if it enlarges, a brain biopsy is performed. This type of approach can delay treatment if the mass is proven to be lymphoma. Advanced imaging techniques described previously can sometimes differentiate these 2 diseases.

Subacute Infarction

Rarely, PCNSL appears as a hypodense mass on CT. Subacute infarcts can have mass effect and show various patterns of contrast enhancement, such as solid, rim, gyriform, or central enhancement.[95] These can occasionally mimic PCNSL if images were acquired during the subacute stage, especially if the patient was not diagnosed or did not present at the time of the acute presentation (**Fig. 15**). Diffusion is also restricted in infarction, although depending on the timing of the infarct, diffusivity can be variable in early subacute infarcts. I-IMP-SPECT, FDP-PET, CT perfusion, and MRI perfusion may offer some help in this setting.

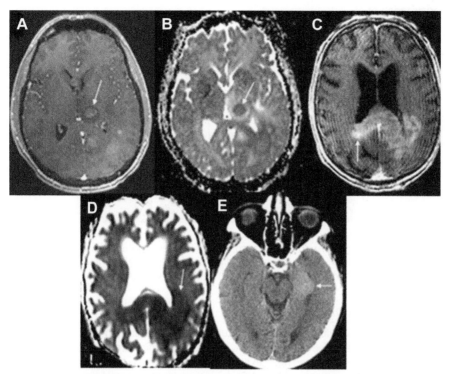

Fig. 13. Hypercellular GBM mimicking PCNSL. Small heterogeneously enhancing lesion in the left thalamus with mild peripheral edema (*A, arrow*) and with restricted diffusion (*B, arrow*). Heterogeneously enhancing mass in splenium of corpus callosum crossing the midline with minimal peripheral edema (*C, arrow*). ADC map demonstrates clear restricted diffusion (*D, arrow*). CT scan without contrast shows a homogenously hyperdense periventricular mass in left medial temporal region (*E, arrow*).

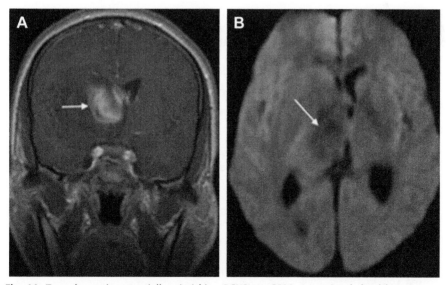

Fig. 14. Toxoplasmosis potentially mimicking PCNSL or GBM. A previously healthy man presenting with headache. Postcontrast T1-weighted imaging shows heterogeneously enhancing mass lesion in the right thalamus (*A, arrow*). DWI, however, shows no restricted diffusion (*B, arrow*). Biopsy showed toxoplasmosis and subsequently patient was diagnosed with AIDS.

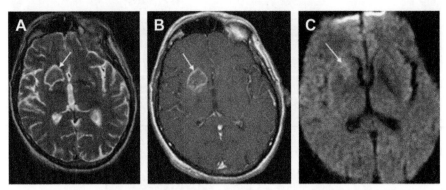

Fig. 15. Subacute infarct potentially mimicking PCNSL in an immunocompromised patient. (*A*) T2-weighted imaging shows an isointense to hypointense lesion in right basal ganglia with a peripheral hyperintense rim (*A, arrow*). (*B*) Postcontrast T1-weighted imaging shows rim enhancement (*B, arrow*). (*C*) DWI showed mild heterogeneous restricted diffusion (*C, arrow*).

Tumefactive Demyelinating Lesions

Patients with PCNSL with atypical MRI features, such as heterogeneous enhancement and absence of mass effect, may be not be easy to differentiate from tumefactive demyelination on conventional imaging.[96] In a retrospective study, Lu and colleagues[96] used MRS to differentiate patients with PCNSL from tumefactive demyelinating lesions and demonstrated higher Cho/Cr ratios, Cho/NAA ratios, and lipid and/or lactate peak grades in atypical PCNSLs when compared with those of tumefactive demyelinating lesions.

SUMMARY

CNS lymphoma is being increasingly diagnosed and can involve multiple areas within the CNS. Lymphoma can have a variable imaging appearance and mimic other brain disorders. Accurate preoperative assessment and imaging diagnosis of lymphoma has an important utility in the overall clinical diagnostic decision making process. Neurologists, neurosurgeons, and neuro-oncologists should be aware of various imaging manifestations of this disease and the imaging workup of these patients.

REFERENCES

1. Koeller KK, Smirniotopoulos JG, Jones RV. Primary central nervous system lymphoma: radiologic-pathologic correlation. Radiographics 1997;17(6):1497–526.
2. Mohile NA, Abrey LE. Primary central nervous system lymphoma. Semin Radiat Oncol 2007;17:223–9.
3. Guzzetta M, Drexler S, Buonocore B, et al. Primary CNS T-cell lymphoma of the spinal cord: case report and literature review. Lab Med 2015;46(2):159–63.
4. Diamond C, Taylor TH, Aboumrad T, et al. Changes in acquired immunodeficiency syndrome-related non-Hodgkin lymphoma in the era of highly active antiretroviral therapy: incidence, presentation, treatment, and survival. Cancer 2006; 106:128–35.
5. Besson C, Goubar A, Gabarre J, et al. Changes in AIDS-related lymphoma since the era of highly active antiretroviral therapy. Blood 2001;98:2339–44.
6. Ferreri AJM. How I treat primary CNS lymphoma. Blood 2011;118(3):510–22.

7. Sobrido Sampedro C, Corroto JD, Arias M, et al. Findings at presentation in primary CNS diffuse large B-cell lymphoma of the brain: a comparison of immunocompetent and immunodeficient patients. J Biomed Graph Comput 2013;3(4): 59–69.

8. Tang YZ, Booth TC, Bhogal P, et al. Imaging of primary central nervous system lymphoma. Clin Radiol 2011;66(8):768–77.

9. Haque S, Law M, Abrey LE, et al. Imaging of lymphoma of the central nervous system, spine, and orbit. Radiol Clin North Am 2008;46(2):339–61.

10. Haldorsen IS, Espeland A, Larsson EM. Central nervous system lymphoma: characteristic findings on traditional and advanced imaging. AJNR Am J Neuroradiol 2011;32(6):984–92.

11. Hill QA, Owen RG. CNS prophylaxis in lymphoma: who to target and what therapy to use. Blood Rev 2006;20:319–32.

12. Cruz AA, Valera FC, Carenzi L, et al. Orbital and central nervous system extension of nasal natural killer/T-cell lymphoma. Ophthal Plast Reconstr Surg 2014; 30(1):20–3.

13. DeAngelis LM, Boutros D. Leptomeningeal metastasis. Cancer Invest 2005;23: 145–54.

14. Gleissner B, Chamberlain M. Treatment of CNS dissemination in systemic lymphoma. J Neurooncol 2007;84:107–17.

15. Bierman P, Giglio P. Diagnosis and treatment of central nervous system involvement in non-Hodgkin's lymphoma. Hematol Oncol Clin North Am 2005;19:597–609.

16. Senocak E, Oguz KK, Ozgen B, et al. Parenchymal lymphoma of the brain on initial MR imaging: a comparative study between primary and secondary brain lymphoma. Eur J Radiol 2011;79(2):288–94.

17. Haldorsen IS, Krakenes J, Krossnes BK, et al. CT and MR imaging features of primary central nervous system lymphoma in Norway, 1989–2003. AJNR Am J Neuroradiol 2009;30:744–51.

18. Buhring U, Herrlinger U, Krings T, et al. MRI features of primary central nervous system lymphomas at presentation. Neurology 2001;57:393–6.

19. Erdag N, Bhorade RM, Alberico RA, et al. Primary lymphoma of the central nervous system: typical and atypical CT and MR imaging appearances. AJNR Am J Neuroradiol 2001;176(5):1319–26.

20. Bataille B, Delwail V, Menet E, et al. Primary intracerebral malignant lymphoma: report of 248 cases. J Neurosurg 2000;92:261–6.

21. Vossough A, Nabavizadeh SA, Pomerentz S, et al. Spectrum of Imaging Findings in Central Nervous System Lymphoma. Radiological Society of North America 2009 Scientific Assembly and Annual Meeting. Chicago; 2009.

22. Kulkarni KM, Sternau L, Dubovy SR, et al. Primary dural lymphoma masquerading as a meningioma. J Neuroophthalmol 2012;32(3):240–2.

23. Rottnek M, Strauchen J, Moore F, et al. Primary dural mucosa-associated lymphoid tissue-type lymphoma: case report and review of the literature. J Neurooncol 2004;68(1):19–23.

24. Iwamoto FM, Abrey LE. Primary dural lymphomas: a review. Neurosurg Focus 2006;21(5):E5.

25. Taylor JW, Flanagan EP, O'Neill BP, et al. Primary leptomeningeal lymphoma: International Primary CNS Lymphoma Collaborative Group report. Neurology 2013;81(19):1690–6.

26. Kuker W, Herrlinger U, Gronewaller E, et al. Ocular manifestation of primary nervous system lymphoma: what can be expected from imaging? J Neurol 2002;249:1713–6.

27. Weller M. Glucocorticoid treatment of primary CNS lymphoma. J Neurooncol 1999;43(3):237–9.
28. Coulon A, Lafitte F, Hoang-Xuan K, et al. Radiographic findings in 37 cases of primary CNS lymphoma in immunocompetent patients. Eur Radiol 2002;12:329–40.
29. Gliemroth J, Kehler U, Gaebel C, et al. Neuroradiological findings in primary cerebral lymphomas of non-AIDS patients. Clin Neurol Neurosurg 2003;105:78–86.
30. Johnson BA, Fram EK, Johnson PC, et al. The variable MR appearance of primary lymphoma of the central nervous system: comparison with histopathologic features. AJNR Am J Neuroradiol 1997;18(3):563–72.
31. Küker W, Nägele T, Korfel A, et al. Primary central nervous system lymphomas (PCNSL): MRI features at presentation in 100 patients. J Neurooncol 2005; 72(2):169–77.
32. Batchelor T, Loeffler JS. Primary CNS lymphoma. J Clin Oncol 2006;24:1281–8.
33. Weaver JD, Vinters HV, Koretz B, et al. Lymphomatosis cerebri presenting as rapidly progressive dementia. Neurologist 2007;13:150–3.
34. Lachenmayer ML, Blasius E, Niehusmann P, et al. Non-enhancing primary CNS lymphoma. J Neurooncol 2011;101:343–4.
35. Jahnke K, Schilling A, Heidenreich J, et al. Radiologic morphology of low-grade primary central nervous system lymphoma in immunocompetent patients. AJNR Am J Neuroradiol 2005;26:2446–54.
36. Raz E, Tinelli E, Antonelli M, et al. MRI findings in lymphomatosis cerebri: description of a case and revision of the literature. J Neuroimaging 2011;21(2):e183–6.
37. Jenkins CN, Colquhoun IR. Characterization of primary intracranial lymphoma by computed tomography: an analysis of 36 cases and a review of the literature with particular reference to calcification haemorrhage and cyst formation. Clin Radiol 1998;53:428–34.
38. Kim IY, Jung S, Jung TY, et al. Primary central nervous system lymphoma presenting as an acute massive intracerebral hemorrhage: case report with immunohistochemical study. Surg Neurol 2008;70:308–11.
39. Schultz CJ, Bovi J. Current management of primary central nervous systemlymphoma. Int J Radiat Oncol Biol Phys 2010;76:666–78.
40. Jahnke K, Thiel E, Martus P, et al. Relapse of primary central nervous system lymphoma: clinical features, outcome and prognostic factors. J Neurooncol 2006;80: 159–65.
41. Schulte-Altedorneburg G, Heuser L, Pels H. MRI patterns in recurrence of primary CNS lymphoma in immunocompetent patients. Eur J Radiol 2012; 81(9):2380–5.
42. Zuckerman D, Seliem R, Hochberg E. Intravascular lymphoma: the oncologist's "great imitator. Oncologist 2006;11(5):496–502.
43. Nakahara T, Saito T, Muroi A, et al. Intravascular lymphomatosis presenting as an ascending cauda equina: conus medullaris syndrome: remission after biweekly CHOP therapy. J Neurol Neurosurg Psychiatry 1999;67:403–6.
44. Calamia KT, Miller A, Shuster EA, et al. Intravascular lymphomatosis. A report of ten patients with central nervous system involvement and a review of the disease process. Adv Exp Med Biol 1999;455:249–65.
45. Vieren M, Sciot R, Robberecht W. Intravascular lymphomatosis of the brain: a diagnostic problem. Clin Neurol Neurosurg 1999;101:33–6.
46. Glass J, Hochberg FH, Miller DC. Intravascular lymphomatosis. A systemic disease with neurologic manifestations. Cancer 1993;71:3156–64.
47. Williams RL, Meltzer CC, Smirniotopoulos JG, et al. Cerebral MR imaging in intravascular lymphomatosis. AJNR Am J Neuroradiol 1998;19:427e31.

48. Iijima M, Fujita A, Uchigata M, et al. Change of brain MRI findings in a patient with intravascular malignant lymphomatosis. Eur J Neurol 2007;15:e4–5.

49. Imai H, Kajimoto K, Taniwaki M, et al. Intravascular large B-cell lymphoma presenting with mass lesions in the central nervous system: a report of five cases. Pathol Int 2004;54:231e6.

50. Kinoshita T, Sugihara S, Matusue E, et al. Intravascular malignant lymphomatosis: diffusion-weighted magnetic resonance imaging characteristics. Acta Radiol 2005;46(3):246–9.

51. Schramm P, Xyda A, Klotz E, et al. Dynamic CT perfusion imaging of intra-axial brain tumours: differentiation of high-grade gliomas from primary CNS lymphomas. Eur Radiol 2010;20(10):2482–90.

52. Weber M-A, Günther M, Lichy MP, et al. Comparison of arterial spin-labeling techniques and dynamic susceptibility-weighted contrast-enhanced MRI in perfusion imaging of normal brain tissue. Invest Radiol 2003;38(11):712–8.

53. Weber MA, Zoubaa S, Schlieter M, et al. Diagnostic performance of spectroscopic and perfusion MRI for distinction of brain tumors. Neurology 2006; 66(12):1899–906.

54. Yamashita K, Yoshiura T, Hiwatashi A, et al. Differentiating primary CNS lymphoma from glioblastoma multiforme: assessment using arterial spin labeling, diffusion-weighted imaging, and ^{18}F-fluorodeoxyglucose positron emission tomography. Neuroradiology 2013;55(2):135–43.

55. Toh CH, Wei KC, Chang CN, et al. Differentiation of primary central nervous system lymphomas and glioblastomas: comparisons of diagnostic performance of dynamic susceptibility contrast-enhanced perfusion MR imaging without and with contrast-leakage correction. AJNR Am J Neuroradiol 2013;34(6):1145–9.

56. Shenkier TN, Blay JY, O'neill BP, et al. Primary CNS lymphoma of T-cell origin: a descriptive analysis from the international primary CNS lymphoma collaborative group. J Clin Oncol 2005;23:2233–9.

57. Liu D, Schelper R, Carter DA, et al. Primary central nervous system cytotoxic/suppressor T-cell lymphoma. Am J Surg Pathol 2003;27:682–8.

58. Kim EY, Kim SS. Magnetic resonance findings of primary central nervoussystem T-cell lymphoma in immunocompetent patients. Acta Radiol 2005;46(2):187–92.

59. Al-Okaili RN, Krejza J, Wang S, et al. Advanced MR imaging techniques in the diagnosis of intraaxial brain tumors in adults. Radiographics 2006;26(Suppl 1):S173–89.

60. Wang S, Kim S, Chawla S, et al. Differentiation between glioblastomas, solitary brain metastases, and primary cerebral lymphomas using diffusion tensor and dynamic susceptibility contrast-enhanced MR imaging. AJNR Am J Neuroradiol 2011;32(3):507–14.

61. Ma WL, Li CC, Yu SC, et al. Adult T-cell lymphoma/leukemia presenting as isolated central nervous system T-cell lymphoma. Case Rep Hematol 2014; 2014:917369.

62. Kickingereder P, Wiestler B, Sahm F, et al. Primary central nervous system lymphoma and atypical glioblastoma: multiparametric differentiation by using diffusion-, perfusion-, and susceptibility-weighted MR imaging. Radiology 2014; 272(3):843–50.

63. Doskaliyev A, Yamasaki F, Ohtaki M, et al. Lymphomas and glioblastomas: differences in the apparent diffusion coefficient evaluated with high b-value diffusion-weighted magnetic resonance imaging at 3T. Eur J Radiol 2012;81(2):339–44.

64. Stadnik TW, Chaskis C, Michotte A, et al. Diffusion-weighted MR imaging of intracerebral masses: comparison with conventional MR imaging and histologic findings. AJNR Am J Neuroradiol 2001;22:969–76.

65. Horger M, Fenchel M, Nägele T, et al. Water diffusivity: comparison of primary CNS lymphoma and astrocytic tumor infiltrating the corpus callosum. AJR Am J Roentgenol 2009;193(5):1384–7.

66. Camacho DLA, Smith JK, Castillo M. Differentiation of toxoplasmosis and lymphoma in AIDS patients by using apparent diffusion coefficients. AJNR Am J Neuroradiol 2003;24(4):633–7.

67. Schroeder PC, Post MJD, Oschatz E, et al. Analysis of the utility of diffusion-weighted MRI and apparent diffusion coefficient values in distinguishing central nervous system toxoplasmosis from lymphoma. Neuroradiology 2006;48(10):715–20.

68. Barajas RF Jr, Rubenstein JL, Chang JS, et al. Diffusion-weighted MR imaging derived apparent diffusion coefficient is predictive of clinical outcome in primary central nervous system lymphoma. AJNR Am J Neuroradiol 2010;31:60–6.

69. Toh CH, Castillo M, Wong AM, et al. Primary cerebral lymphoma and glioblastoma multiforme: differences in diffusion characteristics evaluated with diffusion tensor imaging. AJNR Am J Neuroradiol 2008;29:471–5.

70. Liao W, Liu Y, Wang X, et al. Differentiation of primary central nervous system lymphoma and high-grade glioma with dynamic susceptibility contrast-enhanced perfusion magnetic resonance imaging. Acta Radiol 2009;50(2):217–25 (Stockholm, Sweden: 1987).

71. Nakajima S, Okada T, Yamamoto A, et al. Differentiation between primary central nervous system lymphoma and glioblastoma: a comparative study of parameters derived from dynamic susceptibility contrast-enhanced perfusion-weighted MRI. Clin Radiol 2015;70(12):1393–9.

72. Hartmann M, Heiland S, Harting I, et al. Distinguishing of primary cerebral lymphoma from high-grade glioma with perfusion-weighted magnetic resonance imaging. Neurosci Lett 2003;338:119–22.

73. Pollock JM, Tan H, Kraft RA, et al. Arterial spin-labeled MR perfusion imaging: clinical applications. Magn Reson Imaging Clin N Am 2009;17:315–38.

74. Laissy J-P, Soyer P, Tebboune J, et al. Contrast-enhanced fast MRI in differentiating brain toxoplasmosis and lymphoma in AIDS Patients. J Comput Assist Tomogr 1994;18(5):714–8.

75. Ernst TM, Chang L, Witt MD, et al. Cerebral toxoplasmosis and lymphoma in AIDS: perfusion MR imaging experience in 13 patients. Radiology 1998;208:663–9.

76. Kickingereder P, Sahm F, Wiestler B, et al. Evaluation of microvascular permeability with dynamic contrast-enhanced MRI for the differentiation of primary CNS lymphoma and glioblastoma: radiologic-pathologic correlation. AJNR Am J Neuroradiol 2014;35(8):1503–8.

77. Raizer JJ, Koutcher JA, Abrey LE, et al. Proton magnetic resonance spectroscopy in immunocompetent patients with primary central nervous system lymphoma. J Neurooncol 2005;71(2):173–80.

78. Harting I, Hartmann M, Jost G, et al. Differentiating primary central nervous system lymphoma from glioma in humans using localised proton magnetic resonance spectroscopy. Neurosci Lett 2003;342(3):163–6.

79. Chinn RJ, Wilkinson ID, Hall-Craggs MA, et al. Toxoplasmosis and primary central nervous system lymphoma in HIV infection: diagnosis with MR spectroscopy. Radiology 1995;197(3):649–54.

80. Chang L, Miller BL, McBride D, et al. Brain lesions in patients with AIDS: H-1 MR spectroscopy. Radiology 1995;197:525–31.

81. Lee HY, Kim HS, Park JW, et al. Atypical imaging features of Epstein-Barr virus–positive primary central nervous system lymphomas in patients without AIDS. AJNR Am J Neuroradiol 2013;34(8):1562–7.

82. Radbruch A, Wiestler B, Kramp L, et al. Differentiation of glioblastoma and primary CNS lymphomas using susceptibility weighted imaging. Eur J Radiol 2013;82(3): 552–6.

83. Westwood TD, Hogan C, Julyan PJ, et al. Utility of FDG-PETCT and magnetic resonance spectroscopy in differentiating between cerebral lymphoma and non-malignant CNS lesions in HIV-infected patients. Eur J Radiol 2013;82(8):e374–9.

84. Kosaka N, Tsuchida T, Uematsu H, et al. 18F-FDG PET of common enhancing malignant brain tumors. AJR Am J Roentgenol 2008;190(6):W365–9.

85. Makino K, Hirai T, Nakamura H, et al. Does adding FDG-PET to MRI improve the differentiation between primary cerebral lymphoma and glioblastoma? Observer performance study. Ann Nucl Med 2011;25(6):432–8.

86. Herholz K, Langen K-J, Schiepers C, et al. Brain tumors. Semin Nucl Med 2012; 42(6):356–70.

87. Palmedo H, Urbach H, Bender H, et al. FDG-PET in immunocompetent patients with primary central nervous system lymphoma: correlation with MRI and clinical follow-up. Eur J Nucl Med Mol Imaging 2006;33(2):164–8.

88. Ogawa T, Kanno I, Hatazawa J, et al. Methionine PET for follow-up of radiation therapy of primary lymphoma of the brain. Radiographics 1994;14:101–10.

89. Ruiz A, Ganz WI, Post MJ, et al. Use of thallium-201 brain SPECT to differentiate cerebral lymphoma from toxoplasma encephalitis in AIDS patients. AJNR Am J Neuroradiol 1994;15(10):1885–94.

90. Black KL, Hawkins RA, Kim KT, et al. Use of thallium-201 SPECT to quantitate malignancy grade of gliomas. J Neurosurg 1989;71(3):342–6.

91. Fukahori T, Tahara T, Mihara F, et al. Diagnostic value of high N-isopropyl-p-[123I] iodoamphetamine (IMP) uptake in brain tumors. Nihon Igaku Hoshasen Gakkai zasshi Nippon acta radiologica 1996;56(1):53–9 [in Japanese].

92. Shinoda J, Yano H, Murase S, et al. High 123 I-IMP retention on SPECT image in primary central nervous system lymphoma. J Neurooncol 2003;61(3):261–5.

93. Akiyama Y, Moritake K, Yamasaki T, et al. The diagnostic value of 123 I-IMP SPECT in non-Hodgkin's lymphoma of the central nervous system. J Nucl Med 2000;41(11):1777–83.

94. Naddaf SY, Akisik MF, Aziz M, et al. Comparison between 201Tl-chloride and 99Tc(m)-sestamibi SPET brain imaging for differentiating intracranial lymphoma from non-malignant lesions in AIDS patients. Nucl Med Commun 1998;19(1):47–53.

95. Medina DM, Carmody RF. Stroke. In: Zimmerman RA, Gibby WA, Carmody RF, editors. Neuroimaging: clinical and physical principles. 1st edition. New York: Springer; 2000. p. 786–7.

96. Lu SS, Kim SJ, Kim HS, et al. Utility of proton MR spectroscopy for differentiating typical and atypical primary central nervous system lymphomas from tumefactive demyelinating lesions. AJNR Am J Neuroradiol 2014;35(2):270–7.

Neuroimaging in Leukemia

Seyed Ali Nabavizadeh, MD, Joel Stein, MD, PhD,
Suyash Mohan, MD, PDCC*

KEYWORDS

- Leukemia • Central nervous system • MRI • CT • Neuroimaging • Leukostasis

KEY POINTS

- Localized collection of leukemic cells can present as mass lesions, which can involve multiple organs, including the central nervous system and head and neck, and are called granulocytic sarcoma.
- Granulocytic sarcomas are usually hyperdense on computed tomographic scans due to cellularity and may present as multiple masses.
- On MRI, granulocytic sarcomas are usually isointense to gray matter on T1-weighted sequences and demonstrate homogeneous contrast enhancement. Diffusion restricted may be also seen, indicative of cellularity.
- A variety of cerebrovascular complications can occur in patients with leukemia, including intraparenchymal hemorrhage, leukostasis, and cerebral venous infarctions.

INTRODUCTION

Leukemias are a heterogeneous group of hematologic malignancies that results from uncontrolled neoplastic proliferation of undifferentiated or partially differentiated hematopoietic cells. Patients with acute leukemia can have a variety of craniocerebral complications, which can result from direct leukemic involvement, secondary to cerebrovascular or infectious complications of leukemia, or can be treatment related.

Leukemia is the commonest childhood cancer, accounting for one-fourth to one-third of all childhood malignancy patients. Most cases (75%) of acute leukemia in the pediatric population are acute lymphoblastic leukemia (ALL), with acute myeloid leukemia (AML) accounting for only 20% of cases.[1] Chronic myelogenous leukemia (CML), juvenile myelomonocytic leukemia (JMML), and myelodysplastic myeloproliferative syndrome account for approximately 5% of childhood leukemias.[1] ALL accounts for approximately 15% to 20% of all adult acute leukemias. Central nervous system (CNS) involvement is identified at the time of diagnosis in less than 10% of adult ALL and is not an independent poor prognostic factor; however, leukemic relapse remains a major therapeutic problem, and CNS involvement at the time of relapse, which occurs in 1% to 15% of cases, is associated with poor prognosis.[2]

Department of Radiology, Division of Neuroradiology, Perelman School of Medicine at the University of Pennsylvania, Philadelphia, PA, USA
* Corresponding author.
E-mail address: Suyash.Mohan@uphs.upenn.edu

Hematol Oncol Clin N Am 30 (2016) 823–842
http://dx.doi.org/10.1016/j.hoc.2016.03.006
0889-8588/16/$ – see front matter

CNS involvement in adults with AML is less common when compared with ALL.[3,4] In a study of 395 patients with AML, only 1.8% of patients had initial CNS involvement and 1% suffered an isolated CNS relapse.[5] Several risk factors have been associated with development of CNS leukemia, including age (young adult), mature B-cell ALL, and T-cell leukemia.[6,7]

Although there has been an increase in cure rates of patients with leukemia, secondary to emergence of new treatment modalities, including aggressive chemotherapy, intrathecal prophylaxis, cranial irradiation, and bone marrow transplantation, use of these intensive treatment regimens have also led to new adverse consequences, including neurotoxicity secondary to various chemotherapeutic agents, acute and late effects of CNS radiation, coagulopathy, immunosuppression, and bone marrow suppression.[8,9]

DIRECT LEUKEMIC INVOLVEMENT OF CENTRAL NERVOUS SYSTEM

In leukemia, localized collection of leukemic cells can present as mass lesions, which can involve multiple organs, including the CNS and head and neck. It is more commonly encountered in patients with myeloid leukemia[10] and has been historically called chloroma secondary to greenish hue of the mass on gross specimen secondary to the presence of myeloperoxidase; however, granulocytic sarcoma is considered the preferred terminology because not all lesions are green.[10,11]

Within the head and neck, granulocytic sarcoma can involve skin and subcutaneous tissues, lymph nodes, and calvarium. Additional sites of involvement include orbits, paranasal sinuses, nasopharynx, and temporal bone.[12] In addition, they can involve the intracranial structures including the dura (**Figs. 1** and **2**), with occasional indentation of the subarachnoid space and secondary growth into the brain parenchyma through the perivascular spaces.[11] Granulocytic sarcomas are usually hyperdense on computed tomographic (CT) scan, which results from dense cellularity and may present as single or multiple masses. On MRI, restricted diffusion may be seen, also indicative of cellularity[10] (see **Fig. 1**B, C and **Fig. 2**D, E). Lesions are usually isointense to gray matter on T1-weighted sequences and demonstrate relatively homogeneous enhancement following contrast administration (see **Fig. 1**D). Thus, imaging features are similar to lymphoma. Homogeneous enhancement argues for lymphoma or leukemia and against other enhancing neoplasms, such as solid organ metastases or glioblastoma, which typically show cystic changes or necrosis. Advanced imaging techniques can improve diagnostic certainty. Magnetic resonance spectroscopy demonstrates a neoplastic spectrum with elevated choline indicative of increased cellularity and cell membrane turnover (see **Fig. 1**E). In contrast to metastases and glioblastoma, leukemia (and lymphoma) masses show little elevation of relative cerebral blood volume[10] (see **Fig. 1**F). The differential diagnosis for intraparenchymal granulocytic sarcoma is hemorrhagic infarct, which can result from coagulopathy or can be secondary to leukostasis, which can occur especially when the white blood cell count is greater than $100 \times 10^9/L$ (100,000/µL) in patients with leukemia.[11] On MRI, SWI demonstrating low signal and blooming indicates the presence of hemorrhage. Again, leukemia demonstrates homogeneous enhancement, whereas hematomas demonstrate absent or peripheral enhancement.

In a study of 30 intracranial lesions in patients with adult T-cell leukemia, Kitajima and colleagues[13] demonstrated that the most common intracranial lesions were parenchymal lesions, contrast-enhancing (8 lesions in 4 patients), or nonenhancing (8 lesions in 2 patients), followed by leptomeningeal enhancement (5 cases).

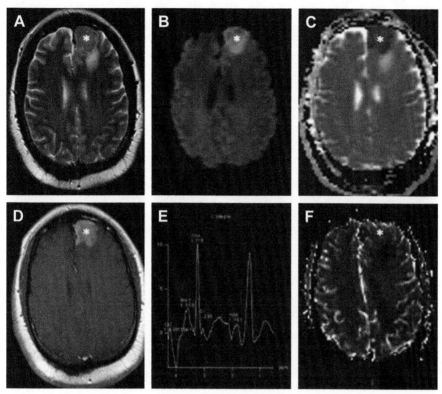

Fig. 1. Frontal dural-based granulocytic carcinoma with advanced imaging in a 52-year-old man with AML. T2-weighted (*A*), diffusion-weighted (*B*), apparent diffusion coefficient map (*C*), and postcontrast T1-weighted (*D*) images demonstrate a dural-based, solid, homogeneously enhancing parasagittal frontal lesion (*asterisks*) with mild adjacent edema, consistent with granulocytic sarcoma. MR spectroscopy (*E*) demonstrates a neoplastic spectrum with elevated choline (Cho), depressed creatinine (Cr), and N-acetylaspartate (NAA), and elevated lipid-lactate. Dynamic susceptibility contrast MR perfusion demonstrates little corresponding elevation of relative cerebral blood volume (*F*), a feature also seen with secondary CNS lymphoma that differentiates from metastases or meningioma.

MENINGEAL LEUKEMIC INFILTRATION

Leukemia can involve the meninges (pachymeninges, leptomeniges, or both, **Figs. 3** and **4**). One of the commonest early manifestations of CNS leukemia is the symptom of increasing intracranial pressure.[14] Additional symptoms could include cranial nerve palsies, vertigo, ataxia, and myelopathy. The differential diagnosis for leptomeningeal enhancement includes leukemic involvement; however, infectious meningitis or chemical meningitis resulting from intrathecal chemotherapy can also have a similar presentation. In addition, extra-axial granulocytic sarcoma can be mistaken for meningiomas, lymphoma, or extra-axial blood.

Leukemic involvement of the orbit can also present as focal intraconal or extraconal masses, which can involve different components of the globe, lacrimal glands, optic nerve, and extra-ocular muscles.[15,16] Granulocytic sarcoma can also involve the skull base[8] (**Fig. 5**) and can present as a paraspinal mass (**Figs. 6** and **7**) with epidural extension and secondary cord compression, although the prevalence is much less

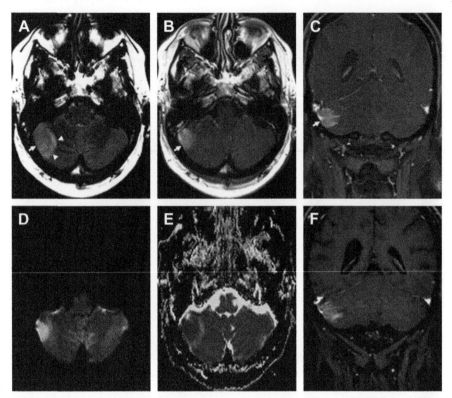

Fig. 2. Extra-axial and intra-axial leukemic lesion in a 49-year-old woman with relapsed ALL. Axial FLAIR (*A*), postcontrast axial (*B*), and coronal (*C*) T1-weighted, axial diffusion-weighted (*D*) and axial apparent diffusion coefficient (ADC) (*E*) images demonstrate an enhancing lesion (*arrows*) involving the lateral right cerebellar hemisphere with restricted diffusion and mild adjacent edema (*arrowheads*). After institution of chemotherapy, a follow-up coronal T1-weighted scan (*F*) 2.5 months later shows decreased enhancement and better reveals a leptomeningeal and subcortical parenchymal pattern. The lesion eventually resolved.

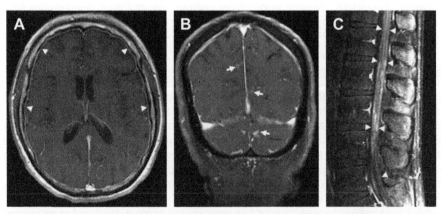

Fig. 3. Leukemic meningitis. Postcontrast axial (*A*) and coronal (*B*) T1-weighted images in a 75-year-old man with AML demonstrates diffuse dural thickening (*arrowheads*) as well as nodular foci of leptomeningeal enhancement (*arrows*). Postcontrast sagittal T1-weighted lumbar spine image (*C*) demonstrates nodular enhancement along the conus and cauda equina nerve roots (*arrowheads*) in a 22-year-old man with AML.

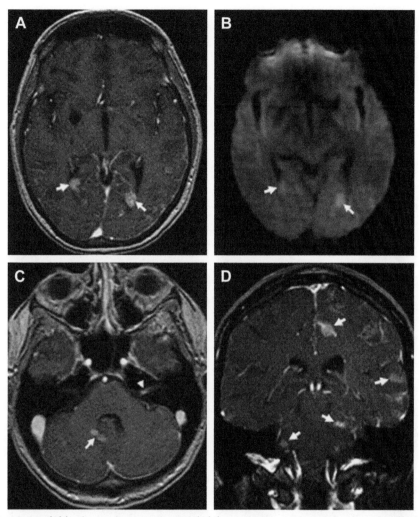

Fig. 4. Myeloblastic carcinomatosis. Axial (*A*) postcontrast T1-weighted and diffusion weighted (*B*) images demonstrate multiple nodular enhancing foci along sulci (*arrows*) consistent with leptomeningeal leukemia in a 59-year-old woman with CML. Additional postcontrast axial (*C*) and coronal (*D*) T1-weighted images demonstrate additional nodular foci of leptomeningeal enhancement in the posterior fossa, including within the left internal auditory canal (*arrows*).

when compared with intracranial involvement.[17,18] Granulocytic sarcoma of the cord is extremely rare; however, it is reported.[19] Meningeal leukemic involvement can also present in the spine as nerve root enhancement and pial enhancement surrounding the cord[17] (see **Fig. 3**; **Fig. 8**).

CENTRAL NERVOUS SYSTEM DISEASE RELATED TO SECONDARY EFFECTS OF MALIGNANCY
Cerebrovascular Complications

A variety of cerebrovascular complications can occur in patients with leukemia, resulting from derangement in hematologic profile, including leukocytosis, thrombocytopenia,

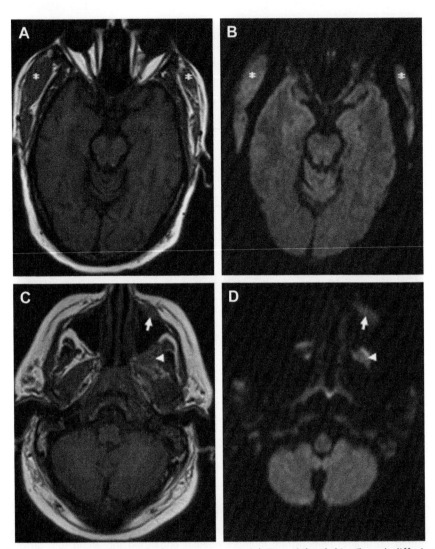

Fig. 5. Facial and skull-base leukemic masses. Axial T1-weighted (*A, C*) and diffusion-weighted (*B, D*) images in a 49-year-old man with CML show leukemic masses involving the temporalis muscles bilaterally (*asterisks*) with additional masses in the left infratemporal fossa (*arrowheads*) and premaxillary space (*arrows*). There was contiguous involvement via the pterygopalatine fossa and infraorbital foramen. Diffusion signal in the right maxillary region is related to incidental sinus disease. This case emphasizes careful evaluation for replacement or asymmetry of fat-containing spaces on head and neck imaging and the utility of diffusion-weighted imaging to increase sensitivity.

coagulopathy, and sepsis.[9] Intraparenchymal hemorrhage is most common in acute leukemia and can be lethal. Patients with acute promyelocytic leukemia are particularly susceptible to disseminated intravascular coagulation during treatment and are susceptible to massive intraparenchymal brain hemorrhage, which also has a high mortality.[9,17] Leukemic patients with a blast crisis are also susceptible to leukostasis within the small arterioles, which can relate to development of hemorrhagic infarcts[11] (**Fig. 9**). Extra-axial

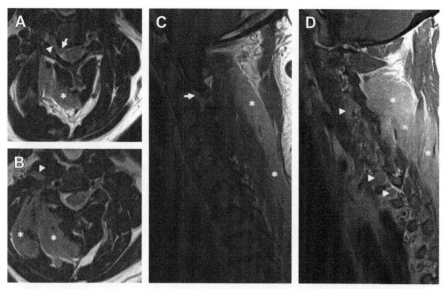

Fig. 6. Paraspinal and intraspinal leukemia. Axial T2-weighted (*A, B*) and sagittal postcontrast T1-weighted images (*C, D*) of the cervical spine in a 52-year-old man with a history of AML show extensive leukemic infiltration of right posterior paraspinal musculature (*asterisks*). Intraspinal tumor is also evident in the right ventral epidural space (*arrows*) with extension along right multiple spinal nerves (*arrowheads*). Note: low marrow signal on the T1-weighted images, obtained without fat suppression, in keeping with AML.

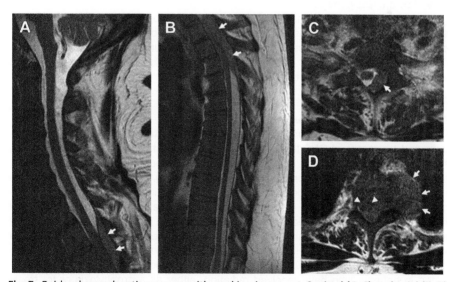

Fig. 7. Epidural granulocytic sarcoma with cord impingement. Sagittal (*A, B*) and axial (*C, D*) T2-weighted images in a 58-year-old man with a history of AML demonstrates an epidural and left paraspinal mass at the T1-T4 levels, filling the spinal canal (*arrows*), displacing and impinging the spinal cord (*arrowheads* in *D*), and extending through multiple left neural foramina.

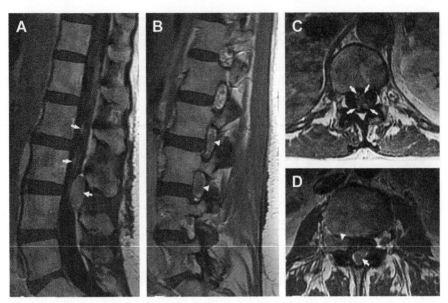

Fig. 8. Leukemic meningitis with intrathecal and epidural involvement. Sagittal (*A, B*) and axial (*C, D*) postcontrast T1-weighted images in a 59-year-old woman with CML and blast crisis demonstrate multiple linear and nodular enhancing lesions along cauda equina nerve roots (*narrow arrows*) as well as in the epidural space, both dorsally (*arrows*) and extending into the neural foramina (*arrowheads*).

hemorrhages (subdural or subarachnoid) can also occur in patients with leukemia; however, they are less common.[20,21]

Cerebral venous infarctions (**Fig. 10**) can also develop in patients with leukemia secondary to venous occlusion/thrombosis from leukostasis, or hypercoagulable state, particularly with the use of certain chemotherapeutic agents, such as L-asparaginase and vincristine.[22,23] Venous thrombosis can also occur because of direct leukemic involvement of the dural sinuses (**Fig. 11**).

Iatrogenic Complications

Direct effect of radiation therapy

Craniospinal irradiation is considered the standard treatment for both CNS prophylaxis and treatment of CNS leukemia.[2] Neurotoxic reactions secondary to radiation therapy can be divided into acute (1–6 weeks after treatment), subacute (3 weeks to several months), and chronic injury (months to years).[24] Acute injury is accompanied by increased capillary permeability and vasodilatation, which can lead to vasogenic edema; however, it is less common with the current radiation therapy regimens.[24] The chronic effects of radiation in the brain include white matter necrosis, demyelination, gliosis, and vasculopathy,[25,26] presenting with focal or multiple white matter lesions, usually in the periventricular distribution with sparing of subcortical U fibers and the corpus callosum.[23] Brain parenchymal volume loss is also noted in patients who have received radiation, either as a prophylaxis or for treatment of CNS disease, and is associated with neurocognitive deficits, especially in younger patients.[23]

Mineralizing microangiopathy is an entity resulting from endothelial proliferation and calcium deposition with hyalinization and fibrinoid necrosis within the small

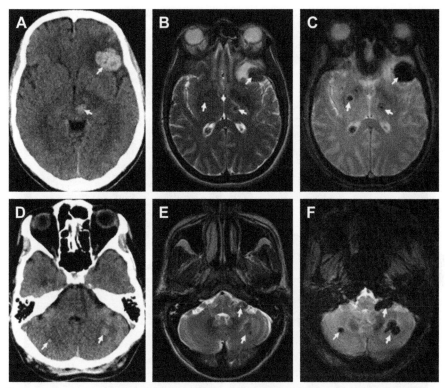

Fig. 9. Leukostasis with multiple hemorrhagic infarcts. Axial unenhanced head CT (*A, D*) in a 52-year-old man with CML shows multiple supratentorial and infratentorial hyperdense masses (*arrows*). The differential diagnosis includes hemorrhagic infarcts, fungal infection or multiple chloromas. Corresponding axial T2-weighted (*B, E*) and gradient-echo (*C, F*) images demonstrate low-signal hemorrhages with susceptibility and adjacent edema (*arrows*). White blood cell count was 66^L 109/L, supporting the diagnosis of leukostasis with hemorrhage.

arteries and arterioles,[17] which usually demonstrates a dystrophic calcification in the basal ganglia and subcortical white matter and is particularly noted in children, who are treated with radiation and intrathecal methotrexate (MTX).[23] Given the nature of this finding, CT scan is the modality of choice; however, mineralizing microangiopathy present on MR has increased T1 signal intensity in the basal ganglia.[27]

Radiation-induced vascular malformations

Radiation-induced vascular injury causes endothelial and basement membrane damage, accelerated atherosclerosis, and telangiectasia formation. So-called radiation-induced cryptic vascular malformations ("cryptic" to angiography, not MR) are predominately capillary telangiectasias ± cavernous angiomas. Lesions tend to be multiple, predominately located in the white matter. T2* gradient echo, and more recently, susceptibility-weighted imaging (SWI) sequences are particularly helpful for identification of these lesions, which result in magnetic field inhomogeneity and signal loss. Patients are usually asymptomatic; however, occasionally lesions can cause focal neurologic signs or seizure, or can present with intracranial hemorrhage.[23]

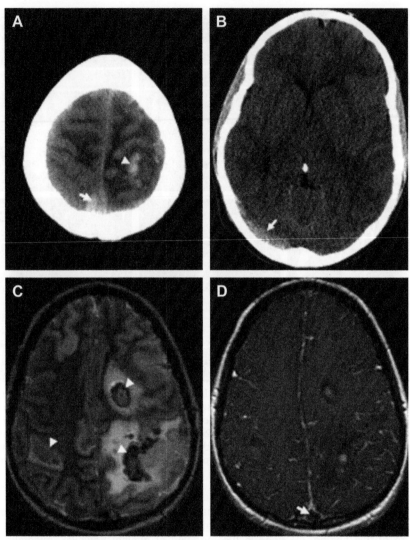

Fig. 10. Sinus thrombosis and venous infarcts. Unenhanced axial CT sections in an 18-year-old man with ALL on chemotherapy show dense thrombus (*arrowhead*) in the superior sagittal sinus (*A*) and right transverse sinus (*B*) along with hemorrhagic left parietal venous infarct (*arrow*). Axial T2-weighted MRI (*C*) shows bilateral venous infarcts manifested by low signal hematoma (*arrowheads*) and surrounding edema. Postcontrast T1-weighted MRI (*D*) shows intrinsic T1-shortening in the areas of hemorrhage and a filling defect in the superior sagittal sinus (*arrow*).

Radiation-induced secondary neoplasms

Brain tumors are the commonest second malignant neoplasms in childhood leukemia survivors and develop in approximately 1% of patients who received cranial radiation.[28] The mean latency for development of a second neoplasm is variable; however, it is reported to be shorter in high-grade gliomas when compared with meningiomas (9 years compared with 19 years).[28] Osteosarcoma is the

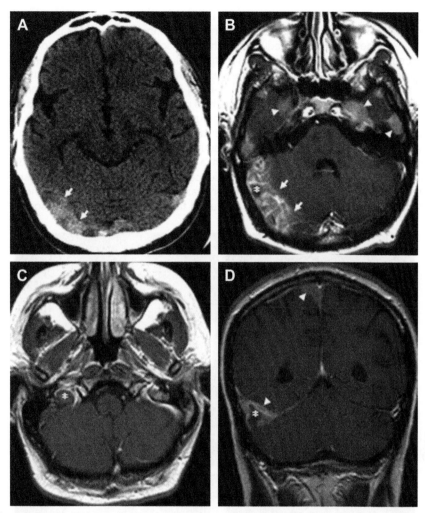

Fig. 11. Dural invasion and thrombosis. Axial unenhanced head CT (*A*) in a 24-year-old man with AML demonstrates hyperattenuation (*arrows*) along the tentorium and right transverse sinus that could represent dural-based leukemia or sinus thrombosis. Axial (*B*, *C*) and coronal (*D*) postcontrast T1-weighted images demonstrate both to be present, with leptomeningeal and dural-enhancing tumor (*arrows*) along and invading the right transverse sinus with associated nonenhancing clot (*asterisk*). Nonocclusive thrombus was present through the sigmoid sinus to the jugular bulb. Note multiple additional dural-based nodules (*arrowheads*) involving the superior sagittal sinus and in the middle cranial fossae.

most common secondary tumor of the skull in children who had underwent cranial irradiation, although benign tumors such as osteoma have also been reported.[14,29]

Effects of chemotherapy

A variety of chemotherapeutic agents can cause cerebral white matter injuries, which are usually nonspecific and can present with diffuse symmetric involvement of periventricular and deep white matter with relative preservation of subcortical U fibers.[25] CNS can be involved by potential toxic effects of chemotherapeutic agents.

The neurotoxic effects of these agents can be caused by crossing the blood-brain barrier or can result from direct injection into the subarachnoid space. MTX is an inhibitor of the enzyme dihydrofolate reductase, which causes blockage of the production of reduced folate, which is necessary for the production of purines and thymidines. Less than 1% of patients with leukemia and lymphoma can present with acute encephalopathy within 2 weeks after receiving high-dose intravenous and/or intrathecal MTX, which can present with a variety of neurologic symptoms, such as strokelike episodes (hemiparesis/dysphasia), confusion, headache, choreoathetosis, and seizure.[30] Restricted diffusion in centrum semiovale on diffusion-weighted image (DWI) is the typical imaging finding of acute MTX encephalopathy (**Fig. 12**) and resolves as clinical status improves; however, subtle abnormalities on T2 and fluid-attenuated inversion recovery (FLAIR) sequences may remain.[30] In a small case series, subsequent intrathecal MTX administration was not associated with recurrence in 4 patients of 6, and the investigators concluded that a single strokelike episode with

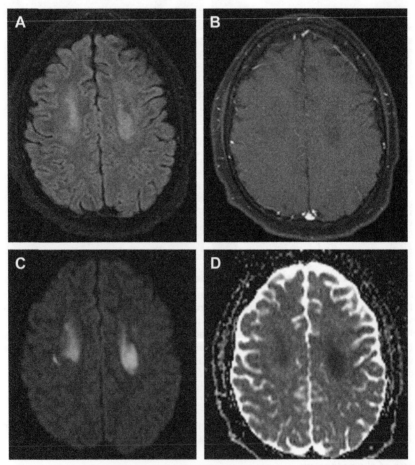

Fig. 12. An 8-year-old patient with ALL who received intrathecal injections of MTX presented with change in mental status. Axial FLAIR images demonstrate hyperintensity in bilateral centrum semiovale (*A*) without enhancement on axial T1 postcontrast images (*B*). Axial diffusion and ADC maps (*C, D*) demonstrate restricted diffusion in these areas. Findings are consistent with acute MTX leukoencephalopathy.

diffusion abnormalities should not necessarily prompt modification of potentially cura-tive chemotherapeutic regimens.[31]

MTX can also cause chronic white matter damage known as MTX leukoencephalop-athy (**Fig. 13**), which demonstrates focal or confluent white matter lesions in peri-ventricular distribution with concomitant brain atrophy.[17,25,26] One of the potential complications of intrathecal MTX administration is anterior lumbosacral radiculopathy, which is attributed to direct toxic effects of MTX, which usually presents as progressive flaccid paralysis of lower extremities. Lumbosacral MRI in these patients usually demon-strates enhancement of the anterior lumbosacral nerve roots.[23,32] The differential diag-noses include leptomeningeal leukemic involvement and Guillain-Barré syndrome[33,34]; however, absence of neoplastic cells in the cerebrospinal fluid and short time interval be-tween MTX administration and development of symptoms help in narrowing the differ-ential diagnosis. Other less common acute complications of MTX include transverse myelopathy[35] and posterior reversible encephalopathy syndrome (PRES).[36]

Cytarabine is a cytosine analogue that inhibits DNA synthesis. It can be given intravenously or intrathecally in patients with leukemia. At high doses, it can cause cerebellar ataxia and encephalopathy. Neuroimaging demonstrates white matter changes and cerebellar atrophy.[37]

Cerebral venous sinus thrombosis is an uncommon complication of treatment of leukemia, which usually occurs in the setting of L-asparaginase therapy in combina-tion with other chemotherapeutic agents.[38] The mechanism is depleting serum levels of several proteins (fibrinogen, plasminogen, proteins C and S, antithrombin III, factors IX and X), which causes an imbalance between clotting and bleeding factors.[38]

Posterior reversible encephalopathy syndrome

PRES is a clinical syndrome that was first described in the context of sudden or pro-longed arterial hypertension with acute neurologic findings, which can include

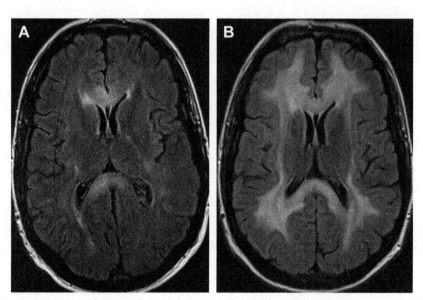

Fig. 13. A 28-year-old man with ALL who received multiple intrathecal injections of MTX in addition to multiagent systemic chemotherapy. Axial FLAIR images 1 week (*A*) and 3 months (*B*) after MTX administration show progressive development of diffuse white matter signal abnormality consistent with MTX leukoencephalopathy.

seizure, altered mental status, cortical blindness, and speech and motor disturbances. It is presumed to result from failure of autoregulatory mechanisms of cerebral vasculature and has also been frequently reported during the course of
chemotherapy in both pediatric and adult leukemia.[23] The spectrum of imaging findings in PRES is wide; however, classic imaging appearance of PRES is vasogenic
edema (hypodensity on CT and hyperintensity on T2-weighted and FLAIR sequences) predominantly in subcortical white matter of posterior parietal, temporal,
and occipital lobes (**Fig. 14A–C**); however, in severe cases, basal ganglia, cerebellar
hemispheres, and brain stem can also be involved. DWI usually demonstrates facilitated diffusion because of the absence of cytotoxic edema; however, restricted
diffusion can be seen in a minority of cases.[39] In addition, up to 22% of patients
with PRES can demonstrate blood products on T2* or SWI sequences[39,40]
(**Fig. 14D–F**).

INFECTIOUS COMPLICATIONS OF LEUKEMIA

Patients with leukemia are particularly susceptible to infectious diseases, resulting
from the underlying disease and complications of treatment, which can result in

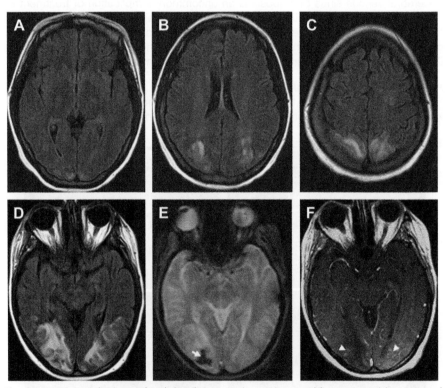

Fig. 14. PRES. Axial T2-weighted (*A–C*) images in a 32-year-old woman with AML and
seizures demonstrate posterior predominant subcortical edema in the bilateral occipital
and parietal lobes with scattered additional foci in the frontal lobes. Axial T2-weighted
(*A*), gradient echo susceptibility-weighted (*B*), and postcontrast T1-weighted (*C*) images in
a 57-year-old woman with AML, periorbital headache, and blurry vision show more extensive bilateral occipital cortical and subcortical edema (*D*) with hemorrhage (*E*) (*arrow*) and
enhancement (*F*).

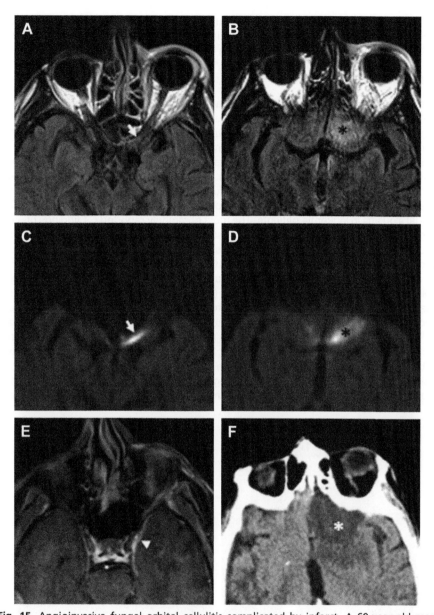

Fig. 15. Angioinvasive fungal orbital cellulitis complicated by infarct. A 69-year-old man with AML on chemotherapy presented with headaches, left eye discomfort, decreased visual acuity, and cranial nerve 3, 4, and 6 palsies. Axial FLAIR (*A, B*) images demonstrate left preseptal periorbital swelling and proptosis, subtle edema in the left prechiasmatic and canalicular optic nerve (*arrow*), and edema in the inferomedial left frontal lobe (*black asterisk*). Corresponding axial diffusion-weighted (*C, D*) images and ADC maps (*not shown*) demonstrate restricted diffusion (*arrow and black asterisk*). Postcontrast T1-weighted image (*E*) shows asymmetric mild fullness and enhancement along the left cavernous sinus suspicious for cavernous sinus involvement (*arrowhead*). Axial unenhanced CT section (*F*) 4 days later shows evolving infarct (*white asterisk*).

immunosuppression, granulocytopenia, mucosal damage, and decreased mucociliary clearance. In the head and neck region, infection can involve the sinuses with the potential to intracranial extension or it can directly involve intracranial structures.

SINUS INFECTIONS

In addition to typical bacterial organisms that affect the paranasal sinuses, patients with leukemia are susceptible to acute invasive fungal rhinosinusitis (AIFR) as one of the most urgent and life-threatening complications with mortalities as high as 50% in the largest published meta-analysis.[41] The causative organisms are usually Aspergillus or Mucor.[23]

Early diagnosis of AIFR is difficult because of similarity of the presenting symptoms with routine viral or bacterial rhinosinusitis. Treatment usually consists of aggressive surgical debridement and intravenous antifungal therapy.[42] CT scan has been demonstrated to be an effective initial imaging modality for screening of aggressive invasive fungal sinusitis in leukemia patients. The most commonly reported CT findings of early aggressive fungal sinusitis include soft tissue infiltration of the maxillary periantral fat and involvement of the pterygopalatine fossa. Osseous dehiscence, orbital invasion, and intracranial extension (**Figs. 15** and **16**) usually indicate advanced disease.[42,43] In a recent study of 42 patients with pathology-proven AIFR, Middlebrooks and colleauges[44] evaluated 7 imaging features (periantral fat, bone dehiscence, orbital invasion, septal ulceration, pterygopalatine fossa, nasolacrimal duct, and lacrimal sac) and demonstrated that the presence of abnormality involving a single variable had 95% sensitivity, and 86% specificity, and abnormality in any of the 2 variables predicted AIFR with 100% specificity and 88.1% sensitivity. MRI can also demonstrate extrasinus extension of infection in addition to focal areas of loss of contrast enhancement of the sinonasal mucosa.[42,45] Existing literature directly comparing MRI and CT found relatively higher sensitivity and positive predictive value (PPV) for AIFR by using

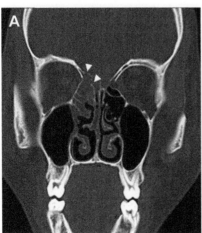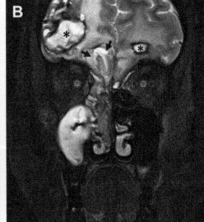

Fig. 16. Angioinvasive fungal sinusitis with cerebritis/abscess and bifrontal hematomas. Coronal unenhanced maxillofacial CT (*A*) in a 19-year-old man with ALL demonstrates partial opacification of the ethmoid air cells with erosions (*arrowheads*) of the cribriform plate and fovea ethmoidalis. Coronal T2-weighted image (*B*) shows the same site of osseous discontinuity at the ventral skull base with overlying frontal lobe edema reflective of cerebritis/abscess formation (*arrows*) and bilateral frontal lobe hematomas with peripheral hemosiderin staining (*asterisks*). High signal filling the right maxillary sinus on the MRI is due to interval surgical exploration; culture yielded Mucormycosis.

MRI.[42] The diagnosis of AIFR needs to be confirmed by histopathology, which usually requires a surgical biopsy, unless the disease process is confined to anterior nasal tissue.[46] One important consideration in patients with suspected AIFR of the sphenoid sinus is performing a vascular study before performing biopsy, because mycotic pseudoaneurysms of the internal carotid artery can bulge into the sphenoid sinus and rupture secondary to biopsy.[47]

INTRACRANIAL INFECTIONS

Intracranial extension of sinonasal fungal infections is one of the most dreadful complications in leukemic patients and is associated with doubling of the mortalities.[41] Angioinvasive aspergillus can also disseminate to the CNS hematogenously, most commonly from the lung, causing acute infarction or intracranial hemorrhage with subsequent development of infectious cerebritis or abscess.[23] The typical manifestations of brain abscesses, such as peripheral enhancement and central restricted diffusion, may not be seen in all patients[48] (**Fig. 17**). In a study of 23 circular lesions in patients

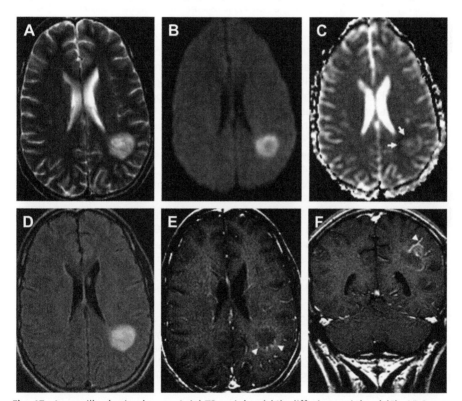

Fig. 17. Aspergillus brain abscess. Axial T2-weighted (A), diffusion-weighted (B), ADC map (C), FLAIR (D), and postcontrast T1-weighted (E) images in a 24-year-old man with ALL demonstrate left parietal parenchymal lesion with internal curvilinear T2 hypointensities, peripheral restricted diffusion (arrows), but central facilitated diffusion and incomplete peripheral enhancement (arrowheads on E). Coronal postcontrast T1-weighted image (F) also demonstrates areas of leptomeningeal enhancement (arrowhead). Lack of surrounding edema, peripheral rather than central restricted diffusion, and incomplete peripheral enhancement favor fungal infection in this immunocompromised patient. Biopsy demonstrated hyphae with 45° branching compatible with Aspergillus.

with brain aspergillosis, restricted diffusion was only seen in 11 cases. In addition, some of the lesions demonstrated peripheral T2 hypointensity on gradient echo sequences, which can be secondary to the presence of metallic elements.[48] Additional organisms, such as cryptococcus, and candida, and bacterial agents, such as Listeria monocytogenes, can also disseminate hematogenously to the CNS.[49,50]

REFERENCES

1. Guillerman RP, Voss SD, Parker BR. Leukemia and lymphoma. Radiol Clin North Am 2011;49(4):767–97.
2. Thomas X, Le QH. Central nervous system involvement in adult acute lymphoblastic leukemia. Hematology 2008;13(5):293–302.
3. Stewart DJ, Keating MJ, McCredie KB, et al. Natural history of central nervous system acute leukemia in adults. Cancer 1981;47(1):184–96.
4. Wolk RW, Masse SR, Conklin R, et al. The incidence of central nervous system leukemia in adults with acute leukemia. Cancer 1974;33(3):863–9.
5. Cheng CL, Li CC, Hou HA, et al. Risk factors and clinical outcomes of acute myeloid leukaemia with central nervous system involvement in adults. BMC Cancer 2015;15:344.
6. Lazarus HM, Richards SM, Chopra M, et al. Central nervous system involvement in adult acute lymphoblastic leukemia at diagnosis: results from the international ALL trial MRC UKALL XII/ECOG E2993. Blood 2006;108:465–72.
7. Hsi AC, Kreisel FH, Frater JL, et al. Clinicopathologic features of adult T-cell leukemias/lymphomas at a North American tertiary care medical center: infrequent involvement of the central nervous system. Am J Surg Pathol 2014; 38(2):245–56.
8. Porto L, Kieslich M, Schwabe D, et al. Granulocytic sarcoma in children. Neuroradiology 2004;46(5):374–7.
9. Ginsberg LE, Leeds EN. Neuroradiology of leukemia. AJR Am J Roentgenol 1995;165:525–34.
10. Hakyemez B, Yildirim N, Taskapilioglu O, et al. Intracranial myeloid sarcoma: conventional and advanced MRI findings. Br J Radiol 2007;80(954):e109–12.
11. Algharras AA, Mamourian A, Coyne T, et al. Leukostasis in an adult with AML presenting as multiple high attenuation brain masses on CT. J Clin Diagn Res 2013; 7(12):3020–2.
12. Lee B, Fatterpekar GM, Kim W, et al. Granulocytic sarcoma of the temporal bone. AJNR Am J Neuroradiol 2002;23(9):1497–9.
13. Kitajima M, Korogi Y, Shigematsu Y, et al. Central nervous system lesions in adult T-cell leukaemia: MRI and pathology. Neuroradiology 2002;44(7):559–67.
14. Porto L, Kieslich M, Schwabe D, et al. Central nervous system imaging in childhood leukaemia. Eur J Cancer 2004;40(14):2082–90.
15. Banna M, Aur R, Akkad S. Orbital granulocytic sarcoma. AJNR Am J Neuroradiol 1991;12(2):255–8.
16. Noh BW, Park SW, Chun JE, et al. Granulocytic sarcoma in the head and neck: CT and MR imaging findings. Clin Exp Otorhinolaryngol 2009;2(2):66–71.
17. Chen C, Zimmerman RA, Faro S, et al. Childhood leukemia: CNS abnormalities during and after treatment. AJNR Am J Neuroradiol 1996;17: 295–310.
18. Baikaidi M, Chung SS, Tallman MS, et al. A 75-year-old woman with thoracic spinal cord compression and chloroma (granulocytic sarcoma). Semin Oncol 2012;39(6):e37–46.

19. Hwang WL, Gau JP, Hu HT, et al. Isolated extramedullary relapse of acute lymphoblastic leukemia presenting as an intraspinal mass. Acta Haematol 1994;91(1):46–8.

20. Kyrnetskiy EE, Kun LE, Boop FA, et al. Types, causes, and outcome of intracranial hemorrhage in children with cancer. J Neurosurg 2005;102(Suppl 1):31–5.

21. Lin CH, Hung GY, Chang CY, et al. Subdural hemorrhage in a child with acute promyelocytic leukemia presenting as subtle headache. J Chin Med Assoc 2005;68(9):437–40.

22. Kingma A, Tamminga RY, Kamps WA, et al. Cerebrovascular complications of L-asparaginase therapy in children with leukemia: aphasia and other neuropsychological deficits. Pediatr Hematol Oncol 1993;10:303–9.

23. Vázquez E, Lucaya J, Castellote A, et al. Neuroimaging in pediatric leukemia and lymphoma: differential diagnosis. Radiographics 2002;22(6):1411–28.

24. Greene-Schloesser D, Robbins ME, Peiffer AM, et al. Radiation-induced brain injury: a review. Front Oncol 2012;19(2):73.

25. Ball WS Jr, Prenger EC, Ballard ET. Neurotoxicity of radio/chemotherapy in children: pathologic and MR evaluation. AJNR Am J Neuroradiol 1992;13:761–76.

26. Edwards-Brown MK, Jakacki RI. Imaging the CNS effects of radiation and chemotherapy of pediatric tumors. Neuroimaging Clin N Am 1999;9:177–93.

27. Shanley DJ. Mineralizing microangiopathy: CT and MRI. Neuroradiology 1995; 37(4):331–3.

28. Walter AW, Hancock ML, Pui CH, et al. Secondary brain tumors in children treated for ALL at St. Jude children's research hospital. J Clin Oncol 1998; 16:3761–7.

29. Kozlowski K, Campbell J, McAlister W, et al. Rare primary cranial vault and base of the skull tumours in children. Report of 30 cases with a short literature review. Radiol Med 1991;81(3):213–24.

30. Inaba H, Khan RB, Laningham FH, et al. Clinical and radiological characteristics of methotrexate-induced acute encephalopathy in pediatric patients with cancer. Ann Oncol 2008;19(1):178–84.

31. Rollins N, Winick N, Bash R, et al. Acute methotrexate neurotoxicity: findings on diffusion-weighted imaging and correlation with clinical outcome. AJNR Am J Neuroradiol 2004;25(10):1688–95.

32. Pascual AM, Coret F, Casanova B, et al. Anterior lumbosacral polyradiculopathy after intrathecal administration of methotrexate. J Neurol Sci 2008;267(1–2):158–61.

33. Gorson KC, Ropper AH, Muriello MA, et al. Prospective evaluation of MRI lumbosacral nerve root enhancement in acute Guillain-Barré syndrome. Neurology 1996;47:813–7.

34. Iwata F, Utsumi Y. MR imaging in Guillain-Barré syndrome. Pediatr Radiol 1997; 27:36–8.

35. Murata KY, Maeba A, Yamanegi M, et al. Methotrexate myelopathy after intrathecal chemotherapy: a case report. J Med Case Rep 2015;9:135.

36. Dicuonzo F, Salvati A, Palma M, et al. Posterior reversible encephalopathy syndrome associated with methotrexate neurotoxicity: conventional magnetic resonance and diffusion-weighted imaging findings. J Child Neurol 2009;24(8):1013–8.

37. Miller L, Link MP, Bologna S, et al. Cerebellar atrophy caused by high-dose cytosine arabinoside: CT and MR findings. AJR Am J Roentgenol 1989;152(2):343–4.

38. Ross CS, Brown TM, Kotagal S, et al. Cerebral venous sinus thrombosis in pediatric cancer patients: long-term neurological outcomes. J Pediatr Hematol Oncol 2013;35(4):299–302.

39. Kasturi O, Schlamann M, Moenninghoff C, et al. Posterior reversible encephalopathy syndrome: the spectrum of MR imaging patterns. Clin Neuroradiol 2015; 25(2):161–71.
40. Junewar V, Verma R, Sankhwar PL, et al. Neuroimaging features and predictors of outcome in eclamptic encephalopathy: a prospective observational study. AJNR Am J Neuroradiol 2014;35(9):1728–34.
41. Turner JH, Soudry E, Nayak JV, et al. Survival outcomes in acute invasive fungal sinusitis: a systematic review and quantitative synthesis of published evidence. Laryngoscope 2013;123:1112–8.
42. Groppo ER, El-Sayed IH, Aiken AH, et al. Computed tomography and magnetic resonance imaging characteristics of acute invasive fungal sinusitis. Arch Otolaryngol Head Neck Surg 2011;137:1005–10.
43. DelGaudio JM, Swain RE Jr, Kingdom TT, et al. Computed tomographic findings in patients with invasive fungal sinusitis. Arch Otolaryngol Head Neck Surg 2003; 129:236–40.
44. Middlebrooks EH, Frost CJ, De Jesus RO, et al. Acute invasive fungal rhinosinusitis: a comprehensive update of CT findings and design of an effective diagnostic imaging model. AJNR Am J Neuroradiol 2015;36(8):1529–35.
45. Safder S, Carpenter JS, Roberts TD, et al. The "Black Turbinate" sign: an early MR imaging finding of nasal mucormycosis. AJNR Am J Neuroradiol 2010; 31(4):771–4.
46. Gillespie MB, Huchton DM, O'Malley BW. Role of middle turbinate biopsy in the diagnosis of fulminant invasive fungal rhinosinusitis. Laryngoscope 2000; 110(11):1832–6.
47. Hurst RW, Judkins A, Bolger W, et al. Mycotic aneurysm and cerebral infarction resulting from fungal sinusitis: imaging and pathologic correlation. AJNR Am J Neuroradiol 2001;22(5):858–63.
48. Charlot M, Pialat JB, Obadia N, et al. Diffusion-weighted imaging in brain aspergillosis. Eur J Neurol 2007;14(8):912–6.
49. Bhatt VR, Viola GM, Ferrajoli A. Invasive fungal infections in acute leukemia. Ther Adv Hematol 2011;2(4):231–47.
50. Bajkó Z, Bălaşa R, Maier S, et al. Listeria monocytogenes meningoencephalitis mimicking stroke in a patient with chronic lymphocytic leukemia. Neurol Ther 2013;2(1–2):63–70.

Imaging of Multiple Myeloma

Barry Amos, DO[a], Amit Agarwal, MD[b], Sangam Kanekar, MD[a,b],*

KEYWORDS

- Imaging • Multiple myeloma • Classification • Treatment • Complications

KEY POINTS

- Diagnosis of multiple myeloma is based on a combination of clinical findings, laboratory studies, bone marrow biopsy, and imaging findings.
- Imaging plays an important role in identifying the extent of the disease, disease process, guiding biopsies, and diagnosing associated spinal and intracranial complications. It also plays an important role in the staging, evaluating response to therapy, and monitoring for recurrence.
- Multiple myeloma and related plasma cell proliferative disorders (PCPDs) have a diverse set of clinicopathologic findings and with those present unique and diverse findings on neuroimaging, not only from the disease itself but from complications of the disease and treatment-related complications. Familiarity with these findings is valuable for clinicians and radiologists alike.
- This article describes the imaging findings associated with common neurologic complications seen with multiple myeloma and related PCPDs.

INTRODUCTION

Multiple myeloma is a malignant neoplasm of plasma cells that produces monoclonal immunoglobulins. Each year in the United States, approximately 20,000 new cases are diagnosed with approximately 11,000 deaths. Most patients are older than 60 years with a median age at diagnosis of 66 years old.[1–3]

Multiple myeloma is a cytogenetically and molecularly diverse neoplasm leading to a wide range of clinical disease. Multiple myeloma is believed to be a progression of a premalignant stage called monoclonal gammopathy of undetermined significance (MGUS).[4–9] Patients present at varying stages from the premalignant MGUS, to an intermediate asymptomatic stage termed smoldering myeloma, to the symptomatic

[a] Department of Radiology, Hershey Medical Center, The Pennsylvania State University, Hershey, PA, USA; [b] Department of Neurology, Hershey Medical Center, The Pennsylvania State University, Hershey, PA, USA
* Corresponding author. Departments of Radiology & Neurology, Hershey Medical Center, The Pennsylvania State University, 500 University Drive, Hershey, PA 17033.
E-mail address: skanekar@hmc.psu.edu

Hematol Oncol Clin N Am 30 (2016) 843–865
http://dx.doi.org/10.1016/j.hoc.2016.03.007
0889-8588/16/$ – see front matter © 2016 Elsevier Inc. All rights reserved.

stage termed multiple myeloma.[4–9] Patients may also present at a stage before multiple myeloma and progress all the way to multiple myeloma at varying rates depending on several cytogenetic and molecular factors.

MGUS is predominantly seen in patients older than 50 years with a prevalence of approximately 3% in the population 50 years and older, 5% in the population 70 years and older, and 7.5% in the population 85 years and older.[1–3]

The purpose of this review article is to describe the imaging findings associated with common neurologic complications seen with multiple myeloma and related plasma cell proliferative disorders (PCPDs). The diagnosis, classification of multiple myeloma and PCPDs, staging and risk stratification, and treatment are briefly described as they pertain to neurologic complications. A brief overview of the imaging of multiple myeloma and then specific imaging findings associated with common neurologic complications seen with multiple myeloma are described.

CLASSIFICATION OF MYELOMA, MONOCLONAL GAMMOPATHY OF UNDETERMINED SIGNIFICANCE, AND RELATED PLASMA-CELL PROLIFERATIVE DISORDERS

The International Myeloma Working Group (IMWG) has set diagnostic criteria for multiple myeloma and MGUS, the most recent revised criteria of 2014 is described in (**Box 1**).[4–9] The IMWG divides the premalignant MGUS and related PCPDs into 6 classes based on several clinicopathologic criteria; non-immunoglobulin (Ig)M MGUS, IgM MGUS, light chain MGUS, solitary plasmacytoma, POEMS syndrome, and systemic amyloid light chain (AL) amyloidosis.[4–9] As previously described, each of these can then progress onto an intermediate stage before becoming multiple myeloma. Also, as described, patients can present at any stage from MGUS to myeloma.[4–9]

IMMUNOGLOBULIN M, NON-IMMUNOGLOBULIN M, AND LIGHT CHAIN MONOCLONAL GAMMOPATHY OF UNDETERMINED SIGNIFICANCE

The first 3 divisions are based on the monoclonal or M-protein, which is secreted by the clonal plasma cells.[4–9] There are the non-IgM MGUS, IgM MGUS, and light chain MGUS. The IgM MGUS is usually compromised of IgG, IgA, and much less frequently IgD and IgE monoclonal gammopathies.[4–9] The PCPD is classified as MGUS when the serum monoclonal protein is present but less than 30 g per liter and clonal bone marrow cells are less than 10%.[4–9] In addition, there must be no end-organ damage from the monoclonal gammopathy such as hypercalcemia, renal insufficiency, anemia, and bone lesions (the so called CRAB features) or amyloidoisis.[4–9] Smoldering myeloma will have a non-IgM serum monoclonal protein more than 30 g per liter

---

Box 1
The International Myeloma Working Group, 2014

Non-IgM MGUS

IgM MGUS

Light chain MGUS

Solitary plasmacytoma

POEMS syndrome

Systemic AL amyloidosis

Data from Refs.[4–9]

and/or clonal bone marrow cells more than 10% but no end-organ damage. Multiple myeloma is diagnosed with evidence of end-organ damage.[4–9]

The diagnosis of IgM MGUS, smoldering IgM myeloma and multiple myeloma (with an IgM monoclonal M-protein) is similar but with an IgM serum monoclonal protein meeting criteria as previously described.[4–9] In addition to smoldering IgM myeloma and multiple myeloma, there are other unique subclassifications of the IgM monoclonal gammopathy termed Waldenström macroglobulinemia (WM) and its associated intermediate form, smoldering WM.[4–9] The diagnosis of smoldering WM and WM requires both serum and bone marrow minimums with distinct cytogenetic of clonal cells, which distinguish it from multiple myeloma[4–9] (**Fig. 1**).

The diagnosis of light chain MGUS is based on an abnormal serum free light chain ratio (<0.26 with elevated lambda light chain or >1.65 with elevated kappa light chain) and no heavy chain immunoglobulin.[4–9] Light chain MGUS also requires less than 10% clonal bone cells, less than 500 mg per 24 hours of urinary monoclonal protein, and lack of end-organ damage.[4–9] The light chain monoclonal gammopathy can progress to an intermediate stage termed idiopathic Bence Jones proteinuria. Idiopathic Bence Jones proteinuria is diagnosed with a urinary monoclonal protein greater than 500 mg per 24 hours without end-organ damage.[4–9] It is termed light chain myeloma with evidence of end-organ damage.[4–9] Progression rates to multiple myeloma have been shown to be about 1% per year for IgM and non-IgM MGUS to multiple myeloma. Light chain progresses less frequently at about 0.3% per year.[4–9]

SOLITARY PLASMACYTOMA, POEMS SYNDROME, AND SYSTEMIC AMYLOID LIGHT CHAIN AMYLOIDOSIS

The last 3 divisions of premalignant disorders are based on other unique clinicopathologic criteria due to distinctness of the disease entity, including disease progression rate and/or prognosis. These include solitary plasmacytoma, POEMS syndrome, and systemic AL amyloidosis.

Solitary plasmacytoma is diagnosed by biopsy of solitary bone or soft tissue lesion (also termed medullary or extramedullary, respectively) demonstrating clonal plasma cells.[4–9] Solitary plasmacytoma must show normal bone marrow without evidence of plasma clonal cells.[4–9] There is a subcategory in which there are less than 10% clonal bone marrow cells, which is termed solitary plasmacytoma with minimal marrow involvement.[4–9] This has a much a higher progression rate to multiple

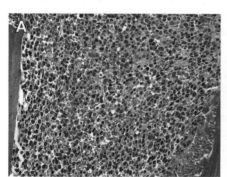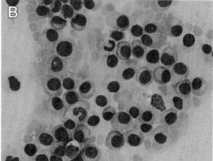

Fig. 1. Multiple myeloma by immunohistochemistry. (*A*) Hematoxylin and eosin-stained bone marrow biopsy with near-complete replacement by plasma cells at 100 × magnification. (*B*) Wright-Giemsa–stained bone marrow aspirate showing abundant plasma cells at 100 × magnification.

myeloma (60% at 3 years) compared with solitary plasmacytoma without marrow involvement (10% at 3 years).[4–9] There must be no other lesions seen on imaging except for the solitary plasmacytoma (**Fig. 2**). There must also be absence of end-organ damage.[4–9]

POEMS syndrome is an acronym for polyneuropathy, organomegaly, endocrinopathy or edema, M-protein, and skin changes. The diagnosis is made by demonstrating the combination of polyneuropathy, a monoclonal PCPD (usually lambda), 1 of 3 major criteria (sclerotic bone lesion, Castleman disease, elevated serum vascular endothelial growth factor [VEGFA] levels), and 1 of 6 minor criteria (organomegaly, volume overload, endocrinopathy, skin changes, papilledema, thrombocytosis or polycythemia).[4–9] Unlike the osteolytic bone lesions seen in multiple myeloma, the bone lesions seen in POEMS syndrome are typically osteoblastic (or sclerotic), which can mimic metastatic prostate cancer and other osteoblastic lesions[10] (**Fig. 3**).

Systemic AL (immunoglobulin light chain) amyloidosis is diagnosed by evidence of an amyloid-related systemic syndrome, such as renal, liver, heart, gastrointestinal, or peripheral nerve involvement.[4–9] There must be positive amyloid staining by Congo red of biopsied tissue and the amyloid must be composed of light chain.[4–9] In addition, there must be evidence of a monoclonal PCPD, as described previously, in light chain MGUS. When patients meet criteria for multiple myeloma and systemic AL amyloidosis they are considered to have both diseases.[4–9]

Plasma cell leukemia is a distinct entity not typically described with MGUS and myeloma, although it will be described here for completeness. This can occur either de novo, in which it is called primary plasma cell leukemia, or it can occur as a relapsed or refractory multiple myeloma, in which it is called secondary plasma cell leukemia.[4–8,10] Plasma cell leukemia is a rare and very aggressive entity distinguished by high levels of plasma cells circulating in the peripheral blood (>2000 per microliter).[4–9,11]

MULTIPLE MYELOMA STAGING AND RISK STRATIFICATION

Multiple myeloma is divided into stage I, II, and III based on 2 classification systems: the International Staging System (ISS) and Durie-Salmon staging (DSS).[4–9] The ISS uses only beta-2 microglobulin and albumin levels to distinguish between the stages. DSS uses hemoglobin levels, calcium levels, serum immunoglobulin levels, urine monoclonal protein levels, and bone lesions seen on imaging to distinguish between stages.[4–9] Bone lesions were historically evaluated with skeletal surveys and divided into no lytic lesions for stage I and advanced lytic lesions for stage III. In the DSS system there are also (a) and (b) subclassifications based on serum creatinine levels.[4–9] In a revised 2006 system of the DSS, termed the DSS Plus, advanced imaging (PET-computed tomography [CT] or MRI) was introduced into the staging to better identify and prognosticate patients who were previously lumped together, yet had distinctly different disease prognostics.[12] Now stage II lesions are better differentiated with this classification as stage I having less than 4 lesions, stage II having 5 to 20 lesions, and stage III having more than 20 seen on advanced imaging.[12]

In addition to staging, there is risk stratification because patients with the same stage, based on the 2 aforementioned staging systems, may have drastic differences in prognosis based on differences in cytogenetics and laboratory values not accounted for.[9]

MULTIPLE MYELOMA TREATMENT

MGUS patients do not meet criteria for treatment.[4–9] Asymptomatic myeloma patients with certain criteria (bone marrow plasmacytosis >60%, markedly elevated serum light

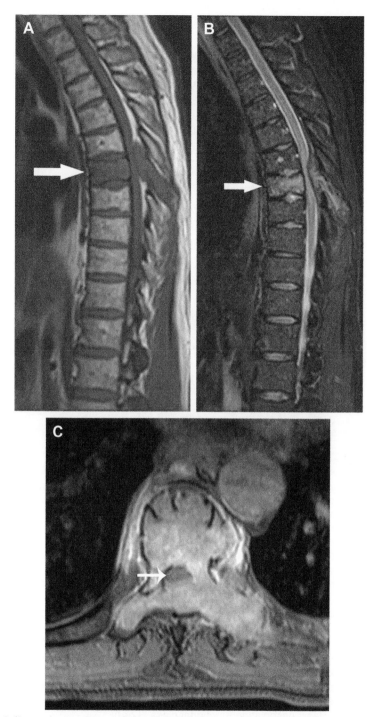

Fig. 2. Solitary plasmacytoma of the thoracic spine. Sagittal T1-weighted (W) (*A*), sagittal T2W (*B*) and postcontrast axial (*C*) images of the thoracic spine reveal a solitary marrow re-placing lesion (*arrow* in *A* and *B*) involving an entire midthoracic vertebra, including the anterior and posterior elements. There is associated enhancing soft-tissue component in the posterior epidural space with cord compression (*arrow* in *C*). There is mild loss of verte-bral body height with preserved adjacent disc spaces.

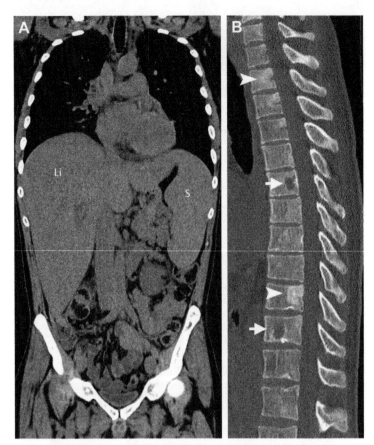

Fig. 3. POEMS syndrome. Coronal body CT (*A*) reveals moderate hepatic and splenic enlargement (organomegaly). Sagittal thoracic spine image (*B*) in the same patient shows numerous lytic (*arrows*) and sclerotic lesions (*arrowheads*) involving multiple thoracic vertebrae.

chain levels, and bone marrow involvement on MRI or CT-PET) may be eligible for treatment, depending on several other patient factors.[4–9]

Solitary plasmacytoma is usually treated with radiation therapy alone to the site with monitoring for progression to multiple myeloma in which the treatment would then progress (see later discussion).[13]

Patients are split into 2 main groups: autologous stem-cell transplant (ASCT)–eligible and non-ASCT–eligible.[9] In the 2013 Updated Mayo Stratification of Myeloma and Risk-Adapted Therapy (mSMART) Consensus Guidelines, "physiologic age less than 70 years old" was used as a cutoff for ASCT eligibility.[7] Other criteria of exclusion commonly used are age greater than 77 years old, direct bilirubin greater than 2.0 mg/dL, Eastern Cooperative Oncology Group (ECOG) performance status 3 or 4, or New York Heart Association functional class III or IV.[4–9]

In the revised mSMART, both ASCT eligible and ineligible patients were classified into standard, intermediate, and high-risk groups to guide therapy.[4–9] High-risk eligible patients receive 4 cycles bortezomib-lenalidomide-dexamethasone (VRD) for induction therapy then go onto ASCT (especially if not in complete remission), with VRD maintenance for a minimum of 1 year.[4–9] Intermediate eligible receive

4 cycles of cyclophosphamide-bortezomib-dexamethasone (CyBorD) then go onto ASCT, followed by bortezomib-based therapy for minimum of 1 year.[4–9] Standard-risk patients receive 4 cycles of dexamethasone (Rd) or CyBorD, then will either go onto ASCT with consideration of lenalidomide maintenance therapy or Rd maintenance alone without ASCT.[4–9] High-risk ineligible patients get VRD. Intermediate ineligible patients receive melphalan-prednisone (MP) plus weekly CyBorD or weekly bortezomib-based therapy, then go onto bortezomib maintenance.[4–9] Standard-risk ineligible patients get Rd or MP plus thalidomide, then go onto observation.[4–9]

These common treatment regimens used in myeloma are important in neurologic imaging because many complications of treatment affect the neurologic system in a specific way and have associated imaging findings.

IMAGING OF MULTIPLE MYELOMA
Radiography

Skeletal survey has historically been the recommended imaging for detecting myeloma bone disease. On radiography, multiple myeloma lesions typically have a punched-out osteolytic appearance. However, at least 50% of the involved trabecular bone needs to be destroyed to be detectable as a lytic lesion on radiography. In some cases, up to 75% of the trabecular bone needs to be destroyed before showing up on radiography.[10,14]

Skeletal lesions can be seen in the spine, pelvis, skull, ribs, sternum, and proximal appendicular skeleton, in order of frequency. Although rare, more distal appendicular skeleton can be affected. Four types of involvement have been described on skeletal radiography: the solitary lesion (plasmacytoma), diffuse skeletal involvement (myelomatosis), the most common diffuse skeletal osteopenia, and the rare presentation of sclerosing myeloma.[10,14]

Computed Tomography

CT compared with radiography is much more sensitive in detecting bone lesions. Lesions with less than 5% of trabecular bone destruction can be detected compared with radiography (**Fig. 4**).[10,14] In addition, CT can be used to evaluate for involvement and compromise of surrounding soft tissues. Body CT can also detect soft tissue extramedullary plasmacytomas. CT is commonly used in guiding biopsies of MRI-detected lesions. Although CT poses higher dose of radiation, low-dose, whole-body CT protocols have been used with similar sensitivities but with a much lower dose of radiation.[10,14]

Nuclear Medicine Studies

Several nuclear medicine studies have been used to evaluate myeloma. Tc-99m bone scans have been attempted but show poor results due to the lack of osteoblastic activity, unless there has been a complication such as a pathologic fracture.[10,14]

Galium-67 (Ga), thallium-201 (Tl), and fluorodeoxyglucose F-18 positron emission tomography (PET) have all been used to detect myeloma. Due to their ability to detect physiologically active disease, these studies were very beneficial not only for detecting disease but for following treatment response.[10,14] However, Ga and Tl are rarely used today due to several technical difficulties that make them obsolete.[10,14] PET-CT on the other hand is becoming more widespread and is supplementing MRI.[10,14] PET-CT can detect active disease and may be better than MRI at monitoring response to therapy. In addition, PET-CT is excellent at evaluating extramedullary disease. Like MRI, PET-CT is included in the DSS Plus system for staging with advanced imaging.[10,12,14]

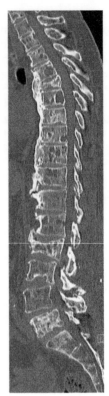

Fig. 4. Multiple myeloma. Sagittal CT image reveals diffuse osteopenia with numerous lytic lesions throughout the thoracolumbar spine along with pathologic collapse of T6 and L2 vertebrae.

MRI

MRI has now become the gold standard for imaging in multiple myeloma. The IMWG released a consensus statement in 2015 stating the indications of MRI in multiple myeloma and PCPDs.[15–18] MRI is very sensitive and specific for detecting bone disease and soft tissue involvement or compromise in myeloma.[10,14]

Detecting myeloma bone disease on MRI is based on replacement of normal bone marrow with neoplastic cells. Normal bone marrow appearance depends on the age of the patient and location of the bone marrow. The axial skeleton is much richer in red marrow than the appendicular skeleton, which is comprised mostly of fatty marrow. As humans age, even the axial skeleton is progressively replaced with fatty marrow. On MRI, this can be seen by the progressive increase in T1-weighted signal intensity in the marrow. The frequency of T1 change from hypointense to iso-hyperintense at different age groups is described by Ricci and colleagues.[15] Most patients with myeloma are more than 50 years old and have fatty replaced marrow, which is T1 hyperintense and hypointense on fluid-sensitive sequences (T2-weighted and short-tau inversion recovery [STIR]).[10,14,19] Therefore, a hypointense lesion on T1 and hyperintense lesion on fluid-sensitive sequences will indicate marrow replacement in this group[10,14,19] (**Fig. 5**). Fluid-sensitive sequences tend to be the most sensitive at detecting lesions, with STIR usually even more so than standard T2 due to fat suppression.[10,14,19] It is important to realize this is a nonspecific sign because this can be seen

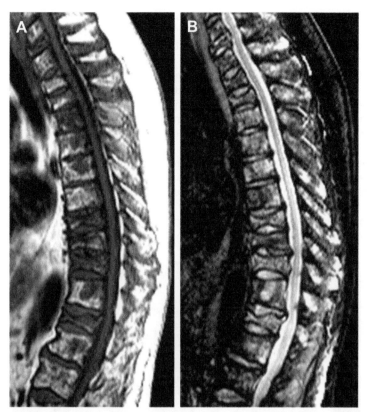

Fig. 5. Multiple myeloma. Sagittal T1W (*A*) and STIR fluid-sensitive (*B*) images reveal numerous focal and diffuse vertebral marrow lesions, which appear hypointense on T1W images with bright signal on the STIR image. Multiple compression deformities are also noted with preservation of the disc space.

in other marrow replacing diseases such as metastatic disease, lymphoma and leukemia. Also, caution must be taken when evaluating diffuse band-like T1 hypointensities, which can be a normal finding in patients more than 60 years of age.[10,14,19]

Many protocols exist for evaluating myeloma with MRI. The 2015 consensus recommends at minimum obtaining T1, T2, and STIR sequences with or without T1-postcontrast imaging of the whole body in axial and sagittal planes, with axial and coronal imaging of the pelvis.[15–18] Considering the high-incidence of renal insufficiency among myeloma patients, the risk of nephrogenic systemic fibrosis has to be considered when considering contrast enhancement. In most cases, contrast enhancement is not necessary because little additional information is gained. If whole-body imaging cannot be performed, whole spine and pelvis imaging should be obtained, which is usually complemented by standard brain MRI imaging. It is important to still obtain appendicular skeletal imaging in the form of a radiographic complete or limited skeletal survey, or alternative cross-sectional imaging of the remaining body. These should be performed with dedicated coils, slice thickness less than 5 mm, and matrix of 512. Most centers meet these requirements and are currently performing similar protocols.[15–18]

The consensus recommends MRI imaging for all patients with newly diagnosed multiple myeloma for prognostic information.[15–18] Some patients previously classified as having smoldering myeloma may be upgraded to having multiple myeloma with MRI showing lesions not previously detectable on radiography. Patients with 1 or more un-equivocal lesions 5 mm or greater on MRI should be classified as having multiple myeloma.[15–18] If there are equivocal lesions, then a repeat MRI should be performed in 3 to 6 months to evaluate for any change in which if there is progression should then be classified as multiple myeloma.[15–18] In patients with MGUS, MRI is not routinely rec-ommended unless there is a high clinical suspicion of more advanced disease. MRI should be used in the evaluation of most symptomatic cases such as painful lesions in myeloma, evaluation of spinal cord involvement, compression fractures, and solitary bone plasmacytoma. MRI is also best to evaluate the head and neck, which are commonly involved.[10,14–18]

Four pathologic patterns of bone marrow involvement on MRI are typically described: solitary lesion ($\geq$5 mm in diameter), homogenous diffuse involvement, combined diffuse and focal lesion, and variegated inhomogeneous involvement with dispersed fat (also termed salt-and-pepper pattern) (**Fig. 6**).[10,12,14–18] The diffuse pattern alone has been shown to have worse prognosis but is not currently used specifically in the staging sys-tems, except being considered stage III in the DSS system.[10,12,14–18]

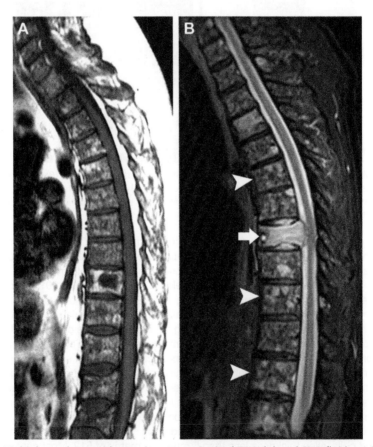

Fig. 6. Multiple myeloma with mosaic pattern. Sagittal T1W (*A*) and STIR fluid-sensitive (*B*) images reveal variegated inhomogeneous involvement of thoracolumbar vertebrae with dispersed fat (salt-and-pepper pattern). There are numerous tiny STIR bright marrow lesions (*arrowheads*) along with diffuse homogenous involvement of a midthoracic vertebra with pathologic collapse and posterior cortical buckling (*arrow*).

Disease response to therapy can be seen with return of fatty marrow signal on T1 and resolution of fluid-sensitive hyperintensities. In addition, lack of enhancement has been shown to be more accurate. However, treated lesions usually take 12 months to appear normal and may continue to appear abnormal for up to 58 months, leading to a high false-positive rate.[10,14] Another appearance of treated myeloma is that of myelofibrosis and amyloidosis. Long-term treatment can lead to diffuse myelofibrosis and/or amyloidosis with focal amyloid deposits.[10,14] Both appear hypointense on both T1 and fluid-sensitive sequences but myelofibrosis will typically have diffuse involvement, whereas amyloidosis tends to have multiple focal lesions.[10,14]

Currently, routine therapy monitoring with MRI is not recommended.[10,12,14–18] PET-CT has been shown to be more accurate in demonstrating response with less false positives (**Fig. 7**). Several centers do perform PET-CT for therapy monitoring; however, there may be more false negatives because the spatial resolution of PET is much lower.[10,12,14–18,20] Like MRI, PET-CT is also not currently recommended for routine imaging.[10,12,14–18,20]

NEUROLOGICAL COMPLICATIONS OF MULTIPLE MYELOMA AND RELATED PLASMA-CELL PROLIFERATIVE DISORDERS

Neurological complications of multiple myeloma may be due to spinal myeloma, skull or intracranial myeloma, cranial nerve involvement; or may be due to metabolic and hematologic complications, or secondary infection related to immunosuppression (**Table 1**).

Spinal Myeloma

Spinal complications in myeloma are common and can be divided into 4 categories: osseous or vertebral involvement, compression of spinal cord, cauda equina syndrome, and/or solitary nerve root compression.[10,14]

Vertebral involvement in myeloma usually manifests clinically as spinal fractures (**Fig. 8**). Spinal fractures in myeloma are a very common cause of morbidity. Vertebral compression fractures occur in approximately 50% of patients diagnosed with multiple myeloma.[10,14] Spinal fractures are thought to be due to 2 main factors: the indirect osteoclast-activating effect of myeloma resulting in osteopenia and direct invasion by focal myeloma lesions. Myeloma cells release several osteoclast-activating tumoral factors that lead to diffuse osteopenia. In addition, several therapies, most notably high-dose steroids, have been associated with insufficiency fractures. Osteopenic insufficiency fractures make up approximately 50% of all fractures.[10,14] When there is a solitary fracture, tumor-infiltrated pathologic fractures make up approximately 80% of fractures but are much less frequent in the case of multiple fractures.[10,14] Differentiating an insufficiency fracture and pathologic fracture can usually be done with MRI. On MRI, insufficiency fractures will tend to have normal T1 marrow signal except for dark fracture lines. Due to edema the fluid-sensitive sequences will be bright. With pathologic fractures, the marrow will usually be replaced on T1 with tumor cells and usually enhance. A confident diagnosis can be made when tumor is seen extending into the epidural space that can be differentiated from retropulsed vertebral elements. The tumor and peritumoral edema will also be bright on fluid-sensitive sequences. Diffusion and opposed-phase imaging may also assist in differentiating insufficiency from pathologic fractures.[10,14]

Bisphosphonate therapy is indicated to decrease bone turnover and prevent fractures in myeloma. Bisphosphonate therapy alone has its own risks, which should be kept in mind during therapy.[10,14,21] Osteonecrosis of the jaw and atypical subtrochanteric fractures are specific complications seen on neuroimaging[10,14,21] (**Fig. 9**).

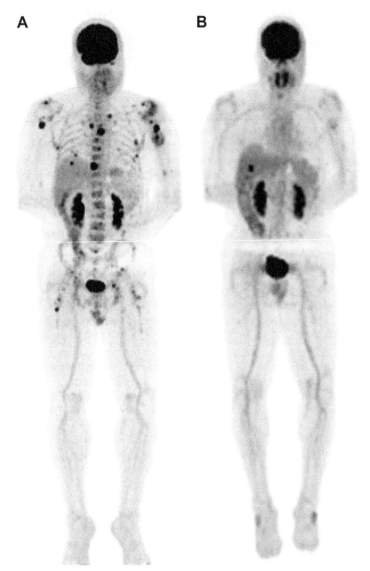

Fig. 7. FDG-PET in multiple myeloma. Pretreatment FDG-PET scan (*A*) shows uptake in multiple vertebrae, ribs, and bones of the extremities. Six-month follow-up FDG-PET scan (*B*) following chemotherapy treatment shows complete resolution of the multiple FDG-avid lesions, suggestive of good response.

In a patient without radiation to the mandibular region or other reason to explain osteonecrosis, osteonecrosis due to bisphosphonates should be considered. Subtrochanteric fractures with bisphosphonate therapy typically occur in the proximal diaphyses, which is an atypical area of hip fracture unless in the setting of specific trauma mechanism to this region.[10,14,21]

Vertebroplasty and kyphoplasty are common treatments for vertebral compression fractures in myeloma. Both help in reducing pain but kyphoplasty has the additional benefit of improving height and posture. The cement will be dense on radiography

Table 1
Neurological complications of multiple myeloma

Spinal myeloma	Osseous or vertebral involvement, compression of spinal cord, cauda equina syndrome, and/or solitary nerve root compression
Extraosseous (Extramedullary) Spinal Myeloma	Contiguous and noncontiguous soft tissue masses, dural myelomatosis, leptomeningeal myelomatosis, and spinal parenchymal myeloma
Skull and Intracranial Myeloma	Calvarium, contiguous extramedullary myeloma, dural myelomatosis, leptomeningeal myelomatosis, and (least common) cerebral parenchymal myeloma
Cranial Nerve Involvement	Dural or leptomeningeal myelomatosis
Metabolic Complications in Myeloma	Hypercalcemia, nephrogenic systemic fibrosis
Immunosuppression and Infectious Complications in Myeloma	Bacterial, fungal, herpes zoster infection
Hematologic Complications in Myeloma	Anemia, diffuse marrow changes, hyperviscosity, venous thromboembolism

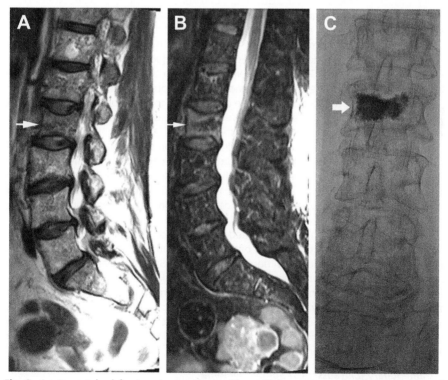

Fig. 8. Acute vertebral fracture in a patient with multiple myeloma. Sagittal T1W (*A*) and STIR fluid-sensitive (*B*) images reveal compression fracture of the L2 vertebral body (*arrows*). Patient was treated with vertebroplasty. Posteroanterior view of the lumbar spine (*C*) shows changes of the vertebroplasty (*arrow*).

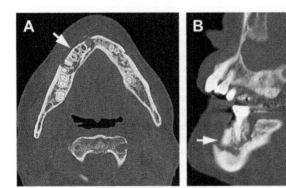

Fig. 9. Bisphosphonate associated mandibular osteonecrosis. Axial (*A*) and sagittal (*B*) CT images reveal fragmentation and sequestrum formation of the right mandibular body (*arrows*). There is associated periosteal reaction and involvement of the alveolar ridge.

and dark on all MRI sequences (see **Fig. 8**). Complications seen on imaging can be due to extruded cement causing pressure on the spinal cord or roots.[10,14] In addition, damage to the roots due to local heat during the procedure may lead to neuropathy.[10,14]

Compression of the spinal cord due to tumor extension or retropulsed fragments can be an urgent or emergent situation. MRI performs extremely well at depicting the extent of disease, degree of spinal canal stenosis, and degree of myelopathy. Tumor can be differentiated from retropulsed fragments, as described previously. Degree of spinal stenosis is best depicted on fluid-sensitive sequences, which can show obliteration of the canal.[10,14] Degree of myelopathy is also best depicted with ill-defined hyperintensities on fluid-sensitive sequences, which represent edema of the cord.[10,14]

Radiation therapy and dexamethasone can be used to treat cord compression and painful lesions. Surgery is usually reserved for refractory cases and fractures with retropulsed bone without tumoral involvement.[10,14,22]

Cauda equina syndrome is a specific clinical syndrome caused by compression of the spinal cord at the conus medullaris. Cauda equina syndrome manifests with the clinical symptoms of perianal and saddle paresthesias with loss of bowel and bladder function. MRI is very useful in depicting the compression of the conus.[10,14,22] This syndrome is an emergent situation and requires surgery within 24 hours.[10,14,22]

Nerve root compression can be isolated but usually occurs with cord compression. MRI can be used to depict the extent of the disease causing the compression and, in addition, demonstrate signs of neuropathy.[10,14,22] Signs of neuropathy on MRI include thickened and enhancing nerves with secondary signs of muscle denervation, which change from the acute or subacute and chronic phases in the denervated muscle groups.[10,14] Many of the myeloma therapies cause neuropathy independent of myeloma. Thalidomide-based therapies and bortezomib have all been associated with neuropathies.[10,14,23,24] These can also manifest with MRI findings of neuropathy but without the tumoral or bone involvement.[10,14,23,24]

Extramedullary (Extraosseous) Spinal Myeloma

Extramedullary myeloma is an uncommon presentation of myeloma.[25–27] However, with advances in therapy leading to longer survival, new presentations of myeloma are being seen as either progression or recurrence of disease. Extramedullary myeloma is only seen in approximately 10% of new myeloma diagnoses but can be seen in up to 20% of patients with progressive disease.[25–27] Approximately, 50% of the cases with extramedullary myeloma are seen in disease recurrence.[25–27] Extramedullary myeloma is considered stage III in the DSS system with a poor prognosis.[12,25–27] MRI and/or PET-CT should be considered in all patients with known or suspected extramedullary disease.[15–18,25–27]

Extramedullary myeloma is divided into contiguous (spreading directly from the bone marrow) and noncontiguous (arising separate from the bone marrow)[25–27] (see **Table 1**). Contiguous extramedullary myeloma makes up approximately 60%, whereas noncontiguous makes up approximately 40%.[25–27] Noncontiguous extramedullary myeloma is believed to be hematogenously spread, affecting the lymph nodes, skin, visceral organs, upper airways, and central nervous system (CNS) parenchyma.[25–27] Contiguous extramedullary myeloma most commonly affects the paraspinal and epidural soft tissues.[25–27] Although paraspinal-epidural masses are more common in the thoracic spine, they can be seen anywhere from the cervical spine to the sacrum.[25–27]

Contiguous extramedullary lesions typically appear iso-hypointense on T1 imaging and iso-hyperintense on fluid-sensitive sequences compared with skeletal muscle, similar to intramedullary lesions (**Fig. 10**).[25–27] Lesions will typically enhance more than skeletal muscle but with varying degrees.[25–27] Noncontiguous extramedullary lesions appear similar on T1 but can have varying degrees of intensity on fluid-sensitive sequences, frequently appearing hypointense similar to lymphoma.[25–27] Noncontiguous lesions also demonstrate some degree of restricted diffusion and increased enhancement compared with skeletal muscle but with varying degrees similar to lymphoma.[25–27] With its similar appearance to lymphoma, it is important to consider this in the differential in the proper setting.[25–27]

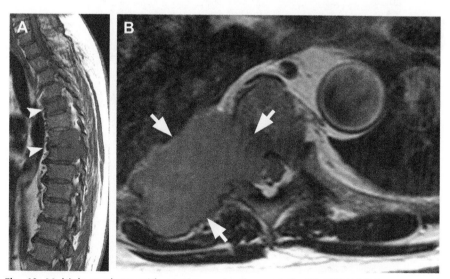

Fig. 10. Multiple myeloma with contiguous involvement. Sagittal T1W (*A*) image reveals contiguous involvement of 2 thoracic vertebrae (*arrowheads*) with T1 hypointense marrow replacement and associated right paraspinal soft tissue mass. Mild enhancement is noted within the large right paraspinal soft tissue mass on the axial postcontrast image (*B*) (*arrows*).

Other less common manifestations of extramedullary spinal myeloma are dural myelomatosis, leptomeningeal myelomatosis, and spinal parenchymal myeloma.[25–29] All are rare and typically occur with other concurrent extramedullary contiguous or noncontiguous disease in the head and/or spine.[25–29] These can affect the entire spine and nerve roots but are more common in the thoracic spine.[25–29] Dural myelomatosis can be either contiguous or noncontigous.[25–29] MRI can show enhancing dural thickening or nodularity (**Fig. 11**).[25–29] Leptomeningeal myelo-matosis is thought to be a result of hematogenous spread and is seen in less than 1% of cases.[25–29] Most commonly, it involves the cranial leptomeninges with or without spinal involvement.[25–29] Rarely, there is isolated spinal leptomeningeal disease. MRI will show linear or nodular leptomeningeal enhancement. Leptomeningeal disease can be confirmed with cerebrospinal fluid analysis and is usually treated with intra-thecal chemotherapy, although the prognosis is poor.[25–29] Spinal parenchymal myeloma is extremely rare and typically appears as focal lesions with T1 hypointense and variable T2 hyperintensity in relation to the cord but almost all enhance compared with the cord.[25–29]

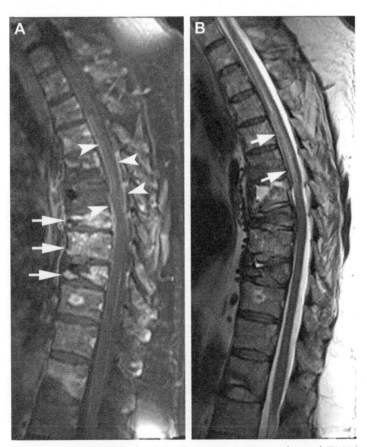

Fig. 11. Multiple myeloma with dural involvement. Contrast-enhanced T1W image (*A*) reveals diffuse dural enhancement (*arrowheads*) in a patient with multiple myeloma. Multiple enhancing vertebral lesions and compression fractures (*arrows*) are also noted. Sagittal T2W image (*B*) in the same patient shows long-segment cord T2 hyperintensity (*arrows*) suggesting cord edema.

Skull and Intracranial Myeloma

The skull is another frequent site of myeloma involvement (see **Table 1**). The appearance on CT and MRI is similar to that seen in the spine (**Fig. 12**).[25–27] Due to the frequency of skull-based myeloma, it is also the second most common site of contiguous extramedullary myeloma (**Fig. 13**).[25–27] Lesions are most commonly located in the anterior cranial fossa and/or skull base.[25–27] These lesions can extend and spread through the scalp, meninges, and even involve the parenchyma.[25–27] Contiguous extramedullary intracranial lesions look similar to those seen in the spine on MRI.[25–27] The dura is the most common involved intracranial structure and usually occurs by direct skull extension.[25–27]

Intracranial myeloma is the most common site of noncontiguous extramedullary myeloma.[25–27] This includes dural myelomatosis, leptomeningeal myelomatosis, and least commonly cerebral parenchymal myeloma (**Fig. 14**).[25–27] As described previously, leptomeningeal myelomatosis is thought to be hematogenously spread and more commonly involves the cranial leptomeninges than spinal leptomeninges.[25–29] Noncontiguous dural myelomatosis and cerebral parenchymal myeloma are also thought to be due to hematogenous seeding of the dura and cerebral parenchyma, respectively.[25–29]

Cranial Nerve Involvement

Cranial nerve involvement like parenchymal involvement can occur due to direct extension from dural or leptomeningeal myelomatosis[27–29] (see **Table 1**). Cranial nerve involvement can also occur due to direct seeding from hematogenous spread. Any of the cranial nerves can be affected, although the most commonly effected cranial nerve is the sixth (abducens) nerve.[27–29] Cranial nerve involvement most commonly occurs from skull base involvement with extension into the anterior or posterior cranial fossa and cavernous sinus (**Fig. 15**).[27–29]

Metabolic Complications in Myeloma

Renal insufficiency and hypercalcemia are common metabolic complications seen in myeloma[4–9] (see **Table 1**). Hypercalcemia does pose several neurologic complications, such as muscle weakness, stupor, or even coma; however, these do not

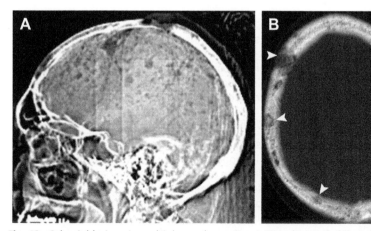

Fig. 12. Calvarial lesions in multiple myeloma. Scout CT radiograph (*A*) and axial CT image (*B*) reveal innumerable lytic lesions (*arrowheads*) of variable sizes involving the calvarium. Many of the lesions are intradiploic and many involve the inner or outer cortical table.

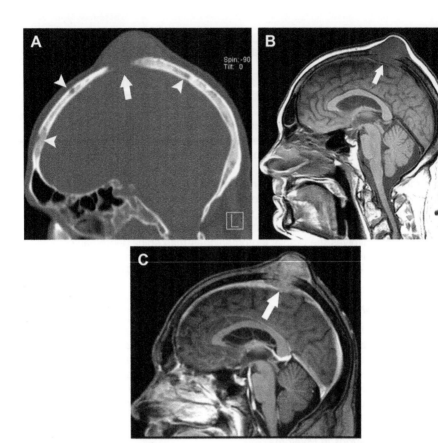

Fig. 13. Extramedullary myeloma. Sagittal CT image (*A*) shows a lytic lesion with large soft tissue component along the vertex (*arrow*). Multiple smaller lytic lesions are also noted (*arrowheads*). Sagittal precontrast (*B*) and postcontrast (*C*) images in the same patient better delineate the large enhancing transcalvarial soft tissue component (*arrows*) with intracranial and extracranial components.

manifest as specific imaging findings.[4–9] Renal insufficiency is important in imaging mainly in consideration of contrast-induced nephropathy with iodinated contrast used in CT and nephrogenic systemic fibrosis with gadolinium-based contrast used in MRI.[4–10,14,30] However, contrast is usually not needed and so can be withheld because it adds little information in most cases.[4–10,14,30]

Immunosuppression and Infectious Complications in Myeloma

Infection is the leading complication seen in myeloma, producing more morbidity and mortality than any other cause.[31,32] It is suggested to have caused approximately 50% of early mortality in myeloma.[31,32] Infections are the result of the patient's health and environment, immunosuppressive effects of myeloma itself, and immunosuppressive effects of the treatment (see **Table 1**). The type of therapy is important to know because certain therapies are associated with increased risk of certain infections.[4–9,31,32]

Most infections are bacterial pneumonia with *Streptococcus pneumoniae*, *Haemophilus influenzae*, and *Escherichia coli* the most common causative agents.[31,32]

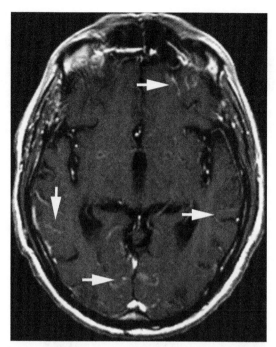

Fig. 14. Leptomeningeal myelomatosis. Axial postcontrast image reveals multiple areas of leptomeningeal enhancement (*arrows*) in a patient with multiple myeloma.

Infections with encapsulated bacteria, for example, *S pneumoniae*, are considered a characteristic infection of myeloma.[31,32]

Bacterial CNS infections can be due to direct seeding of the blood from vascular lines, in which *Staphylococcus aureus* is a common causative agent, or seeding from other infections, mainly respiratory, in which the 3 agents described previously are common.[31,32] CNS infections most commonly involve the meninges leading to meningitis. However, due to immunosuppression, contiguous or noncontiguous spread leading to cerebritis, cerebral abscess, and/or ventriculitis may often occur.[4–9,31,32]

Fungal infections due to immunosuppression include aspergillosis, cryptococcosis, mucormycosis, and candidiasis.[4–9,31,32] These can have distinct presentations but most commonly, like bacterial disease, cause meningitis.[4–9,31,32] They will also have contiguous or noncontiguous spread, causing cerebritis, cerebral abscesses, and/or ventriculitis.[4–10,14,31,32]

Herpes zoster is the most common viral agent, which usually affects the peripheral nerves; however, it may cause an encephalomyelitis and cranial nerve involvement.[4–10,14,31,32] Herpes simplex and cytomegalovirus (CMV) are common causes of CNS viral infections.[4–10,14,31,32] Herpes simplex encephalitis has a typical distribution involving the medial temporal lobes and inferolateral frontal lobes with sparring of the basal ganglia.[4–10,14,31,32] CMV typically causes a meningoencephalitis with periventricular parenchymal involvement with or without ventriculitis.[4–10,14,31,32]

Prophylaxis with pneumococcal vaccines, antibiotics, intravenous immunoglobulin, and antivirals are common practice to help prevent such complications.[4–10,14,31,32]

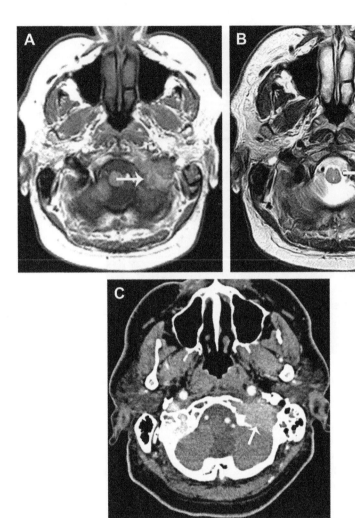

Fig. 15. Cranial nerve involvement in myeloma. Axial T1 (*A*) and T2W (*B*) images through the posterior fossa show a large lytic lesion with soft tissue component involving the left skull base with obliteration of the hypoglossal canal (*arrows*). CT in the same patient (*C*) better reveals the lytic bony changes along the left skull base (*arrow*).

Another uncommon neurologic presentation associated with immunosuppressives such as bortezomib and thalidomide-based therapies is posterior reversible encephalopathy syndrome (PRES). PRES is thought to represent an inability to autoregulate the posterior cerebral circulation. PRES is typically seen as bilateral confluent parietal-occipital lobe intensities with fluid-sensitive sequences on MRI.[10,14]

Hematologic Complications in Myeloma

Anemia, hyperviscosity, and less frequently thrombosis are hematologic complications seen in myeloma[4–9] (see **Table 1**). Anemia is important because rebound marrow stimulation from severe anemia can sometimes simulate diffuse marrow involvement by myeloma on MRI.[10,14] Hyperviscosity may have several neurologic symptoms such as blurred vision and neuropathy, although it typically has no neuroimaging findings.[4–9] Thrombosis can be a complication of the disease itself or of treatment such as thalidomide or lenalidomide-based regimens among others.[4–9] There is a much higher risk of venous thromboembolism than arterial thromboembolism.[4–9] Although uncommon, neuroimaging can demonstrate cerebral venous thrombosis (ie, dural venous sinus) or much less frequently cerebral arterial thromboembolism. Venous and arterial thromboembolisms have distinct imaging findings on MRI, including vessel with intraluminal clot, restricted diffusion territory, and hemorrhage in venous thromboembolism.[4–10,14]

SUMMARY

Multiple myeloma is the most common bone malignancy. Diagnosis of multiple myeloma is based on a combination of clinical findings, laboratory studies, bone marrow biopsy, and imaging findings. Imaging plays an important role in identifying the extent of the disease, disease process, guiding biopsies, and diagnosing associated spinal and intracranial complications. It also plays an important role in the staging, evaluating response to therapy, and monitoring for recurrence. Multiple myeloma and related PCPDs have a diverse set of clinicopathologic findings, which present unique and diverse findings on neuroimaging, not only from the disease itself but from complications of the disease and treatment-related complications. Familiarity with these findings is valuable for clinicians and radiologists alike.

REFERENCES

1. Jemal A, Siegel R, Ward E, et al. Cancer statistics. CA Cancer J Clin 2009;59(4): 225–49.
2. Kaya H, Peressini B, Jawed I, et al. Impact of age, race and decade of treatment on overall survival in a critical population analysis of 40,000 multiple myeloma patients. Int J Hematol 2012;95(1):64–70.
3. Kyle RA, Rajkumar SV. Epidemiology of the plasma cell disorders. Best Pract Res Clin Haematol 2007;20(4):637–64.
4. Palumbo A, Rajkumar SV, San Miguel JF, et al. International Myeloma Working Group consensus statement for the management, treatment, and supportive care of patients with myeloma not eligible for standard autologous stem-cell transplantation. J Clin Oncol 2014;32(6):587–600.
5. Rajkumar SV, Dimopoulos MA, Palumbo A, et al. International Myeloma Working Group updated criteria for the diagnosis of multiple myeloma. Lancet Oncol 2014;15(12):538–48.
6. Bird JM, Owen RG, D'Sa S, et al. Guidelines for the diagnosis and management of multiple myeloma 2011. Br J Haematol 2011;154(1):32–75.
7. Bird J, Behrens J, Westin J, et al. UK Myeloma Forum (UKMF) and Nordic Myeloma Study Group (NMSG): guidelines for the investigation of newly detected M-proteins and the management of monoclonal gammopathy of undetermined significance (MGUS). Br J Haematol 2009;147(1):22–42.
8. Kyle RA, Child JA, Anderson K, et al. Criteria for the classification of monoclonal gammopathies, multiple myeloma and related disorders: a report of the International Myeloma Working Group. Br J Haematol 2003;121(5):749–57.
9. Mikhael JR, Dingli D, Roy V, et al. Management of newly diagnosed symptomatic multiple myeloma: updated Mayo Stratification of Myeloma and Risk-Adapted Therapy (mSMART) consensus guidelines 2013. Mayo Clin Proc 2013;88(4): 360–76.

10. Hanrahan CJ, Carl RC, Julia RC. Current concepts in the evaluation of multiple myeloma with MR imaging and FDG PET/CT 1. Radiographics 2010;30(1):127–42.
11. De Larrea CF, Kyle RA, Durie BG, et al. Plasma cell leukemia: consensus statement on diagnostic requirements, response criteria and treatment recommendations by the International Myeloma Working Group. Leukemia 2013;27(4):780–91.
12. Durie BG. The role of anatomic and functional staging in myeloma: description of Durie/Salmon plus staging system. Eur J Cancer 2006;42(11):1539–43.
13. Kilciksiz S, Karakoyun-Celik O, Agaoglu FY, et al. A review for solitary plasmacytoma of bone and extramedullary plasmacytoma. ScientificWorldJournal 2012. http://dx.doi.org/10.1100/2012/895765.
14. Angtuaco EJ, Fassas AB, Walker R, et al. Multiple myeloma: clinical review and diagnostic imaging 1. Radiology 2004;231(1):11–23.
15. Ricci C, Cova M, Kang Y, et al. Normal age-related patterns of cellular and fatty bone marrow distribution in the axial skeleton: MR imaging study. Radiology 1990;177(1):83–8.
16. Dimopoulos M, Terpos E, Comenzo RL, et al. International myeloma working group consensus statement and guidelines regarding the current role of imaging techniques in the diagnosis and monitoring of multiple Myeloma. Leukemia 2009; 23:1545–56.
17. Hillengass J, Landgren O. Challenges and opportunities of novel imaging techniques in monoclonal plasma cell disorders: imaging "early myeloma". Leuk Lymphoma 2013;54(7):1355–63.
18. Regelink JC, Minnema MC, Terpos E, et al. Comparison of modern and conventional imaging techniques in establishing multiple myeloma-related bone disease: a systematic review. Br J Haematol 2013;162:50–61.
19. Dimopoulos MA, Hillengass J, Usmani S, et al. Role of magnetic resonance imaging in the management of patients with multiple myeloma: a consensus statement. J Clin Oncol 2015;33(6):657–64.
20. Shortt CP, Gleeson TG, Breen KA, et al. Whole-body MRI versus PET in assessment of multiple myeloma disease activity. AJR Am J Roentgenol 2009;192(4):980–6.
21. Vogel MN, Weise K, Maksimovic O, et al. Pathologic fractures in patients with multiple myeloma undergoing bisphosphonate therapy: incidence and correlation with course of disease. AJR Am J Roentgenol 2009;193(3):656–61.
22. Rades D, Hoskin PJ, Stalpers LJ, et al. Short-course radiotherapy is not optimal for spinal cord compression due to myeloma. Int J Radiat Oncol Biol Phys 2006; 64(5):1452–7.
23. Ravaglia S, Corso A, Piccolo G, et al. Immune-mediated neuropathies in myeloma patients treated with bortezomib. Clin Neurophysiol 2008;119(11):2507–12.
24. Facon T, Mary JY, Hulin C, et al. Melphalan and prednisone plus thalidomide versus melphalan and prednisone alone or reduced-intensity autologous stem cell transplantation in elderly patients with multiple myeloma (IFM 99–06): a randomised trial. Lancet 2007;370(9594):1209–18.
25. Tirumani SH, Shinagare AB, Jagannatha JP, et al. MRI features of extramedullary myeloma. AJR Am J Roentgenol 2014;202(4):803–10.
26. Shpilberg KA, Esses SJ, Fowkes ME, et al. Imaging of extraosseous intracranial and intraspinal multiple myeloma, including central nervous system involvement. Clin Imaging 2015;39(2):213–9.
27. Lasocki A, Gangatharan S, Gaillard F, et al. Intracranial involvement by multiple myeloma. Clin Radiol 2015;70(8):890–7.
28. Schluterman KO, Fassas AB, Van Hemert RL, et al. Multiple myeloma invasion of the central nervous system. Arch Neurol 2004;61(9):1423–9.

29. Chang H, Bartlett ES, Patterson B, et al. The absence of CD56 on malignant plasma cells in the cerebrospinal fluid is the hallmark of multiple myeloma involving central nervous system. Br J Haematol 2005;129(4):539–41.
30. Pahade JK, LeBedis CA, Raptopoulos VD, et al. Incidence of contrast-induced nephropathy in patients with multiple myeloma undergoing contrast-enhanced CT. AJR Am J Roentgenol 2011;196(5):1094–101.
31. Nucci M, Anaissie E. Infections in patients with multiple myeloma in the era of high-dose therapy and novel agents. Clin Infect Dis 2009;49(8):1211–25.
32. Teh BW, Harrison SJ, Worth LJ, et al. Risks, severity and timing of infections in patients with multiple myeloma: a longitudinal cohort study in the era of immuno-modulatory drug therapy. Br J Haematol 2015;171(1):100–8.

Venous Thrombosis
Causes and Imaging Appearance

Andrew Steven, MD[a],*, Prashant Raghavan, MD[a], Wilson Altmeyer, MD[b],
Dheeraj Gandhi, MD[a]

KEYWORDS

- Venous thrombosis • Dural sinus thrombosis • Dural venous sinus thrombosis
- Sinus thrombosis • Cortical vein thrombosis • MRV • Venography

KEY POINTS

- CVT can be an elusive clinical diagnosis because of the varied and nonspecific presenting symptoms. A high index of suspicion is required for clinicians and radiologists, especially for the detection of isolated cortical vein thrombosis.

- A noncontrast head computed tomography is fairly insensitive for the detection of cerebral vein thrombosis (CVT), and a normal study does not exclude the diagnosis. Additional imaging is warranted when CVT is suspected.

- MRI/magnetic resonance venography is an excellent, noninvasive technique for diagnosing CVT. Newer sequences, including susceptibility-weighted imaging and postcontrast 3-dimensional gradient echo T1, allow for improved diagnostic sensitivity and specificity compared with traditional protocols.

- Most patients recover with medical management. Endovascular thrombectomy should be considered for patients with contraindication to heparin, with high morbidity/mortality risk factors, and those who progress despite conservative therapy.

INTRODUCTION

Thrombosis of intracranial veins and the dural venous sinus system has long been a diagnostic dilemma because of its protean, nonspecific clinical manifestations and subtle appearance on traditional imaging modalities. However, this complex condition has become increasingly recognized in recent years, particularly with the advance of MRI.

It is estimated that the annual incidence of CVT is between 2 and 7 cases per million people and that a typical tertiary-care center will see between 5 and 8 cases of CVT per year.[1] These numbers are likely underestimated as sensitivity for detection of this disease has improved significantly in recent years. The disease affects a wide

Disclosures: The authors have nothing to disclose.
[a] Department of Diagnostic Radiology, University of Maryland Medical System, 22 South Green Street, Baltimore, MD 21201, USA; [b] Department of Radiology, University of Texas Health Science Center at San Antonio, 7703 Floyd Curl Drive, San Antonio, TX 78229-3900, USA
* Corresponding author.
E-mail address: asteven@umm.edu

hemonc.theclinics.com

age group from newborn through elderly. Although there is no specific age demographic, it is well established that CVT preferentially affects women (by a ratio of approximately 3 to 1).

The exact cascade of events that result in CVT is not entirely understood, but predisposing conditions may include an underlying hypercoagulable state, mechanical obstruction, venous stasis, or some combination thereof. There are a wide variety of known risk factors, and most patients with CVT will have one or more. Intrinsic and acquired coagulopathies seem to be the most important factor, associated with up to 70% of cases.[2]

Cancer is an important cause of venous thromboembolism and accounts for approximately 20% of all cases of this entity. Venous thrombosis is the second leading cause of death in patients with cancer. Thrombotic events in patients with cancer usually manifest as extremity deep venous thrombosis or pulmonary embolism but can also occur in the cerebral circulation.[3–6]

The most common cancers associated with venous thrombosis involve the prostate, colon, lung, and brain in men and the breast, lung, and ovary in women.[6] Importantly, idiopathic thromboembolic disease may be a predictor of the presence of occult malignancy; cancers in such patients are associated with an advanced stage and a poor prognosis.[3,7]

The cause of venous thrombosis in malignancy is complex and incompletely understood. It is now thought that almost all types of tumor cells are capable of activating the clotting pathway, causing thrombosis by their ability to produce and release procoagulant substances and inflammatory cytokines and through their interaction with leucocytes, endothelial, and platelet host cells. In cancer, there seems to be a shift to a prothrombotic state, achieved by disruption of the fine balance between the coagulation and fibrinolytic systems that normally exist. This shift may occur either as a result of an excess of procoagulant proteins (s tissue factor, fibrinogen, and plasminogen activator inhibitor) or as a consequence of deficiency in other molecules (antithrombin III, proteins C and S, and tissue plasminogen activator).[8] In addition, venous thrombosis may also occur as a consequence of chemotherapy, as is well known with L-asparaginase in patients with acute lymphoblastic leukemia[9] and possibly with agents such as cisplatin, etoposide, medroxyprogesterone acetate, and tamoxifen. Also, factors such as surgery and postoperative immobility and placement of venous catheters play an important role in the predisposition to thrombosis.

Unlike deep vein thrombosis seen in the upper or lower extremities, external compression is typically not an issue for the cerebral venous sinus system. However, mechanical obstruction may occur from intracranial masses, such as a meningioma or focal disruption/distortion of the sinus as seen in a temporal bone fracture.

Venous stasis is another potential contributing factor in the development of CVT. Dehydration, hypovolemia, and intracranial hypotension are associated with thrombosis. The veins and dural sinuses distend in this setting as a compensatory reaction to decreased cerebrospinal fluid (CSF).[10] This distention and associated delayed venous transit time may promote thrombus formation.

Alteration or obstruction of normal venous drainage from CVT results in increased venous and capillary blood pressure, which in turn can disrupt the blood-brain barrier. Depending on the severity and duration of this disruption, CVT can cause vasogenic edema, cytotoxic edema (venous infarction), and/or hemorrhage. The acuity of the venous thrombosis also seems to play a significant role in the development of edema and hemorrhage, likely related to the development of venous collateral system. For example, dural sinuses that become occluded over the course of months to years from slow-growing meningiomas rarely induce brain parenchymal injury, whereas those ligated during surgery commonly do.

In addition to localized venous hypertension, dural sinus thrombosis may result in elevated intracranial pressure. The choroid plexus produces CSF at a rate of approximately 500 mL/d, and resorption is thought to occur at the level of the dural venous sinuses through arachnoid granulations and arachnoid villi. Disruption of this homeostasis from thrombosis may result in hydrocephalus and increased intracranial pressure; symptoms and outcomes from CVT vary widely.[11]

Patients will most commonly present complaining of a headache. This headache may be seen in isolation or with additional symptoms of intracranial hypertension, such as vomiting and visual disturbance. The features of the headache are not specific and may mimic other headache syndromes, such as migraine or subarachnoid hemorrhage. Headaches may be gradual in onset or acute, localized, or diffuse.

In addition to headaches, patients may develop focal neurologic deficits from vasogenic or cytotoxic edema. Motor and sensory deficits are the most commonly described, but verbal and visual defects also occur. As with most diseases affecting the brain, symptomatology is determined by the specific site and extent of involvement. Many neurologic deficits resolve with treatment; however, those patients who experience infarction or hemorrhage may never recover. CVT may cause focal or generalized seizures. Profound cases of CVT can cause encephalopathic symptoms, including disturbances of consciousness, cognitive dysfunction, and even coma.

CVT places patients at risk for the later development of dural arteriovenous fistulas.[12] The exact mechanism for which is not entirely understood, but localized venous hypertension may result in enlargement of physiologic arteriovenous shunts or promote neoangiogenesis. The development of these abnormal shunts between dural arteries and venous sinuses can lead to delayed complications from venous hypertension.

PREIMAGING PLANNING

An understanding of venous anatomy is necessary for accurate image interpretation.[13] The supratentorial venous system is traditionally divided into superficial and deep drainage. The deep venous system drains deep gray and white matter structures in a centripetal fashion collecting in the paired internal cerebral veins and basal veins of Rosenthal, which lead to the vein of Galen and straight sinus. The superficial cerebral veins drain the cortex and subcortical white matter in a centrifugal fashion, collecting in the dural venous sinuses (superior sagittal sinus, transverse sinuses). (**Fig. 1**) Infratentorial veins may drain into the vein of Galen, the petrosal sinuses, or the dural venous sinuses. The superficial and deep venous systems coalesce at the torcula herophili, which is formed at confluence of the superior sagittal sinus, straight sinus, and transverse sinuses. Extracranial drainage is through the internal jugular veins via the sigmoid sinuses (see **Fig. 1**).

Venous anatomy is highly variable. Superficial cortical veins vary in size and number among patients and are asymmetric, complicating imaging interpretation. Because of the expected variation from one side to another and between patients, absent signal from a thrombosed vessel can easily be overlooked. One of the most commonly confusing anatomic variations is the difference in the size of the transverse sinuses, occurring in almost 50% of people. In 20% of cases, the smaller sinus (typically left sided) is atretic or absent[14] (**Fig. 2**). This anatomic variation may lead to a false-positive result for inexperienced readers who assume absent enhancement equals thrombosis.

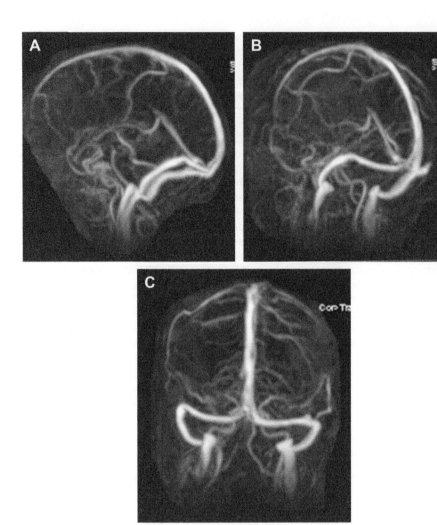

Fig. 1. Rotating maximum-intensity-projection images (*A–C*) from a magnetic resonance venogram demonstrating normal venous anatomy.

Developmental venous anomalies (DVAs) are the most commonly occurring vascular malformations. These variations occur as a primary dysplasia of normal venous drainage, which results in a radiating collection of small medullary veins that converge on a solitary transcerebral vein[15] (**Fig. 3**). Although thought to be benign entities composed of mature vascular elements, numerous cases of isolated DVA thrombosis with or without infarction and hemorrhage have been reported. Many investigators think that these structures have abnormal elevated venous pressures and associated vascular stasis.

DIAGNOSTIC IMAGING TECHNIQUE AND INTERPRETATION/ASSESSMENT OF CLINICAL IMAGES

Imaging protocol for patients with suspected CVT typically requires evaluation of the brain parenchyma as well as the intracranial vasculature.

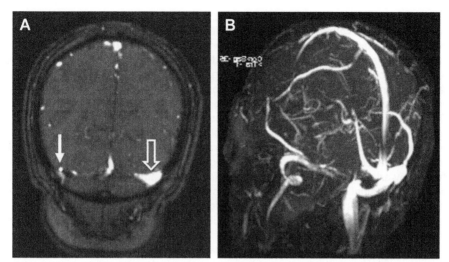

Fig. 2. Coronal source image from a 2-dimensional time-of-flight magnetic resonance venogram in a patient without sinus thrombosis (*A*) shows a dominant left transverse sinus (*open arrow*) that is significantly larger than the right (*arrow*). A 3-dimensional maximum-intensity-projection image (*B*) confirms the developmental asymmetry.

Computed Tomography

A noncontrast head computed tomography (CT) often serves as the initial imaging modality for most cases of CVT, as it is fast, widely available, and helpful at excluding other acute intracranial processes, such as hemorrhage, infarct, and space-occupying lesions. Unfortunately, a noncontrast head CT is relatively insensitive for CVT as findings may be subtle or nonexistent.

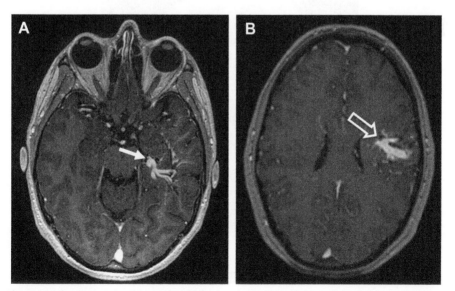

Fig. 3. Axial postcontrast T1-weighted MRI (*A, B*) demonstrating sizable DVAs in 2 different patients. Patient in (*A*) has a large left temporal DVA (*arrow*). The DVA in (*B*) drains the opercular left frontal lobe (*open arrow*).

The most direct and reliable finding of CVT is increased attenuation (usually >70 HU) within the thrombosed vessel. When viewed perpendicular to the plane of imaging, as is the case for portions of the superior sagittal sinus on most routine axial images, this creates a "dense triangle sign"[16] (**Fig. 4**). Cortical vein thrombosis manifests as curvilinear high attenuation structures overlying the cerebral convexities, referred to as a "cord sign" (**Fig. 5**). In addition to the increased attenuation, an acutely thrombosed sinus will tend to be distended. The typically concave margins of the sinus (when viewed in plane) will appear convex when the sinus is expanded by thrombosis. Venous structures are slightly increased in attenuation relative to the brain parenchyma (assuming a normal hematocrit level), should be uniform throughout, and identical in attenuation to the nearby arteries. Any asymmetry or focal increase in attenuation among the dural sinuses or cortical veins should raise suspicion for CVT. Acute thrombi are hyperattenuating compared with flowing blood (**Fig. 6**). However, they decrease in attenuation with age making identification of subacute or chronic thrombi difficult or impossible without contrast.

Indirect signs may include vasogenic edema, cytotoxic edema, or intracranial hemorrhage.[17,18] Naturally the location of brain edema and infarction will correspond with the site of venous thrombosis (**Fig. 7**). Frontal, parietal, and occipital lesions suggest superior sagittal sinus or cortical vein thrombosis, especially when bilateral. Temporal lobe lesions may implicate the vein of Labbé, transverse sinus, or sigmoid sinus. Deep parenchymal lesions, classically bilateral thalamic edema, hemorrhage, or infarction, correspond to the deep cerebral veins. A good rule of thumb is that infarction or hemorrhage in a nonarterial distribution should raise suspicion for CVT and warrant vascular imaging.

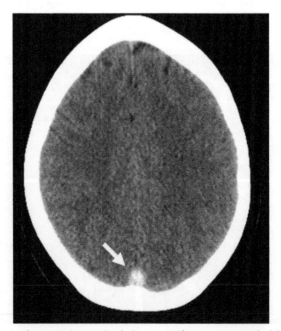

Fig. 4. Thrombus in the superior sagittal sinus manifests as a rounded hyperattenuating focus when viewed in cross section on this noncontrast CT examination (*arrow*). This focus is the classic dense triangle sign of dural sinus thrombosis.

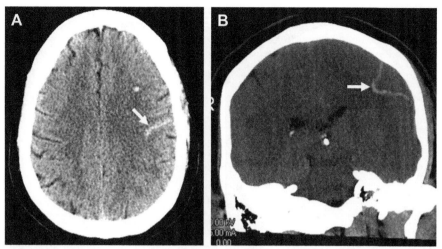

Fig. 5. (A) Axial noncontrast CT image exhibits a curvilinear hyperattenuating focus in a left frontal sulcus (*arrow*) corresponding to a thrombosed cortical vein, consistent with a cord sign. (B) The value of a multiplanar reconstruction, in this case an oblique coronal, to confirm the lesion is indeed vascular in cause (*arrow*).

Intracranial hemorrhage may be intraparenchymal or subarachnoid in location and should be near the site of thrombosis. Intraparenchymal hemorrhage tends to be cortical or subcortical in nature, and both petechial hemorrhage and/or frank hematomas may occur. These foci tend to have more surrounding edema than other common hemorrhagic lesions (eg, hypertensive hemorrhage, cerebral amyloid angiopathy).

CT Venography

CT angiography requires a large bolus of iodinated contrast administered intravenously to allow for opacification of the vessels.[19,20] The more commonly performed

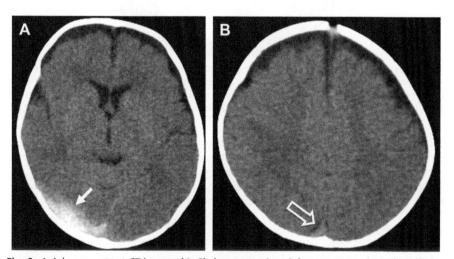

Fig. 6. Axial noncontrast CT images (A, B) demonstrating right transverse sinus thrombosis. Note the relative increase in attenuation of the thrombosed sinus (*arrow*) in (A) compared with the normal superior sagittal sinus (*open arrow*) in (B).

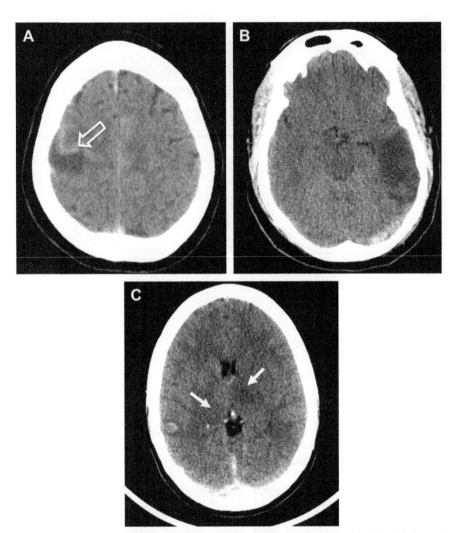

Fig. 7. Three patterns of edema in CVT on axial noncontrast CT images. (*A*) High right parietal edema (*open arrow*) and adjacent subarachnoid hemorrhage in a patient with superior sagittal sinus thrombosis. (*B*) Left temporal lobe in a patient with transverse sinus thrombosis. (*C*) Bilateral thalamic edema (*arrows*) in a patient with thrombus in the straight sinus.

CT arteriography involves a short delay between the intravenous bolus injection and image acquisition to allow time for the contrast to pass from the systemic veins through the pulmonary circulatory system into the systemic arteries. CT venography (CTV) is performed with a slightly longer delay to allow for preferential enhancement of the venous system and is the preferred study for the diagnosis of CVT. CTV has a reported sensitivity approaching 95%, much higher than a noncontrast examination[21] (**Fig. 8**).

Contrast opacification of the dural sinuses should result in a nonenhancing filling defect referred to as the "Empty Delta Sign."[22] Enhancement surrounding the thrombus may reflect intraluminal contrast in the setting of a partially occlusive thrombus, dural enhancement from localized venous congestion, or small collateral vessels.

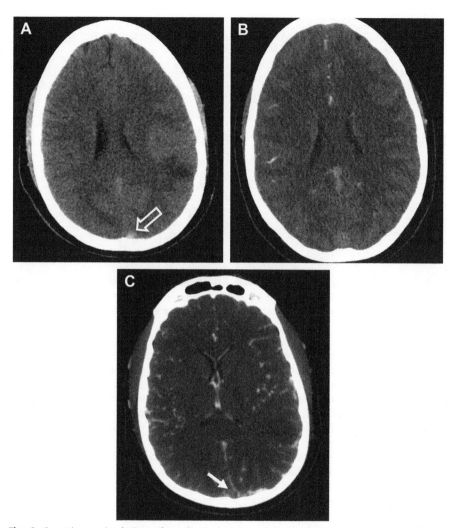

Fig. 8. Superior sagittal sinus thrombosis (*open arrow*) is subtle on noncontrast CT (*A*). Thrombus is inconspicuous on the CT arteriogram (*B*) as it is essentially isodense to the poorly opacified veins. The finding is more readily apparent on CT venogram (*C*) as a filling defect or empty delta sign (*arrow*).

Not all filling defects in the dural sinuses represent thrombus. Arachnoid granulations, small brain herniations, and fat may all present as focal areas of nonenhancement.[13,23] Reliable differentiation from CVT can be made based on the size, morphology, distribution, and imaging characteristics of these lesions. Arachnoid granulation defects tend to be round, focal, and well defined as opposed to linear thrombi. They also tend to occur in predictable locations (most commonly the lateral transverse sinuses)[13] and should be identical to CSF in CT attenuation and magnetic resonance (MR) signal (**Fig. 9**).

Modern CT techniques, using helical multidetector systems, allow isotropic volume acquisition that can be reconstructed in any orthogonal plane without sacrificing imaging quality. Reviewing examinations in the coronal or sagittal plane may

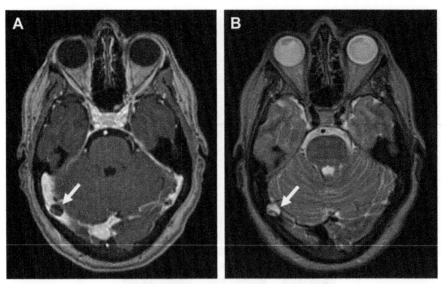

Fig. 9. Axial T1-weighted postcontrast (*A*) and T2-weighted (*B*) MRI of an arachnoid granulation (*arrows*). The rounded filling defect in the right transverse sinus follows CSF signal on all pulse sequences.

be helpful for confirming or excluding suspected findings found on the traditional axial display. This information is particularly helpful for assessing the transverse sinuses as they are oriented parallel to the plane of imaging on axial images and may suffer from volume averaging artifact. Thin-section imaging with 1-mm thick slices or less is possible on most modern scanners and can be very helpful in the evaluation of small sinuses and cortical veins, which may only measure 2 or 3 mm maximally.

Appropriate windowing is essential to distinguish between contrast-opacified venous structures and the adjacent high-attenuation calvarium. Multiplanar reformats are typically used over maximum-intensity projections and help avoid confounding artifacts from the adjacent bone.[21] Both 2-dimensional (2D) and 3-dimensional (3D) reconstruction techniques are available, and many modern postprocessing formats allow for automated or semiautomated bone removal to facilitate 3D volume rendering of the superficial venous system.[19]

MRI

The advent of MRI as a routine imaging modality has aided greatly in the diagnosis of CVT. Traditional T1- and T2-weighted sequences may be all that is required to alert a reader to the presence of CVT. On spin-echo techniques, flowing blood should create a low-signal-intensity flow void. The presence of altered signal intensity with loss of this expected flow void is highly suspicious for thrombus (**Fig. 10**). Unfortunately, slow-flowing blood can also cause loss of the expected flow void, so the finding is not entirely specific.

Thrombi can demonstrate a wide variety of signal intensities on T1- and T2-weighted sequences depending on the time of imaging from the age of the thrombus due to evolution and breakdown of the hemoglobin molecule. Of note, subacute blood products are typically T1 hyperintense, which can be a striking finding on a noncontrast study or a potential pitfall on postcontrast imaging. Acute thrombi may

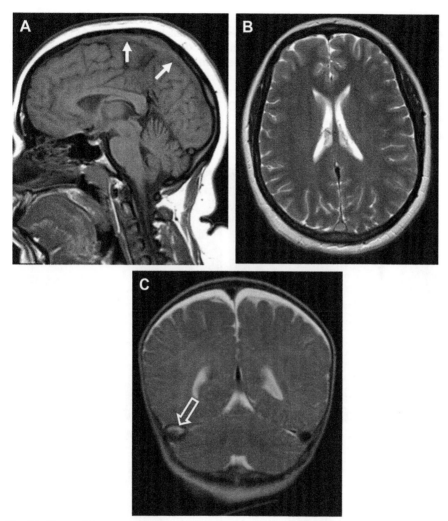

Fig. 10. Three different patients exhibiting loss of the normal flow void indicating dural sinus thrombosis. Sagittal T1-weighted image (*A*) demonstrates the intermediate signal intensity of an acute thrombus within the superior sagittal sinus (*arrows*). Axial T2-weighted image (*B*) shows increased signal in an expanded superior sagittal sinus. Coronal T2-weighted image (*C*) shows mixed signal intensity (*open arrow*) in the thrombosed right transverse sinus. Compare that with the dark flow void in the normal left transverse and superior sagittal sinuses.

be T2 hypointense, mimicking a flow void and creating a false-negative study. Because these findings are not entirely specific or sensitive, additional confirmatory sequences are helpful.

Gradient echo T2*-weighted sequences aid in the diagnostic sensitivity of MRI and are routinely performed in brain imaging protocols at most imaging centers. These techniques identify areas of hemorrhage or calcification as they induce localized alterations in the magnetic field. Paramagnetic substances such as those found in blood products (deoxyhemoglobin and methemoglobin) manifest as a large areas of signal void or blooming artifact. The more recently developed susceptibility-weighted imaging (SWI) sequence is another heme-sensitive sequence that has been shown to further increase sensitivity for the detection of hemorrhage and blood products compared with traditional T2* sequences. This sequence has been shown to be particularly useful in the acute phase of CVT and for identifying isolated cortical vein thrombosis (**Fig. 11**).[24]

Secondary signs of CVT, including cerebral edema, infarction, and hemorrhage, should all be more readily apparent on MRI than CT (**Fig. 12**). Vasogenic and cytotoxic edema should present as regional areas of increased signal on T2-weighted and fluid-attenuation inversion recovery (FLAIR) sequences. Associated lesions on

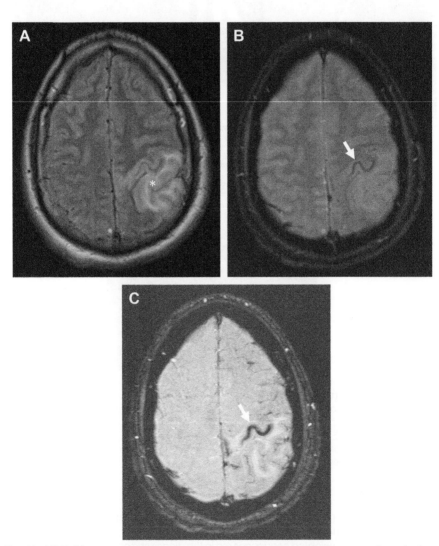

Fig. 11. (A) Fluid-attenuation inversion recovery image demonstrating parenchymal edema and subarachnoid hemorrhage centered in the left parietal lobe (*asterisk*). T2* gradient recalled echo (B) and SWI (C) images at the same level exhibit curvilinear focus of susceptibility corresponding to a thrombosed cortical vein (*arrows*). Note the increased conspicuity of the vessel and adjacent petechial hemorrhage on SWI.

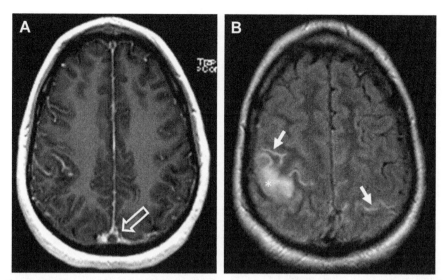

Fig. 12. Edema and hemorrhage associated with superior sagittal sinus thrombosis. Axial T1-weighted postcontrast image (*A*) demonstrates a thrombosis in the superior sagittal sinus (*open arrow*). Corresponding fluid-attenuation inversion recovery image (*B*) shows right parietal edema (*asterisk*). High signal is the cerebral sulci bilaterally (*arrows*), which reflects subarachnoid hemorrhage.

diffusion-weighted imaging (DWI) may indicate ischemia or irreversible infarction (**Fig. 13**). DWI may also help identify thrombi in the dural venous sinuses or cortical veins. Hematomas may restrict diffusion as reflected by high signal on DWI images, which is easily identifiable as flowing blood in vascular structures should result in no signal (**Fig. 14**).

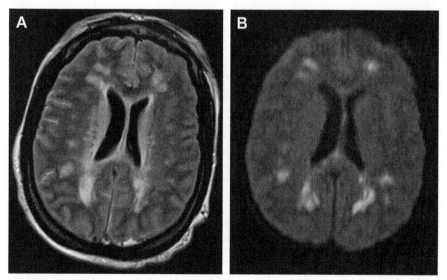

Fig. 13. Axial FLAIR image (*A*) in an encephalopathic patient with extensive dural sinus thrombosis. Increased signal surrounding the dilated ventricles is consistent with edema. Corresponding DWI image (*B*) shows patchy foci of diffusion restriction that may indicate irreversible infarction.

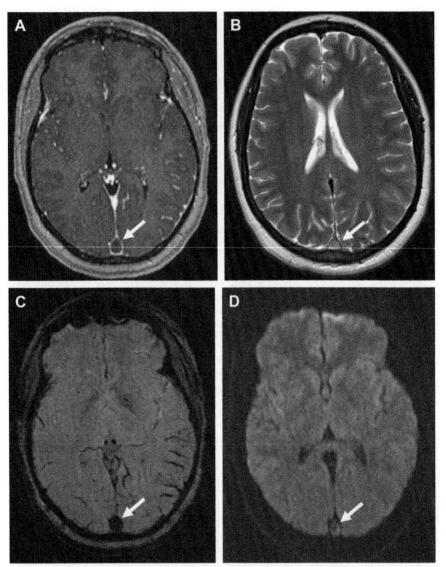

Fig. 14. Superior sagittal sinus thrombosis (*arrows*) manifesting as an empty delta sign on a T1-weighted image (*A*), loss of the normal flow void on a T2-weighted image (*B*), blooming artifact on SWI (*C*), and increased signal on DWI (*D*).

Magnetic Resonance Venography

There are a variety of MR venography (MRV) techniques available, but the most commonly used in clinical practice is a noncontrast time-of-flight (TOF) MRV. This sequence visualizes protons that move into a slice in a specified direction, creating a so-called flow-related signal. Two-dimensional source images are typically combined to create a 3D maximum-intensity reconstruction of the entire venous system, which can be reviewed in multiple projections. Thrombosis will manifest as loss of flow-related signal or complete absence of a vessel.[25] It is important to note that this sequence works well for vessels oriented perpendicular to the plane of imaging, but saturation artifact results in decreased signal in blood flowing parallel to the plane of imaging. Some centers perform imaging in 2 or 3 different complimentary planes (ie, coronal and sagittal) to account for this known pitfall.

Reviewing the source images from the MRV in conjunction with brain MRI is essential for accurate diagnosis. Because these sequences are T1-weighted, high signal from a subacute hematoma may mimic flow-related enhancement resulting in a false-negative interpretation. A developmentally atretic or absent transverse sinus can result in a false-positive interpretation.

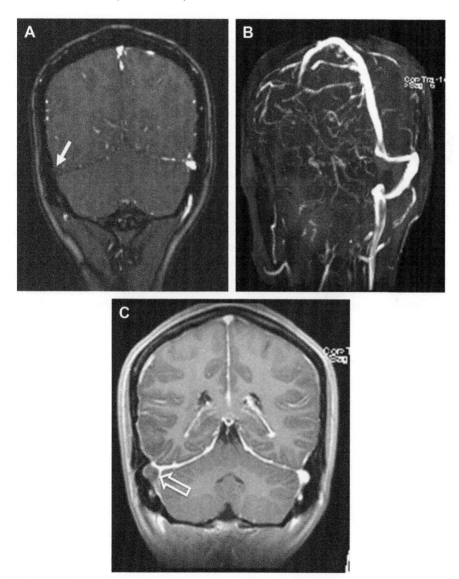

Fig. 15. A 2D source image in the coronal plane (*A*) and a 3D maximum-intensity-projection reconstruction (*B*) from a time of MRV demonstrating absent flow-related signal in the right transverse sinus (*arrow*). A coronal reconstruction of a postcontrast T1-weighted image (*C*) offers direct visualization of the corresponding thrombus (*open arrow*).

A thin-section postcontrast gradient echo T1-weighted sequence (ie, T1 MP-RAGE [magnetization prepared rapid acquisition gradient echo]) has proven well suited for the evaluation of the dural sinuses.[26,27] The rapid echo time eliminates the flow void found on traditional spin-echo sequences. Although technically not considered a venogram, this sequence allows for excellent spatial resolution and contrast between the dural sinuses and adjacent structures and isotropic acquisition allows for reconstruction of the image in any plane. Several studies suggest greater performance than TOF MRV or digitally subtracted angiographic (DSA) for the diagnosis of CVT (**Fig. 15**).

Digitally Subtracted Angiographic

Catheter-based angiography with DSA images is the traditional gold standard for evaluation of the intracranial vasculature. The techniques require percutaneous arterial access, with advancement of a small catheter to the vessel of interest. This technique offers several major advantages, including a dynamic assessment of cerebral blood flow in arterial, capillary, and venous phases as well as high spatial resolution compared with CT or MRI. Filling defects within a sinus or failure of the sinus to appear are the most direct angiographic findings on DSA. Secondary findings may include venous congestion, enlarged collateral veins, or reversal of normal venous flow (**Fig. 16**).[28]

Venography can also be performed through a catheter-placed dural venous system via percutaneous access of the common femoral vein or internal jugular vein. This technique offers a direct visualization of the venous system and the additional benefit of direct venous pressure measurements.

Despite their advantages, DSA (arteriography and venography) are rarely performed as a primary means of investigation because of the risks associated with the invasive nature of the technique and the insensitivity for assessment of associated parenchymal lesions.[29] DSA can be performed for confirmatory purposes on equivocal cases, to assess the degree of collateral vessel formation, identify or exclude associated arteriovenous shunting, and when an endovascular intervention is being considered.

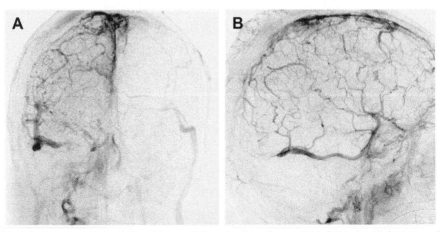

Fig. 16. Anteroposterior (*A*) and lateral (*B*) projections from a DSA following right internal carotid artery injection demonstrating occlusion of the right transverse sinus and distal superior sagittal sinus. There are prominent collateral veins with drainage through alternate venous pathways.

OPTIONS/PATHWAYS FOR SURGICAL INTERVENTION

Although most patients with CVT are left with minimal or no deficits, approximately 15% become severely disabled and the mortality rate approaches 10%. Risk factors associated with poor outcomes include male sex, increased age, coma or alteration in mental status, and the presence of intracranial hemorrhage.

Treatment remains controversial because of the unforeseeable evolution and general lack of data regarding outcomes. Early intervention with medical management is recommended in virtually all cases.[29,30] Treatment should include hydration, anticoagulation with heparin, and intracranial pressure monitoring. Stable or improved patients may go on to continued oral anticoagulation for months or indefinitely depending on the detection of an underlying cause or hypercoagulable condition.

Repeat imaging is recommended in patients with neurologic deterioration despite appropriate medical treatment. Patients with intracranial hemorrhage or severe mass effect may benefit from a decompressive craniectomy. Placement of an

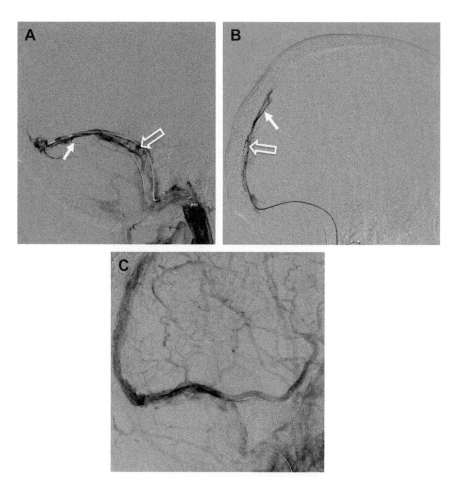

Fig. 17. Right anterior oblique views from a DSA during thrombectomy. Note the microcatheter (*arrow*) in the transverse sinus in (*A*) and in the superior sagittal sinus in (*B*). Direct injection of the sinus exhibits numerous filling defects (*open arrow*) and decreased caliber of these vessels. There is improved opacification of these sinuses following thrombectomy and thrombolysis (*C*).

intraventricular drainage catheter or monitoring device can be useful in managing intracranial pressure. Endovascular treatment with mechanical thrombectomy or localized fibrinolytic therapy is reserved for symptomatic patients unresponsive to medical therapy and those with high mortality risk (seizure, encephalopathy, coma) **(Fig. 17)**.[31]

SUMMARY

CVT is an elusive but increasingly recognized disorder that may incur serious neurologic complications. Most affected patients will have at least one known risk factor, including cancer or other prothrombotic state. Both CT and MRI are excellent noninvasive diagnostic studies that can identify the extent and severity of clot burden as well as associated parenchymal injury, such as edema, infarction, or hemorrhage. Prompt diagnosis and appropriate medical management are sufficient treatments for most patients, with endovascular therapy reserved for refractory and high-risk cases.

ACKNOWLEDGMENTS

Special thanks to Brigitte Pocta, MLA for assistance in the preparation of this article.

REFERENCES

1. Masuhr F, Mehraein S, Einhaupl K. Cerebral venous and sinus thrombosis. J Neurol 2004;251(1):11–23.
2. Poon CS, Chang J-K, Swarnkar A, et al. Radiologic diagnosis of cerebral venous thrombosis: pictorial review. AJR Am J Roentgenol 2007;189(Suppl 6):S64–75.
3. Lip GYH, Chin BSP, Blann AD. Cancer and the prothrombotic state. Lancet Oncol 2002;3(1):27–34.
4. Hickey WF, Garnick MB, Henderson IC, et al. Primary cerebral venous thrombosis in patients with cancer–a rarely diagnosed paraneoplastic syndrome. Report of three cases and review of the literature. Am J Med 1982;73(5): 740–50.
5. Liu PG, Jacobs JB, Reede D. Trousseau's syndrome in the head and neck. Am J Otolaryngol 1985;6(5):405–8.
6. Lee AYY, Levine MN. Venous thromboembolism and cancer: risks and outcomes. Circulation 2003;107(23 Suppl 1):I17–21.
7. Sorensen HT, Mellemkjaer L, Olsen JH, et al. Prognosis of cancers associated with venous thromboembolism. N Engl J Med 2000;343(25):1846–50.
8. De Cicco M. The prothrombotic state in cancer: pathogenic mechanisms. Crit Rev Oncol Hematol 2004;50(3):187–96.
9. Priest JR, Ramsay NK, Steinherz PG, et al. A syndrome of thrombosis and hemorrhage complicating L-asparaginase therapy for childhood acute lymphoblastic leukemia. J Pediatr 1982;100(6):984–99.
10. Farb RI, Forghani R, Lee SK, et al. The venous distension sign: a diagnostic sign of intracranial hypotension at MR imaging of the brain. AJNR Am J Neuroradiol 2007;28(8):1489–93.
11. Ferro JM, Canhao P, Stam J, et al. Prognosis of cerebral vein and dural sinus thrombosis: results of the international study on cerebral vein and dural sinus thrombosis (ISCVT). Stroke 2004;35(3):664–70.
12. Gandhi D, Chen J, Pearl M, et al. Intracranial dural arteriovenous fistulas: classification, imaging findings, and treatment. AJNR Am J Neuroradiol 2012;33(6): 1007–13.

13. Leach JL, Fortuna RB, Jones BV, et al. Imaging of cerebral venous thrombosis: current techniques, spectrum of findings, and diagnostic pitfalls. Radiographics 2006;26(Suppl 1):S19–41 [discussion: S42–3].

14. Zouaoui A, Hidden G. Cerebral venous sinuses: anatomical variants or thrombosis? Acta Anat (Basel) 1988;133(4):318–24.

15. Lee C, Pennington MA, Kenney CM 3rd. MR evaluation of developmental venous anomalies: medullary venous anatomy of venous angiomas. AJNR Am J Neuroradiol 1996;17(1):61–70.

16. Garetier M, Rousset J, Pearson E, et al. Value of spontaneous hyperdensity of cerebral venous thrombosis on helical CT. Acta Radiol 2014;55(10):1245–52.

17. Anderson B, Sabat S, Agarwal A, et al. Diffuse subarachnoid hemorrhage secondary to cerebral venous sinus thrombosis. Pol J Radiol 2015;80:286–9.

18. Boukobza M, Crassard I, Bousser M-G, et al. Radiological findings in cerebral venous thrombosis presenting as subarachnoid hemorrhage: a series of 22 cases. Neuroradiology 2016;58(1):11–6.

19. Rodallec MH, Krainik A, Feydy A, et al. Cerebral venous thrombosis and multidetector CT angiography: tips and tricks. Radiographics 2006;26(Suppl 1):S5–18 [discussion: S42–3].

20. Khandelwal N, Agarwal A, Kochhar R, et al. Comparison of CT venography with MR venography in cerebral sinovenous thrombosis. AJR Am J Roentgenol 2006; 187(6):1637–43.

21. Wetzel SG, Kirsch E, Stock KW, et al. Cerebral veins: comparative study of CT venography with intraarterial digital subtraction angiography. AJNR Am J Neuroradiol 1999;20(2):249–55.

22. Lee EJY. The empty delta sign. Radiology 2002;224(3):788–9.

23. Battal B, Castillo M. Brain herniations into the dural venous sinuses or calvarium: MRI of a recently recognized entity. Neuroradiol J 2014;27(1):55–62.

24. Idbaih A, Boukobza M, Crassard I, et al. MRI of clot in cerebral venous thrombosis: high diagnostic value of susceptibility-weighted images. Stroke 2006; 37(4):991–5.

25. Ayanzen RH, Bird CR, Keller PJ, et al. Cerebral MR venography: normal anatomy and potential diagnostic pitfalls. AJNR Am J Neuroradiol 2000;21(1):74–8.

26. Sari S, Verim S, Hamcan S, et al. MRI diagnosis of dural sinus - cortical venous thrombosis: immediate post-contrast 3D GRE T1-weighted imaging versus unenhanced MR venography and conventional MR sequences. Clin Neurol Neurosurg 2015;134:44–54.

27. Liang L, Korogi Y, Sugahara T, et al. Evaluation of the intracranial dural sinuses with a 3D contrast-enhanced MP-RAGE sequence: prospective comparison with 2D-TOF MR venography and digital subtraction angiography. AJNR Am J Neuroradiol 2001r;22(3):481–92.

28. Saposnik G, Barinagarrementeria F, Brown RDJ, et al. Diagnosis and management of cerebral venous thrombosis: a statement for healthcare professionals from the American Heart Association/American Stroke Association. Stroke 2011;42(4):1158–92.

29. Heiserman JE, Dean BL, Hodak JA, et al. Neurologic complications of cerebral angiography. AJNR Am J Neuroradiol 1994;15(8):1401–7 [discussion: 1408–11].

30. Schwarz S, Daffertshofer M, Schwarz T, et al. Current controversies in the diagnosis and management of cerebral venous and dural sinus thrombosis. Nervenarzt 2003;74(8):639–53 [in German].

31. Tsai FY, Kostanian V, Rivera M, et al. Cerebral venous congestion as indication for thrombolytic treatment. Cardiovasc Intervent Radiol 2007;30(4):675–87.

Central Nervous System Complications of Hematopoietic Stem Cell Transplant

Faiz I. Syed, MD, MS[a], Daniel R. Couriel, MD, MS[b],
David Frame, PharmD[c], Ashok Srinivasan, MBBS, MD[d],*

KEYWORDS

- Stem cell transplant • CNS complications • CNS drug toxicity • PRES
- CNS infection

KEY POINTS

- Central nervous system (CNS) complications in patients with stem cell transplants result in high morbidity.
- Major CNS complications include drug toxicity, infection, and cerebrovascular diseases, and occur most often during the first year after transplant.
- There is an increased risk of CNS cancers 5 or more years after allogeneic SCT.

INTRODUCTION

Hematopoietic stem cell transplantation (SCT) is used to treat several hematologic and nonhematologic diseases, and involves transfer of stem cells from a donor to a recipient.[1] Although autologous transplants involve the collection of a patient's own hematopoietic cells to be reinfused later, allogeneic SCT involves transplantation of cells from a healthy related or unrelated donor. Syngeneic transplants are uncommon and are taken from a genetically identical twin donor.[2]

   Stem cells can be harvested from bone marrow, umbilical cord, or peripheral blood. For autologous transplantation, hematopoietic stem cells are usually frozen and used

[a] Division of Neuroradiology, Department of Radiology, VA Ann Arbor Health System, University of Michigan Health System, 1500 East Medical Center Drive, Ann Arbor, MI 48109, USA; [b] BMT Program, Huntsman Cancer Center, University of Utah, 2000 Circle of Hope. Office #2151, Salt Lake City, UT 84112, USA; [c] Department of Pharmacy, University of Michigan Health System, 1500 East Medical Center Drive, Ann Arbor, MI 48109, USA; [d] Division of Neuroradiology, Department of Radiology, University of Michigan Health System, 1500 East Medical Center Drive, Ann Arbor, MI 48109, USA
* Corresponding author.
E-mail address: ashoks@med.umich.edu

Hematol Oncol Clin N Am 30 (2016) 887–898
http://dx.doi.org/10.1016/j.hoc.2016.03.009
0889-8588/16/$ – see front matter © 2016 Elsevier Inc. All rights reserved.

within a few weeks. This can be used in older patients because it does not induce graft-versus-host disease (GVHD). Hence, mortality is significantly lower with autologous transplantation compared with allogeneic transplantation; however, the absence of graft-versus-tumor activity in autologous transplantation reduces its effectiveness.[3]

The purpose of conditioning regimens before transplantation is to eradicate cancer and, in allogeneic transplantation, to induce immunosuppression that permits engraftment. Regimens typically involve both radiation and chemotherapy. A better understanding of graft-versus-tumor biology has led to the development of reduced-intensity regimens that are primarily immunosuppressive and depend on the graft to eradicate cancer. For patients with advanced hematologic cancer, however, the low mortality rate associated with reduced-intensity preparative regimens may be offset by high relapse rates.[3] Chemotherapeutic agents in conditioning regimens may include cyclophosphamide, busulfan, and fludarabine.[4] The incidence and severity of rejection and GVHD increase with human leukocyte antigens mismatch.[2] Although cyclosporin A (CsA), tacrolimus, mycophenolate, methotrexate, and antithymocyte globulin can be used for GVHD prophylaxis, infection prophylaxis may include routine use of antibiotics, antifungal, and antiviral agents.[4]

CENTRAL NERVOUS SYSTEM COMPLICATIONS

Central nervous system (CNS) complications after allogeneic hematopoietic SCT are common and life-threatening.[1] Recent studies have shown the incidence of significant CNS complications in 9% to 14% of SCT subjects.[1,4-6] In an autopsy study[7] of 180 subjects who underwent bone marrow transplant, 90.55% of subjects were found to have CNS abnormalities. However, these complications were the cause of death in only 31 subjects (17%). In another study of 128 subjects, 32% demonstrated structural abnormalities on brain imaging.[8]

CNS complications may be of infectious, vascular, toxic, immune-mediated, or metabolic origin.[1,4,6,8,9] Disease relapse in the CNS[6] and secondary malignancies can also occur.[10] Neuroimaging is crucial for early diagnosis and treatment of CNS complications, with MRI significantly more likely than computed tomography (CT) to provide specific imaging diagnosis of cerebral lesions.[8]

Drug-Related Toxicity

Busulfan and fludarabine are used in conditioning regimens. Although busulfan has been associated with seizures, in a large study of 954 pediatric subjects, the investigators demonstrated that the incidence of seizures was very low (1.3%) when it was administered along with seizure prophylaxis.[11]

Significant dose-related neurotoxicity has been described with fludarabine including cortical blindness, altered mental status, and generalized seizure with the toxicity seen several weeks after intravenous infusion.[12,13] In a study of 1596 subjects, 39 subjects (2.4%) were reported to have fludarabine-related neurotoxicity with different manifestations, including posterior reversible encephalopathy syndrome (PRES), acute toxic leukoencephalopathy, and other leukoencephalopathy syndromes. Acute toxic leukoencephalopathy can manifest as fluid-attenuated inversion recovery (FLAIR) hyperintensity and restricted diffusion in the periventricular white matter with no enhancement. Prognosis is poor with fludarabine-related neurotoxicity, with decreased median time of survival.[14]

Calcineurin inhibitors (CsA and tacrolimus [also known as FK506]) are often used for GVHD prophylaxis. In a retrospective study evaluating tacrolimus CsA in 87 SCT subjects, the investigators showed no significant differences in neurotoxicity between the drugs in the first 100 days after transplantation. Seizures were noted in 5 out of 87 subjects and altered mental status occurred in the presence of significant metabolic abnormalities and infection.[15] In another prospective study of 294 subjects undergoing solid organ transplants, major neurotoxicity related to tacrolimus was reported in 16 subjects (5.4%). The common presentations included encephalopathy, seizures, and focal deficits.[16]

The major neurotoxicity associated with calcineurin inhibitors is PRES.[17,18] Hypertension is commonly associated with CsA, whereas PRES occurs in about 10% of patients who receive CsA.[19] In 1 study, subjects had been taking CsA between 6 days and 5 years before symptom onset. The symptoms included headache, seizures, and visual abnormalities.[19] In another study, 6 of 129 subjects (4.6%) undergoing allogeneic transplants developed CsA-related PRES with the toxicity appearing 3 to 37 days after initiating CsA.[20] PRES secondary to CsA has also been reported in a study of 239 subjects undergoing bone marrow transplants in which 10 subjects (4.2%) developed the syndrome characterized by hypertension, visual disturbances, and seizures.[21]

However, in patients with tacrolimus-associated encephalopathy, there is no association with hypertension. Also, serum levels of tacrolimus are found to be elevated in patients with encephalopathy.[17,18] **Fig. 1** shows an example of tacrolimus-associated PRES in a 55-year-old man who developed seizures on day 1 after undergoing allogeneic SCT.

Ictal electroencephalograph in patients with PRES may show rhythmic spikes involving parieto-occipital or temporal-occipital regions. Imaging may be characterized by a posterior-predominant pattern of cortical-subcortical involvement by increased T2 signal and no enhancement. However, frontal and temporal lobes, cerebellum, and basal ganglia may also be involved. Rarely, intraparenchymal hemorrhage may be seen.[22]

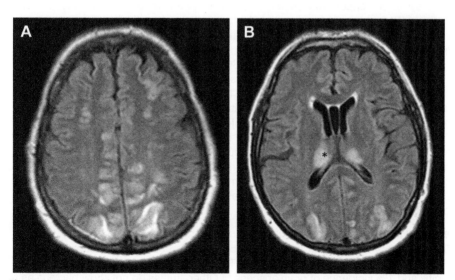

Fig. 1. A 55-year-old man with myelofibrosis developed seizures 1 day before allogeneic peripheral blood SCT. (*A*) MRI shows hyperintensity in the bilateral frontal, parietal, and occipital white matter on FLAIR sequence with (*B*) signal abnormality also involving the thalami (*asterisk*). A diagnosis of tacrolimus-associated PRES was made. Subsequently, tacrolimus was discontinued and the patient was switched to CsA. No further seizures were recorded. However, the patient developed grade IV GVHD and died 1 month later.

Acute toxic leukoencephalopathy has also been described with CsA, 5-fluorouracil, and methotrexate, among other causes.[23]

Infection

In a study of 655 subjects who had undergone allogeneic, syngeneic, or autologous SCT, all CNS infections occurred in allogeneic hematopoietic SCT subjects with a 4% incidence. The most common infections were toxoplasma and aspergillus. Overall mortality of subjects with opportunistic CNS infections was 67%.[24]

Fungal infection

In a study of 230 autologous and allogeneic SCT subjects, 12 subjects were found to have a fungal brain abscess with the most common organism being *Aspergillus*. The median time of symptom onset was 117 days, with all subjects demonstrating an abnormal CT or MRI.[25] Other studies have shown similar times of onset of cerebral aspergillosis at a median of 110 days (mean 143 ± 94). Lesions related to *Aspergillus* were located cortically, subcortically, in the basal ganglia and cerebellum, with MRI demonstrating large lesions with intermediate T2 signal, rim enhancement, and associated vasogenic edema.[24]

A study of subjects, most with aspergillus infections, showed that infections in the early post-transplantation period do not show significant vasogenic edema or enhancement when the white blood cell count is low, whereas there is increase in vasogenic edema and associated enhancement as the white blood cell counts increase.[26]

Toxoplasma infection

The incidence of toxoplasma in allogeneic SCT subjects has been variably reported in a range from 0.2% to 3% in different studies.[24,27,28] In 1 study, the median symptom onset was 84 days post-transplant (range 51–184 days).[28] The typical MRI features include multiple lesions in the subcortical white matter, basal ganglia, and cerebellum, with focal nodular or rim enhancement present in some lesions.[27,28]

In an older study of 655 hematopoietic SCT subjects, toxoplasma was diagnosed in 20 subjects with median onset of 72.5 days (mean of 123 ± 150 days). Two subgroups of subjects were identified in this study. The first group showed supratentorial and infratentorial T2-hyperintense lesions with minimal mass effect and no contrast enhancement. The infection in these subjects manifested itself from day 14 to day 75 (mean 45 ± 22) with a mortality rate of 71%. In the second group, the typical MRI appearances were the presence of multiple T2-hyperintense lesions with associated vasogenic edema, mass effect, and rim enhancement. The disease onset in the latter group was between 62 to 689 days (mean 180 ± 184.4 days) with a mortality rate of 36%. The most common locations of lesions were in the subcortical white matter, basal ganglia, and cerebellum.[24]

Bacterial infection

Brain abscess is a rare but severe CNS complication of SCT. In a large study from Brazil of 1000 subjects who underwent SCT, there was 3% incidence of bacterial meningitis and 1% incidence of brain abscess.[29] Other studies do not show bacteria as a significant burden of CNS infection in these subjects,[1,4,24] suggesting decreasing incidence of bacterial brain abscess and meningoencephalitis. Similar to aspergillus and toxoplasma infections, bacterial abscesses may not show significant mass effect or enhancement.[30] These atypical imaging characteristics of a brain abscess may portend a poor prognosis.[31]

Viral infection

In a prospective study of 281 subjects who underwent allogeneic SCT, the incidence of herpes virus–associated encephalitis or myelitis was 6.3% with the median time of disease onset being 65 days (range: 22–542) post-transplantation. Causative viruses included herpes simplex virus 1, cytomegalovirus (CMV), varicella-zoster virus, and Epstein-Barr virus (EBV).[6,32] In another study, the incidence of EBV-associated CNS disease, including encephalitis or myelitis, has been reported to be 3.4%, with the median time of disease onset being 49 days (22–184) post-transplant.[33] Although MRI of the brain may be normal in these subjects, focal or diffuse signal FLAIR hyperintensities or space-occupying lesions may also be seen.

Human herpesvirus (HHV)-6–associated encephalitis in the SCT transplant population is reported to have an incidence of 4% with the median time to initial symptoms being 18 to 21 days (range 6 to 145 days).[34,35] Patients may present with headaches, altered mental status, and amnesia, with seizures sometimes seen during the disease course. Although the brain MRI within 7 days may be normal, the most common imaging pattern is FLAIR hyperintensity involving the mesial temporal lobes during the early phase, with subsequent hippocampal atrophy.[34,35] **Fig. 2** shows a 55-year-old woman who underwent allogeneic SCT and developed HHV-6 encephalitis 3 months later, with prominent involvement of the mesial temporal lobes on MRI. Nonspecific white matter signal abnormality can also be seen with some patients, demonstrating persistent long-term memory deficits.[34,35]

CMV encephalitis after allogeneic hematopoietic SCT is a late-onset disease (median time of onset: 210 days) with CT or MRI showing changes suggestive of encephalitis or ventriculoencephalitis.[36] Diffuse white matter signal abnormality with punctate foci of restricted diffusion in the subependymal, periventricular, and corpus callosum white matter may be present, and is thought to be highly suggestive of CMV encephalitis.[37]

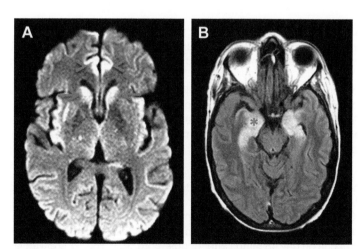

Fig. 2. A 55-year-old woman who underwent allogeneic cord blood SCT developed HHV-6 encephalitis 3 months after the transplant. Patient presented at this time with significant memory impairment and altered consciousness. Restricted diffusion in the (A) caudate nuclei (*arrows*) and cingulate gyri (*arrow heads*) were seen with prominent FLAIR hyperintensity (*asterisk*) noted in (B) the mesial temporal lobes. The patient was started on foscarnet without improvement in mentation and died a few days later. This example illustrates the high mortality associated with CNS complications after SCT and emphasizes the need for increased awareness of these complications.

Infection along the ventricular margin can be seen on imaging as abnormal ependymal enhancement.[38] The disease-associated mortality is very high with CMV encephalitis. Therefore, appropriate therapy needs to be instituted in a timely fashion.[36]

Progressive multifocal leukoencephalopathy (PML), a demyelinating encephalopathy caused by the JC virus,[39] is a rare but serious complication of bone marrow transplantation.[40] Lesions involve the lobar white matter with involvement of the subcortical U-fibers. Lesions are hypoattenuating on CT and hyperintense on T2-weighted MRI without mass effect or enhancement. There may be diffusion restriction at the margins of the lesions.[39] **Fig. 3** shows a 69-year-old man who presented with worsening mental status on day 98 after allogeneic SCT. Successive brain MRIs showed worsening patchy nonenhancing areas of FLAIR hyperintensity in the subcortical white matter.

Metabolic

Metabolic encephalopathy may clinically manifest as altered mental status and seizures, commonly secondary to electrolyte imbalances, acid-base disturbances, or hepatic or renal insufficiency.[29]

Wernicke encephalopathy is a rare complication and may develop secondary to thiamine deficiency from total parenteral nutrition (TPN).[9,29] Patients on long-term TPN and intravenous glucose solutions have a higher thiamine requirement and may rapidly deplete thiamine stores. The classic clinical triad is altered mental status, ocular findings, and ataxia,[9] with the periventricular structures in the brain stem, hypothalamus, and thalamus demonstrating petechial hemorrhage, neuronal loss, and gliosis. Typical MRI findings include T2-FLAIR hyperintensity in these locations, including the region of the mammillary bodies. There may be enhancement in the acute phase.[41]

Vascular

Extra-axial hemorrhage

Subarachnoid hemorrhage (SAH) or subdural hematoma (SDH) can occur in the post-SCT setting but has a low incidence and is not associated with increased patient mortality.[9,42–44]

In a prospective study of 50 SCT subjects, subdural hygromas were seen in 9 (18%) subjects (8 in allogeneic, 1 in autologous), with all of them resolving within 60 days. Although these complications were not associated with thrombocytopenia, there was association with lumbar puncture and intrathecal methotrexate administration.[45]

Stroke

Intraparenchymal hemorrhage is reported to have an incidence of 1.1% to 2.4% posttransplant with a median onset time after transplant of 122 days.[43,46] In contrast to SDH and SAH, the mortality is high after intraparenchymal hemorrhage.[42,43] **Fig. 4** illustrates an example of a 57-year-old man who was found to have hypertension and severe headache on day 48 status after double-cord SCT. The CT showed large intraparenchymal hemorrhage as well as SAH and SDH. Compared with SAH, SDH, and intraparenchymal hemorrhages, ischemic infarcts are rarer and have been reported in only 9 out of 1245 SCT subjects in a study published by Coplin and colleagues[46] in 2001.

Vasculitis has been rarely reported secondary to chronic GVHD.[47] Imaging of vasculitis may reveal periventricular white matter lesions, infarction, leukoencephalopathy, or hemorrhage, with occasional presence of leptomeningeal involvement.[48,49]

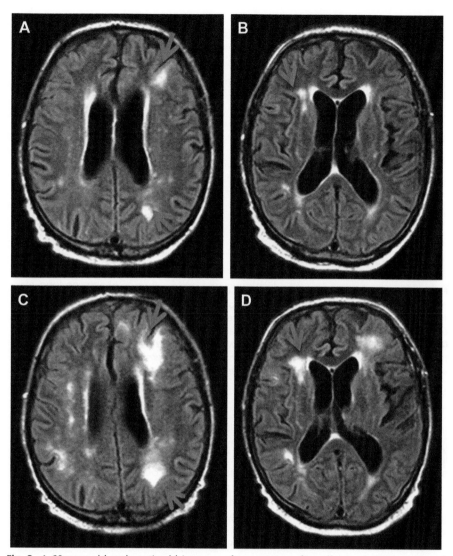

Fig. 3. A 69-year-old male retired history professor status after allogeneic SCT presented on day 98 with 1 to 2 week history of worsening altered mental status, word-finding difficulties, and episodes of confusion. A brain MRI (*A, B*) demonstrated patchy areas of nonenhancing FLAIR hyperintensity in the left frontal and parietal subcortical white matter (*arrows*) as well as the right subinsular subcortical white matter (*arrow*). JC virus was detected in the cerebrospinal fluid. Patient was readmitted with continued worsening of mental status 2 weeks later and at this time was inappropriately answering questions. (*C, D*) A repeat brain MRI at this time showed progression of patchy areas of FLAIR hyperintensity (*arrows*) without significant mass effect (*arrow*). A diagnosis of PML was made. All immunosuppressive agents were withheld and Mirtazapine was administered. The patient died 5 weeks after initial presentation. Autopsy confirmed the diagnosis of PML.

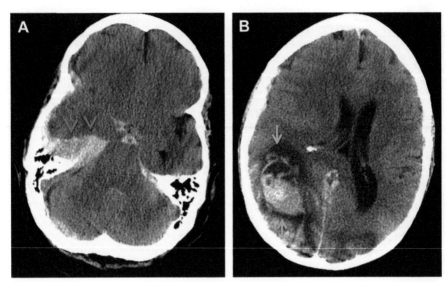

Fig. 4. A 57-year-old man with double-cord SCT developed a severe headache and lethargy on day 48. Clinical and laboratory examinations revealed hypertension (systolic blood pressure 180s–200s) and thrombocytopenia (platelets = 26,000/mm³). (*A*) A non-contrast head CT showed subdural hemorrhage (*arrow heads*) along the right tentorial leaflet and SAH (*asterisk*) in the basilar cisterns. (*B*) There was a large intraparenchymal hemorrhage in the right posterior cerebrum (*arrows*) with subfalcine herniation. The family declined aggressive measures. The patient died on the same day.

Neoplastic Disease After Transplantation

In a large study of 18,014 subjects published in 1999, the risk of post-transplant lymphoproliferative disorder (PTLD) was noted as 1% at 10 years, with the highest incidence in the first year after transplant.[10,50] However, more recent, albeit smaller, studies show the incidence of EBV-associated PTLD to be higher at 3% to 4%.[6,32,33]

Increased incidence of cancers after allogenic transplantation, including those involving the CNS, has also been observed in a large study of 19,229 subjects in which the investigators noted the risk to be higher 5 or more years after transplantation. This increased risk was thought to be likely related to conditioning with radiation, altered immune function, and prior treatment of the primary disease.[10]

Miscellaneous

Encephalitis and GVHD
There have been rare reports of encephalitis associated with chronic GVHD, with involvement of the cerebral white matter, brain stem, and cortical atrophy.[47]

Demyelinating disease
In a small histopathologic study of 14 subjects, there were higher numbers of cluster of differentiation CD3+ and CD8+ cytotoxic T cells, and higher scores of CD68+ microglia or macrophages in active multiple sclerosis (MS) lesions compared with lesions that were not active or normal-appearing white matter. Although subjects without MS who underwent transplantation demonstrated higher numbers of CD3+ and CD8+ cytotoxic T cells, and higher scores of CD68+ microglia or macrophages, no demyelination was identified in these non-MS samples. This showed that

transplantation did not halt demyelination in subjects with MS.[51] Demyelination has also been rarely reported to occur during chronic GVHD.[49]

Morbidity and mortality

In a study of 191 subjects with allogeneic SCT, the nonrelapse mortality at 1 year was 42% in subjects with CNS complications compared with 20% in subjects without CNS involvement. The overall survival at 4 years was 33% in subjects with CNS complications compared with 45% without CNS involvement, thereby emphasizing the long-term implications of encountering CNS complications.[1] In another study, the overall mortality of subjects who developed CNS infections was 57.9% and 66.7% of those died of CNS complications.[6] It is apparent from these studies that the overall mortality is significantly higher for patients who develop CNS complications and, hence, timely detection and management of these complications is paramount for improving patient survival.[4,6]

SUMMARY

In conclusion, although SCTs are increasingly commonly used to combat a variety of conditions and have improved patient outcomes, the increased mortality when encountering CNS complications remains an important concern. Early clinical detection with appropriate recognition of features on neuroimaging can help reduce the overall morbidity and mortality associated with these complications, and help institute earlier appropriate treatment.

REFERENCES

1. Barba P, Pinana JL, Valcarcel D, et al. Early and late neurological complications after reduced-intensity conditioning allogeneic stem cell transplantation. Biol Blood Marrow Transplant 2009;15(11):1439–46.
2. Bashir Q, Champlin R. Hematopoietic stem cell transplantation. In: Niederhuber JE, Armitage JO, Doroshow JH, et al, editors. Abeloff's clinical oncology. Clinical oncology. 5th edition. Philadelphia: Elsevier; 2014. p. 485–592.
3. Copelan EA. Hematopoietic stem-cell transplantation. N Engl J Med 2006; 354(17):1813–26.
4. Bhatt VR, Balasetti V, Jasem JA, et al. Central nervous system complications and outcomes after allogeneic hematopoietic stem cell transplantation. Clin Lymphoma Myeloma Leuk 2015;15(10):606–11.
5. Uckan D, Cetin M, Yigitkanli I, et al. Life-threatening neurological complications after bone marrow transplantation in children. Bone Marrow Transplant 2005; 35(1):71–6.
6. Cao XY, Wu T, Lu Y, et al. A study of the central nervous system complications after hematopoietic stem cell transplantation. Zhonghua Nei Ke Za Zhi 2010;49(1):42–4.
7. Bleggi-Torres LF, de Medeiros BC, Werner B, et al. Neuropathological findings after bone marrow transplantation: an autopsy study of 180 cases. Bone Marrow Transplant 2000;25(3):301–7.
8. Chen BT, Ortiz AO, Dagis A, et al. Brain imaging findings in symptomatic patients after allogeneic haematopoietic stem cell transplantation: correlation with clinical outcome. Eur Radiol 2012;22(10):2273–81.
9. Bleggi-Torres LF, de Medeiros BC, Ogasawara VS, et al. Iatrogenic Wernicke's encephalopathy in allogeneic bone marrow transplantation: a study of eight cases. Bone Marrow Transplant 1997;20(5):391–5.

10. Curtis RE, Rowlings PA, Deeg HJ, et al. Solid cancers after bone marrow transplantation. N Engl J Med 1997;336(13):897–904.

11. Caselli D, Rosati A, Faraci M, et al. Risk of seizures in children receiving busulphan-containing regimens for stem cell transplantation. Biol Blood Marrow Transplant 2014;20(2):282–5.

12. Warrell RP Jr, Berman E. Phase I and II study of fludarabine phosphate in leukemia: therapeutic efficacy with delayed central nervous system toxicity. J Clin Oncol 1986;4(1):74–9.

13. Lee MS, McKinney AM, Brace JR, et al. Clinical and imaging features of fludarabine neurotoxicity. J Neuroophthalmol 2010;30(1):37–41.

14. Beitinjaneh A, McKinney AM, Cao Q, et al. Toxic leukoencephalopathy following fludarabine-associated hematopoietic cell transplantation. Biol Blood Marrow Transplant 2011;17(3):300–8.

15. Woo M, Przepiorka D, Ippoliti C, et al. Toxicities of tacrolimus and cyclosporin A after allogeneic blood stem cell transplantation. Bone Marrow Transplant 1997; 20(12):1095–8.

16. Eidelman BH, Abu-Elmagd K, Wilson J, et al. Neurologic complications of FK 506. Transplant Proc 1991;23(6):3175–8.

17. Singh N, Bonham A, Fukui M. Immunosuppressive-associated leukoencephalopathy in organ transplant recipients. Transplantation 2000;69(4):467–72.

18. Mammoser A. Calcineurin inhibitor encephalopathy. Semin Neurol 2012;32(5): 517–24.

19. Schwartz RB, Bravo SM, Klufas RA, et al. Cyclosporine neurotoxicity and its relationship to hypertensive encephalopathy: CT and MR findings in 16 cases. AJR Am J Roentgenol 1995;165(3):627–31.

20. Trullemans F, Grignard F, Van Camp B, et al. Clinical findings and magnetic resonance imaging in severe cyclosporine-related neurotoxicity after allogeneic bone marrow transplantation. Eur J Haematol 2001;67(2):94–9.

21. Reece DE, Frei-Lahr DA, Shepherd JD, et al. Neurologic complications in allogeneic bone marrow transplant patients receiving cyclosporin. Bone Marrow Transplant 1991;8(5):393–401.

22. Cordelli DM, Masetti R, Zama D, et al. Etiology, characteristics and outcome of seizures after pediatric hematopoietic stem cell transplantation. Seizure 2014; 23(2):140–5.

23. McKinney AM, Kieffer SA, Paylor RT, et al. Acute toxic leukoencephalopathy: potential for reversibility clinically and on MRI with diffusion-weighted and FLAIR imaging. AJR Am J Roentgenol 2009;193(1):192–206.

24. Maschke M, Dietrich U, Prumbaum M, et al. Opportunistic CNS infection after bone marrow transplantation. Bone Marrow Transplant 1999;23(11): 1167–76.

25. Baddley JW, Salzman D, Pappas PG. Fungal brain abscess in transplant recipients: epidemiologic, microbiologic, and clinical features. Clin Transplant 2002; 16(6):419–24.

26. Yuh WT, Nguyen HD, Gao F, et al. Brain parenchymal infection in bone marrow transplantation patients: CT and MR findings. AJR Am J Roentgenol 1994; 162(2):425–30.

27. Matsuo Y, Takeishi S, Miyamoto T, et al. Toxoplasmosis encephalitis following severe graft-vs.-host disease after allogeneic hematopoietic stem cell transplantation: 17 yr experience in Fukuoka BMT group. Eur J Haematol 2007;79(4): 317–21.

28. Hakko E, Ozkan HA, Karaman K, et al. Analysis of cerebral toxoplasmosis in a series of 170 allogeneic hematopoietic stem cell transplant patients. Transpl Infect Dis 2013;15(6):575–80.

29. Teive HA, Funke V, Bitencourt MA, et al. Neurological complications of hematopoietic stem cell transplantation (HSCT): a retrospective study in a HSCT center in Brazil. Arq Neuropsiquiatr 2008;66(3B):685–90.

30. Nishiguchi T, Mochizuki K, Shakudo M, et al. CNS complications of hematopoietic stem cell transplantation. AJR Am J Roentgenol 2009;192(4):1003–11.

31. Enzmann DR, Brant-Zawadzki M, Britt RH. CT of central nervous system infections in immunocompromised patients. AJR Am J Roentgenol 1980;135(2):263–7.

32. Wu M, Huang F, Jiang X, et al. Herpesvirus-associated central nervous system diseases after allogeneic hematopoietic stem cell transplantation. PLoS One 2013;8(10):e77805.

33. Liu QF, Ling YW, Fan ZP, et al. Epstein-Barr virus (EBV) load in cerebrospinal fluid and peripheral blood of patients with EBV-associated central nervous system diseases after allogeneic hematopoietic stem cell transplantation. Transpl Infect Dis 2013;15(4):379–92.

34. Bhanushali MJ, Kranick SM, Freeman AF, et al. Human herpes 6 virus encephalitis complicating allogeneic hematopoietic stem cell transplantation. Neurology 2013;80(16):1494–500.

35. Sakai R, Kanamori H, Motohashi K, et al. Long-term outcome of human herpesvirus-6 encephalitis after allogeneic stem cell transplantation. Biol Blood Marrow Transplant 2011;17(9):1389–94.

36. Reddy SM, Winston DJ, Territo MC, et al. CMV central nervous system disease in stem-cell transplant recipients: an increasing complication of drug-resistant CMV infection and protracted immunodeficiency. Bone Marrow Transplant 2010;45(6):979–84.

37. Battiwalla M, Paplham P, Almyroudis NG, et al. Leflunomide failure to control recurrent cytomegalovirus infection in the setting of renal failure after allogeneic stem cell transplantation. Transpl Infect Dis 2007;9(1):28–32.

38. Seo SK, Regan A, Cihlar T, et al. Cytomegalovirus ventriculoencephalitis in a bone marrow transplant recipient receiving antiviral maintenance: clinical and molecular evidence of drug resistance. Clin Infect Dis 2001;33(9):e105–8.

39. Bag AK, Cure JK, Chapman PR, et al. JC virus infection of the brain. AJNR Am J Neuroradiol 2010;31(9):1564–76.

40. Amend KL, Turnbull B, Foskett N, et al. Incidence of progressive multifocal leukoencephalopathy in patients without HIV. Neurology 2010;75(15):1326–32.

41. Zuccoli G, Gallucci M, Capellades J, et al. Wernicke encephalopathy: MR findings at clinical presentation in twenty-six alcoholic and nonalcoholic patients. AJNR Am J Neuroradiol 2007;28(7):1328–31.

42. Bleggi-Torres LF, Werner B, Gasparetto EL, et al. Intracranial hemorrhage following bone marrow transplantation: an autopsy study of 58 patients. Bone Marrow Transplant 2002;29(1):29–32.

43. Najima Y, Ohashi K, Miyazawa M, et al. Intracranial hemorrhage following allogeneic hematopoietic stem cell transplantation. Am J Hematol 2009;84(5):298–301.

44. Colosimo M, McCarthy N, Jayasinghe R, et al. Diagnosis and management of subdural haematoma complicating bone marrow transplantation. Bone Marrow Transplant 2000;25(5):549–52.

45. Staudinger T, Heimberger K, Rabitsch W, et al. Subdural hygromas after bone marrow transplantation: results of a prospective study. Transplantation 1998; 65(10):1340–4.
46. Coplin WM, Cochran MS, Levine SR, et al. Stroke after bone marrow transplantation: frequency, aetiology and outcome. Brain 2001;124(Pt 5):1043–51.
47. Saad AG, Alyea EP, Wen PY, et al. Graft-versus-host disease of the CNS after allogeneic bone marrow transplantation. J Clin Oncol 2009;27(30): e147–9.
48. Padovan CS, Bise K, Hahn J, et al. Angiitis of the central nervous system after allogeneic bone marrow transplantation? Stroke 1999;30(8):1651–6.
49. Grauer O, Grauer O, Wolff D, et al. Neurological manifestations of chronic graft-versus-host disease after allogeneic haematopoietic stem cell transplantation: report from the Consensus Conference on Clinical Practice in chronic graft-versus-host disease. Brain 2010;133(10):2852–65.
50. Curtis RE, Travis LB, Rowlings PA, et al. Risk of lymphoproliferative disorders after bone marrow transplantation: a multi-institutional study. Blood 1999;94(7): 2208–16.
51. Lu JQ, Joseph JT, Nash RA, et al. Neuroinflammation and demyelination in multiple sclerosis after allogeneic hematopoietic stem cell transplantation. Arch Neurol 2010;67(6):716–22.

Central Nervous System Complications of Oncologic Therapy

Ellen G. Hoeffner, MD

KEYWORDS

- Neurotoxicity • Chemotherapy • Radiation therapy • Magnetic resonance imaging
- Cancer

KEY POINTS

- Neurotoxicity related to cancer treatment is increasing in frequency related to improvements in cancer treatment and patients surviving longer.
- Neurotoxicity is a widely recognized adverse effect of cancer treatment and can result from radiation therapy, traditional chemotherapeutic agents, and newer biologic and immunotherapeutic agents used to treat cancer.
- MRI is the main imaging modality used to assess patients with cancer with new symptoms referable to the CNS.
- CNS complications of oncologic treatment can have variable imaging appearances and in some cases mimic cancer progression or recurrence.

INTRODUCTION

Neurotoxicity is a widely recognized adverse effect of cancer treatment and can result from radiation therapy (RT), traditional chemotherapeutic agents, and newer biologic and immunotherapeutic agents used to treat cancer.[1] Although the exact incidence of treatment-related neurotoxicity is unknown, its frequency is thought to be increasing.[2] Higher doses of chemotherapeutic agents are being administered because of advances in supportive care, with escalating doses resulting in neurotoxicity. Additionally, improvements in cancer treatment have led to patients with cancer living longer. Thus, treatment-related neurotoxicity with a long latency between treatment and symptom onset is increasingly recognized.[2] After myelosuppression, neurotoxicity is the most common dose-limiting factor of cancer treatment.[3] It was once thought that the blood-brain and blood-cerebrospinal fluid barriers and the

No disclosures.
Department of Radiology, University Hospital, University of Michigan, #UH-B2 A209, 1500 East Medical Center Drive, Ann Arbor, MI 48109-0030, USA
E-mail address: hoeffner@med.umich.edu

nondividing central nervous system (CNS) cells would protect the CNS from the toxic effects of RT and chemotherapy. However, it is now known that the CNS contains stem cells that replenish some neuron populations and that glial cells do divide. Although the pathophysiologic mechanisms are not fully known, traditional chemotherapeutic agents and RT can directly damage neural structures and cause indirect damage through injury to the vasculature. Newer immune and biologic agents can affect the CNS through a heightened immune response or cross reactivity with nervous system cells.[1] When patients with cancer develop new neurologic symptoms it is important to distinguish symptoms related to the cancer itself from those related to other causes, such as paraneoplastic syndromes, infection, or treatment-related toxicity. Although attributing symptoms to neurotoxicity is generally a diagnosis of exclusion, it is important to recognize so that further injury is prevented by dose adjustment or treatment cessation.[1,4] MRI is the main imaging modality used to assess patients with cancer with new symptoms referable to the CNS. It is important to be aware of the common neurotoxic syndromes that can occur as a result of cancer treatment, the agents responsible for them, and the imaging findings to allow prompt diagnosis.

RADIATION-INDUCED CENTRAL NERVOUS SYSTEM COMPLICATIONS

RT to the brain and spinal cord is used to treat a variety of primary and metastatic tumors and may be administered prophylactically to prevent the development of metastases. The brain may also be included in the RT port of patients with other cancers, notably head and neck cancers.[5] Injury to the CNS can occur after whole brain RT, involved field RT, or focal RT, such as stereotactic radiosurgery and brachytherapy.[5,6] Radiation can directly affect the CNS or indirectly induce vasculopathy, endocrinopathy, or carcinogenesis.[4,5,7] Risk factors associated with radiation-induced injury include energy of radiation, total dose, fraction size, time between fractions, treatment volume, and previous or concurrent chemotherapy.[4,5,8,9] Patient-specific factors, including age, sex, genetic predisposition, pre-existing CNS damage, systemic disease, and lifestyle choice, also impact the risk of radiation-induced injury.[5,7]

Radiation injury to the brain is typically classified into three phases based on the time of onset after radiation. Acute injury occurs during or shortly after radiation, subacute or early delayed injury occurs weeks to months after radiation, and late-delayed occurs months to years after radiation.[10]

Acute injury presents clinically with headache, nausea, vomiting, lethargy, and worsening of pre-existing neurologic symptoms.[11,12] This is most commonly seen following large fractions (>3 Gy) delivered to large brain volumes in patients with increased intracranial pressure. The pathogenesis is likely related to disruption of the blood-brain barrier by endothelial apoptosis leading to increased edema and possibly an increase in intracranial pressure.[13,14] The incidence and severity of this type of injury has decreased with prophylactic steroid use, surgical debulking, and careful treatment planning with conventional fractionation (1.8–2 Gy per fraction) and the symptoms are usually reversible.[6,8,11,15] Although acute brain swelling has been reported, typically no computed tomography (CT) or MRI findings are present with this type of injury.[16,17]

In patients receiving RT for high-grade gliomas, particularly in combination with temozolamide (Temodar), a temporary increase in brain edema and enhancement in the RT treatment volume can occur that is believed to be an early delayed effect of treatment. This usually occurs on the first MRI done within 2 to 3 months after treatment and has been termed "pseudoprogression," because the imaging findings mimic tumor progression on MRI, but stabilize or improve spontaneously over the following 4 to 6 months (**Fig. 1**).[17,18] Thus pseudoprogression is a clinical diagnosis, not a pathologic one.[19] Overall it is currently estimated that 50% of patients with high-grade gliomas have early posttherapy MRI findings concerning for progressive disease; approximately 40% of these changes (or 20% of all patients with high-grade glioma) are caused by pseudoprogression.[19] Patients with methylated O6-methyl guanine-DNA methyltransferase are twice as likely to manifest pseudoprogression in comparison with patients with nonmethylated O6-methyl guanine-DNA methyltransferase.[20,21] Pseudoprogression is less likely to be associated with clinical symptoms than early progression. Approximately one-third of patients with pseudoprogression have symptoms compared with 50% to 67% of patients with early progression.[19–21] The pathophysiology is not fully understood but may relate to killing of tumor cells and endothelial cells leading to abnormal vessel permeability and edema. Additionally, in patients who have undergone biopsy for progressive changes in the first 6 months after combined chemoradiotherapy with temozolamide a high incidence of necrosis has been reported.[17,22]

Conventional MRI techniques cannot reliably differentiate pseudoprogression from true early progression. A recent study indicated that subependymal enhancement on the initial post-RT MRI was the only conventional MRI feature predictive for early progression, but the negative predictive value was only 41%. Other features including various patterns of enhancement, increasing peritumoral T2 abnormality, cystic or necrotic change, and restricted diffusion had no predictive value.[23] Advanced imaging techniques, such as MR spectroscopy, diffusion-weighted imaging, and MR perfusion imaging, are being investigated to differentiate pseudoprogression from early progression (**Table 1**). These techniques have shown promise but further prospective studies are needed for validation.[19,24–31] Similar progression of imaging findings can occur in a one-third to one-half of patients treated with radiosurgery for brain metastases. The increase in lesion size can begin at 6 weeks postradiosurgery and last for up to 15 months.[32] A recent study evaluated 67 patients who underwent radiosurgery for brain metastases followed by histopathologic evaluation via biopsy or surgery in the setting of imaging findings concerning for disease progression versus radiation change. A total of 28% of patients had only necrosis on pathology, 11% had mixed necrosis and viable tumor, 60% had tumor progression, and 2% were indeterminate. There were no MRI criteria that could distinguish among these entities.[33]

Late-delayed radiation injury manifests as radiation necrosis or diffuse leukoencephalopathy.[4,34] Radiation necrosis occurs following external beam RT or radiosurgery for primary and metastatic brain tumors. It may also occur in patients with extracranial tumors, particularly head and neck cancers, where the brain is included in the radiation field.[4,34] The incidence varies from 5% to 24% for metastatic tumors and is approximately 5% for primary brain tumors.[4] Symptoms include focal neurologic deficit, seizure, headache, and cognitive impairment and may mimic those of the original tumor.[4,6] Direct injury to the vasculature and to neuronal and glial structures has been implicated in the pathology of radiation necrosis.[35] Rim-enhancing or nodular-enhancing lesions with varying degrees of surrounding hyperintensity on T2-weighted and fluid-attenuated inversion recovery (FLAIR) images and mass effect are seen on MRI, often at the site of the previous tumor.[36–38] Cystic changes may also be seen and are thought to reflect late stages of tissue necrosis (**Fig. 2**).[38,39] Imaging findings of necrosis are not readily distinguishable from those of recurrent tumor. As with pseudoprogression, advance imaging techniques, such as MR spectroscopy, diffusion-weighted imaging, and MR perfusion, may help in differentiating radiation necrosis from tumor, but biopsy remains the gold standard.[28,30]

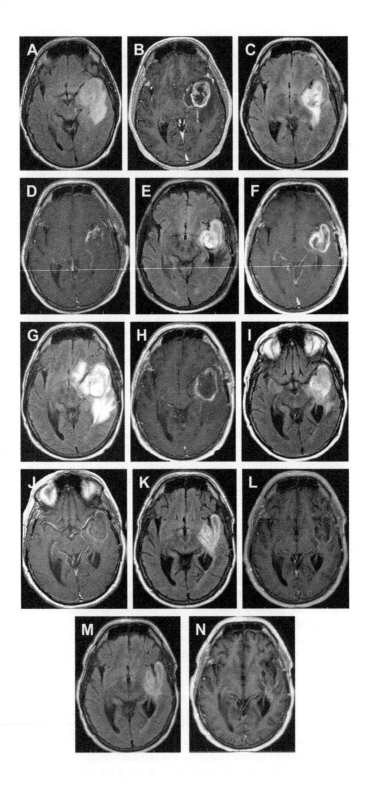

Table 1
Overview of advanced MRI techniques used to distinguish PD from RI

Technique	Supporting Studies	Findings Associated with PD (Compared with RI)	Limitations
Diffusion-weighted MRI	19,24–26	Lower mean ADC values and ADC ratios	Overlap between recurrence and radiation change; ADC value dependent on sampling method
MR perfusion	19,27–29	Higher rCBV	Overlap between recurrence and radiation change; rCBV cutoff values vary by study, technique; vascular leak problematic
MR spectroscopy	19,30,31	Higher choline/creatine and choline/N-acetylaspartate	Overlap between recurrence and radiation change; cutoff values vary by study; problems when both recurrence and postradiation change present

Abbreviations: ADC, apparent diffusion coefficient; PD, progressive disease; rCBV, relative cerebral blood volume; RI, radiation injury.

Leukoencephalopathy with brain volume loss is the other common late-delayed effect of radiation, often following whole brain radiation for therapy or prophylaxis.[7,12] Concomitant chemotherapy can enhance the process and intensify clinical and radiographic severity.[6,7] Patients typically have cognitive deficits consisting of impairments in learning, memory, executive function, attention, and concentration. Less commonly patients may have dementia, gait abnormalities, and urinary incontinence.[6,40] The underlying pathophysiology is not fully known but may relate to direct damage to neurons and neuron precursors, demyelination, and impairments in hippocampal

Fig. 1. Pseudoprogression. A 63-year-old man with glioblastoma multiforme. Imaging at time of diagnosis. (A) Axial fluid-attenuated inversion recovery (FLAIR) image shows hyperintense signal related to tumor and surrounding tumoral edema in left temporal lobe with significant mass effect. (B) Axial T1-weighted postcontrast image shows heterogeneous mass with nodular peripheral enhancement. Images obtained 2 days following biopsy and tumor debulking. (C) Axial FLAIR image shows persistent abnormal FLAIR signal but improved mass effect. (D) Axial T1-weighted postcontrast image shows decreased size of mass including enhancing component. Patient treated with temozolamide and RT. Imaging obtained 1 month following completion of RT. (E) Axial FLAIR image shows some improvement in abnormal signal. (F) Axial T1-weighted postcontrast image shows increased enhancement. Imaging obtained 3 months following completion of RT. (G) Axial FLAIR image shows significant increase in abnormal signal and mass effect. (H) Axial T1-weighted postcontrast image shows increase in size of enhancing mass. Concern for pseudoprogression versus true progression. Dexamethasone dose was increased at this time. Imaging repeated 4 months later following a decrease in dose of dexamethasone. (I) Axial FLAIR image shows improvement in left temporal signal changes and mass effect. (J) Axial T1-weighted postcontrast image shows decreased size of mass and diminished enhancement. Imaging repeated 3 months later. (K) Axial FLAIR image shows further decrease in left temporal signal changes. (L) Axial T1-weighted postcontrast image shows further decrease in size of mass with persistent peripheral enhancement. Imaging repeated 4 months later. (M) Axial FLAIR image shows stable signal changes. (N) Axial T1-weighted postcontrast image shows slight decrease in size of mass with stable enhancement.

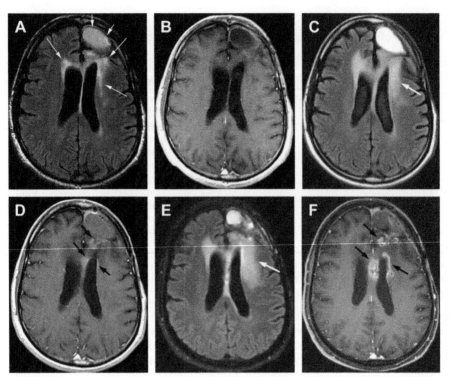

Fig. 2. Radiation necrosis. A 46-year-old man with history of left frontal oligodendroglioma with two prior recurrences treated with resection, radiation, and multiple chemotherapeutic agents. MRI obtained 9 months following most recent resection and 6 months following completion of reirradiation. (*A*) Axial FLAIR image shows resection cavity in left frontal region (*short arrows*) and nonspecific hyperintensities in periventricular and deep white matter (*long arrows*). (*B*) Axial T1-weighted postcontrast image shows posttreatment changes with no enhancement. MRI repeated 3 months later. (*C*) Axial FLAIR image shows increasing hyperintense signal in left frontal lobe (*arrow*). (*D*) Axial T1-weighted postcontrast image shows new foci of enhancement in the left frontal lobe and along the margins of left frontal horn (*arrows*). MRI obtained 3 months later. (*E*) Axial FLAIR image shows further progression of left frontal hyperintensities (*arrow*). (*F*) Axial T1-weighted postcontrast image shows further increase in the enhancement (*arrows*). Subsequent biopsy of left frontal lobe revealed posttreatment changes only including areas of necrosis.

neurogenesis.[7,41] On MRI there are symmetric, confluent white matter hyperintensities on T2-weighted and FLAIR images without enhancement. There is often associated atrophy with enlarged sulci and ventricles (**Fig. 3**).[6,12,37,42]

Radiation to the spine or spinal cord can result in toxicity that presents as an early delayed or late-delayed myelopathy. Patients with early delayed myelopathy typically present 2 to 4 months after radiation with Lhermitte sign, a nonpainful, unpleasant electric shock-like sensation that shoots down the spine during neck flexion. MRI is usually normal in these patients and symptoms usually completely resolve.[7,43] With late-delayed myelopathy symptoms can vary from minor motor and sensory deficits to a Brown-Séquard syndrome. Disruption of blood–spinal cord barrier leads to edema and demyelination that may progress to necrosis. Damage to the vasculature also occurs.[44] Acutely, MRI may be normal or show swelling, hyperintensity on

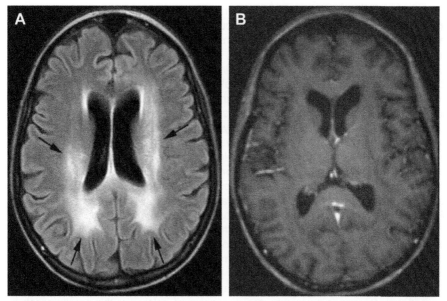

Fig. 3. Radiation leukoencephalopathy. A 27-year-old woman who had total brain RT for leukemia. (*A*) Axial FLAIR image shows bilateral periventricular and deep white matter hyperintensities (*arrows*) with no mass effect. (*B*) Axial T1-weighted postcontrast image shows no enhancement. There is mild, diffuse brain volume loss.

T2-weighted images, and enhancement that is often patchy. In later stages the cord appears atrophic. Identification of hyperintensity in the vertebral bodies on T1-weighted MRIs often helps to outline the radiation portal. Over time atrophy of the cord can develop (**Fig. 4**).[7,45]

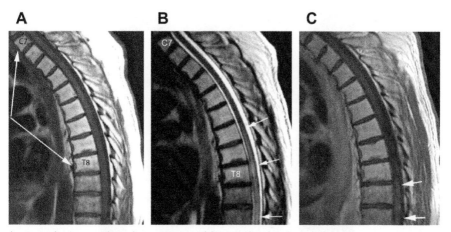

Fig. 4. Radiation myelopathy. A 53-year-old man who developed lower extremity numbness and weakness 7 months following chest RT for small cell lung cancer. (*A*) Sagittal T1-weighted precontrast image of thoracic spine shows hyperintense marrow from C7 through T8 (*arrows*) compatible with postradiation change. (*B*) Sagittal T2-weighted image shows increased signal in thoracic cord from T6 through T12 (*arrows*). (*C*) Sagittal T1-weighted postcontrast image shows cord enhancement in lower thoracic region (*arrows*). After extensive negative neurologic work-up findings were attributed to radiation myelopathy.

Radiation to the brain can also result in indirect injury to the CNS through radiation-induced vasculopathy or tumors. Cavernous malformations can develop in the CNS after RT and are more common in children and males. The latency period can range from 2 to 10 years or more after radiation. They can lead to hemorrhage or seizures, although most are asymptomatic.[46,47] On MRI they have a variable appearance because of the nature of hemoglobin breakdown products. Centrally they may have heterogeneous signal with a hypointense rim on T2-weighted images or may be hypointense on all sequences. Additional lesions may be seen on gradient echo sequences or susceptibility-weighted sequences as hypointense foci, presumably related to prior hemorrhage (**Fig. 5**).[47–49] Large vessel vasculopathy can also develop related to intimal proliferation, thrombosis, and accelerated atherosclerosis. The latency period ranges from 4 months to 20 years. The common and internal carotid arteries are the most vulnerable vessel of neurologic interest.[50–53] CT angiography, MR angiography, or catheter angiography can be used to diagnose vessel narrowing. The diagnosis of RT-induced stenosis or occlusion is suggested when the carotid artery was included in the RT field and the site of stenosis is different from its usual location at the carotid bifurcation in nonirradiated patients. Stenotic lesions tend to be longer after RT and the maximum stenosis is often at the end of the stenotic area (**Fig. 6**). Multiple moyamoya-like collaterals may be seen, particularly if the intracranial arteries are involved (**Fig. 7**).[7,51,53] Mineralizing microangiopathy is a frequent finding in children treated with RT and is caused by the deposition of calcium within small vessels of the irradiated brain parenchyma. It usually occurs in conjunction with chemotherapy, but may occur after RT alone. The relationship to clinical symptoms is unclear. It is best seen on CT as multiple, punctate calcifications that most frequently involve the basal ganglia and less commonly the cortex or brainstem (**Fig. 8**).[37] Finally, neoplasms can develop as a consequence of RT to the CNS. These tumors probably result from radiation damage to DNA with abnormal repair, with biologic variables also playing a

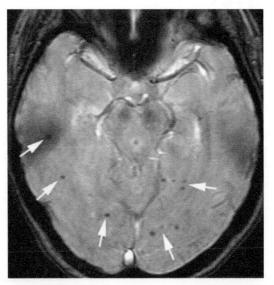

Fig. 5. Cavernous malformation. A 43-year-old woman treated 8 years previously with resection, chemotherapy, and craniospinal RT for a medulloblastoma. Axial susceptibility-weighted image shows multiple punctate foci of hypointense signal (*arrows*) compatible with cavernous malformations.

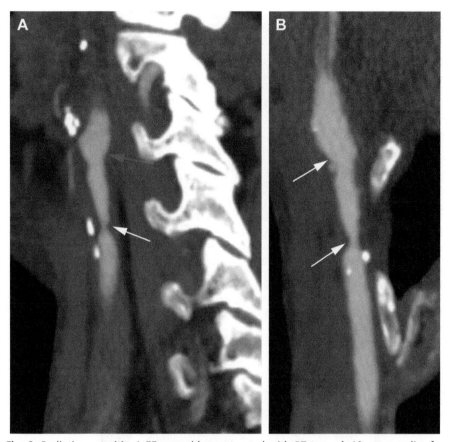

Fig. 6. Radiation arteritis. A 55-year-old man treated with RT to neck 10 years earlier for head and neck cancer. (*A*) Sagittal reformatted image from neck CT angiogram shows a long segment stenosis in distal common carotid artery (*white arrow*) extending to carotid bulb (*red arrow*), which is of normal caliber. (*B*) Coronal reformatted image from neck CT angiogram shows stenosis (*arrows*) extending to normal caliber carotid bulb. The location is unusual for atherosclerotic steno-occlusive disease and narrowing believed to be related to prior RT.

role. This is a particular problem in children who are more susceptible and have longer survival after treatment of their initial neoplasm. The latency period is generally many years after initial radiation.[7] In adults meningiomas are the commonest radiation-induced tumor followed by sarcomas and gliomas. In children malignant gliomas are more common followed by meningiomas, low-grade astrocytomas, and sarcomas.[54,55] The imaging appearance of these tumors does not differ from those not associated with radiation. However, radiation-induced meningiomas are more likely to be atypical or anaplastic, occur in younger patients, have a more equal gender distribution, and have a tendency for multiplicity and recurrence than those that are not radiation-induced (**Fig. 9**).[56]

CHEMOTHERAPY-INDUCED CENTRAL NERVOUS SYSTEM COMPLICATIONS

Compared with radiation-induced CNS complications, the neurotoxic effects of chemotherapy are less well-characterized, but are increasingly being recognized.

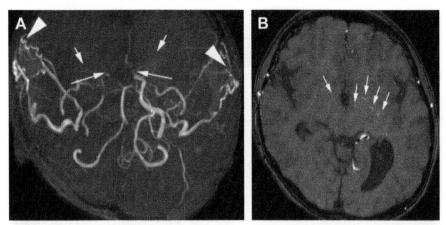

Fig. 7. Radiation arteritis with moyamoya disease. A 15-year-old boy treated with resection and RT for a posterior fossa ependymoma diagnosed at age 11 months. (*A*) Maximum intensity projection image from an MR angiogram of the head shows stenosis and occlusion of distal internal carotid arteries (*long arrows*) with multiple small moyamoya collaterals (*short arrows*). Findings were believed secondary to prior RT. The patient had undergone bilateral encephaloduroarteriomyosynangiosis for the occlusions (*arrowheads*). (*B*) Axial MRA source image shows the multiple small collaterals in cross-section (*arrows*).

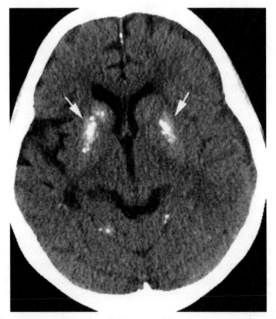

Fig. 8. Mineralizing microangiopathy. A 19-year-old woman treated with surgery, chemotherapy, and craniospinal RT at age 4 years for a right frontal primitive neuroectodermal tumor. Axial CT image shows multiple calcifications in the basal ganglia (*white arrows*) and additional calcifications in the cerebellum (*red arrows*) compatible with mineralizing microangiopathy.

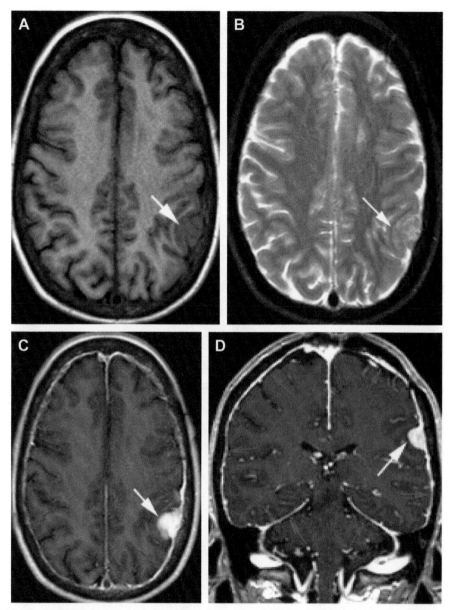

Fig. 9. Radiation-induced meningiomas. A 50-year-old woman diagnosed at age 19 years with a medulloblastoma that was treated with surgery and craniospinal RT. (*A*) Axial T1-weighted precontrast image shows an isointense, extra-axial, dural-based mass in left parietal region (*arrow*). (*B*) Axial T2-weighted image shows mass is isointense to brain parenchyma (*arrow*). (*C*) Axial T1-weighted postcontrast image shows mass homogeneously enhancing (*white arrow*). There is more diffuse dural enhancement (*red arrows*). (*D*) Coronal T1-weighted postcontrast image shows an additional mass over left temporal convexity (*white arrow*) with diffuse dural enhancement again seen (*red arrows*). Masses compatible with radiation-induced meningiomas. Diffuse dural enhancement is also a common post-treatment finding.

The toxicity of a given drug depends on a variety of factors including total dose, route of administration, interactions with other drugs, presence of structural brain lesions, exposure to prior or concurrent RT, and individual patient vulnerability.[1,57] Toxicity may be related to direct injury to neurons or glia or indirectly, such as with a coagulopathy or metabolic disturbances.[1,3] Toxicity may occur acutely, during or shortly

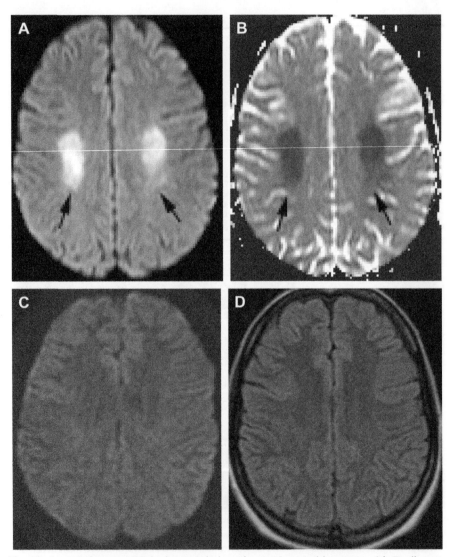

Fig. 10. Acute/subacute MTX leukoencephalopathy. A 16-year-old woman with T-cell acute lymphoblastic leukemia who developed left-sided weakness and numbness, dysarthria, and incoordination 12 days after receiving intravenous and intrathecal MTX. (*A*) Axial diffusion-weighted image shows oval areas of high signal in bilateral centrum semiovale (*arrows*). (*B*) Axial apparent diffusion coefficient image shows corresponding areas of hypointense signal (*arrows*). Findings compatible with areas of restricted diffusion from MTX. (*C*) Follow-up axial diffusion-weighted image shows resolution of abnormal signal. (*D*) Axial FLAIR image from follow-up MRI shows no residual signal abnormalities.

after administration of chemotherapeutic agent, or in a delayed manner and may occur following systemic or intrathecal chemotherapy. Clinical neurotoxic syndromes do not always correlate well with findings on neuroimaging studies.[1,3,6]

Multiple chemotherapeutic agents can cause a leukoencephalopathy, either alone or in combination with RT.[1,2,4,6,58] Methotrexate (MTX) is one of the most common and well-documented agents causing a leukoencephalopathy, occurring in approximately 10% of patients after systemic therapy and up to 40% after intrathecal administration.[59] Neurotoxicity related to MTX is acute, subacute, or chronic. Acutely and subacutely, patients most commonly experience a chemical meningitis. Less frequently they present with somnolence, confusion, seizures, encephalopathy, and focal neurologic deficits, the latter of which may mimic a stroke.[2,57,59] Risk factors for MTX neurotoxicity include high-dose treatment, intrathecal administration, young age, and associated cranial RT. Areas of restricted diffusion have been reported in patients with acute and subacute MTX toxicity. These changes are often in the white matter of the centrum semiovale and round to oval in shape. The symptoms and imaging changes are often transient, although some white matter abnormalities may persist, appearing as areas of increased signal on T2-weighted and FLAIR images on follow-up imaging (**Fig. 10**).[60,61] A chronic leukoencephalopathy can develop months to years after intravenous or intrathecal MTX. Patients usually develop mild to moderate neurocognitive deficits, although in extreme cases dementia can occur. Pathology in chronic cases reveals necrosis and demyelination.[2] Diffuse, symmetric white matter abnormalities of high signal on T2-weighted and FLAIR images, often sparing the subcortical fibers, are typical MRI findings (**Fig. 11**). There may be associated brain volume loss. Mass effect and enhancement may be present.[4,6,57,62,63]

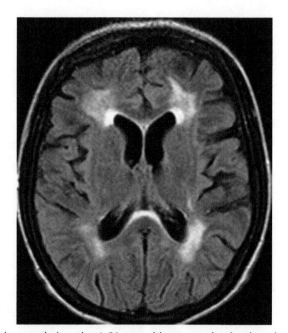

Fig. 11. MTX leukoencephalopathy. A 64-year-old woman who developed progressive white matter changes following MTX-based treatment of lymphoblastic lymphoma with involvement of the cerebrospinal fluid. Axial FLAIR image shows fairly symmetric signal hyperintensities in the periventricular and deep white matter (*arrows*).

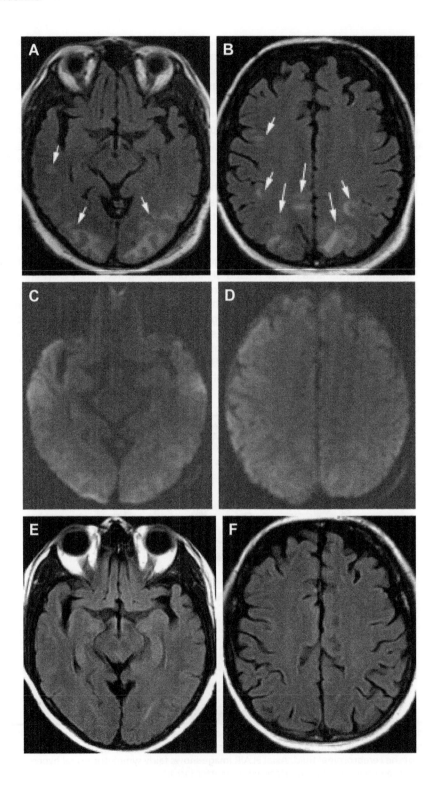

Posterior reversible encephalopathy syndrome has been associated with many chemotherapeutic agents. Common symptoms are headache, confusion, visual changes including cortical blindness, and seizures. The symptom onset is variable but usually shortly after treatment with the offending agent.[1,4,64] The cause of posterior reversible encephalopathy syndrome is uncertain, but thought to be related to failure of autoregulation of cerebral blood pressure and/or endothelial dysfunction resulting in breakdown of the blood-brain barrier and vasogenic edema.[65,66] Typical MRI findings include areas of T2 and FLAIR prolongation in the subcortical white matter and cortex, often in the parietal, occipital, and posterior temporal lobes. There is usually no restricted diffusion, supporting the hypothesis that changes are related to vasogenic edema. Less commonly abnormalities may be seen in the frontal lobes, deep white matter, basal ganglia, brainstem, and cerebellum. Areas of restricted diffusion, hemorrhage, and enhancement are uncommon. In most patients the imaging findings and symptoms resolve with discontinuation of the causative agent and control of blood pressure (**Fig. 12**). Hemorrhage and restricted diffusion is associated with a worse outcome.[6,67,68]

Cerebrovascular disease, including ischemic stroke, cerebral venous sinus thrombosis, and intracranial hemorrhage, is associated with a variety of antineoplastic agents. The exact mechanism that results in ischemic stroke is unknown.[69–73] Newer antiangiogenic agents used to target vascular endothelial growth factor and its receptor, such as bevacizumab (Avastinn), sunitinib (Sutent), and sorafenib (Nexavar), have an increased risk of intracranial hemorrhage, including intratumoral hemorrhage.[74–78] Finally, L-asparaginase, used to treat acute lymphoblastic leukemia, is associated with coagulation defects and can lead to venous sinus thrombosis.[79,80] The symptoms of these cerebrovascular complications are variable depending on the part of the brain affected. The imaging findings in these cerebrovascular complications are the same as those in the general population (**Figs. 13** and **14**).

A cerebellar syndrome can occur in up to 10% to 20% of patients undergoing systemic treatment with cytosine arabinoside (ara-C; Cytosar-U or Depocyt). Patients present with ataxia, dysmetria, gait imbalance, and nystagmus. Ara-C is directly toxic to the Purkinje cells of the cerebellum. Most patients recover when the drug is discontinued. Imaging is usually normal initially with cerebellar atrophy developing months after treatment (**Fig. 15**). Fluoruracil can also cause a cerebellar syndrome.[81–83]

Patients receiving intrathecal chemotherapy, including MTX and ara-C, can develop a myelopathy. Patients typically present with low-back pain and Lhermitte sign, followed by ascending flaccid paraparesis, sensory deficits, and sphincter dysfunction. Cessation of chemotherapy is generally indicated and most patients recover completely.[84] Imaging may initially be normal; however, reported MRI findings include cord swelling, areas of spinal cord hyperintensity on T2-weighted images, and cord enhancement. Over time atrophy of the cord may develop.[85–88] In children receiving

◀──

Fig. 12. Posterior reversible encephalopathy syndrome. A 58-year-old man with diffuse large B-cell lymphoma who presented with a seizure 9 days following intrathecal MTX and 7 days following start of first cycle of R-CHOP. (A) Axial FLAIR image shows foci of increased signal in subcortical white matter of right posterior temporal and bilateral occipital lobes (*arrows*). (B) More superior axial FLAIR image shows similar signal changes in subcortical white matter of posterior frontal and parietal lobes (*short arrows*) with some cortical involvement (*long arrows*). (C, D) Corresponding axial diffusion-weighted images show no foci of restricted diffusion. (E, F) Follow-up axial FLAIR images show signal changes have completely resolved.

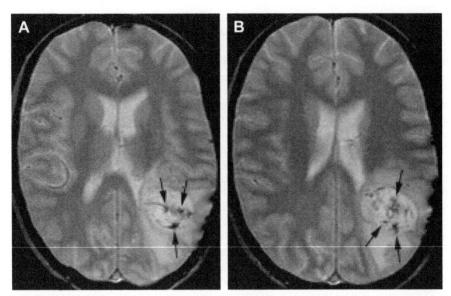

Fig. 13. Bevacizumab-related intratumoral hemorrhage. A 20-year-old woman with left tempoparietal oligoastrocytoma with multiple recurrences being treated with bevacizumab. (*A, B*) Axial gradient-echo T2-weighted images show foci of hypointense signal (*arrows*) within the mass concerning for new areas of hemorrhage.

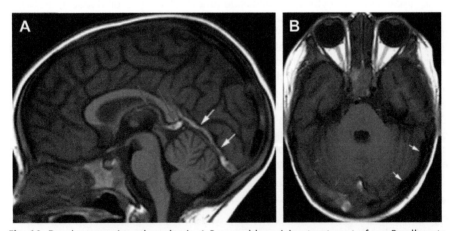

Fig. 14. Dural venous sinus thrombosis. A 2 year old receiving treatment of pre-B-cell acute lymphoblastic leukemia, including pegasparaginase. (*A*) Sagittal T1-weighted precontrast image shows increased signal with loss of normal flow void in the internal cerebral vein (*short red arrow*), vein of Galen (*long red arrow*), and straight sinus (*white arrows*). (*B*) Axial T1-weighted precontrast image shows increased signal with loss of normal flow void in the right transverse sinus (*red arrows*). Normal flow void is seen in the left transverse sinus (*white arrows*). Dural venous sinus thrombosis was attributed to the pegasparaginase treatment.

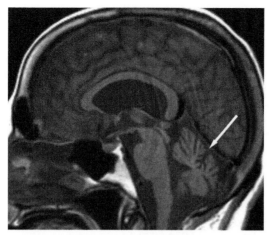

Fig. 15. Cerebellar atrophy. A 62-year-old woman with acute myelomonocytic leukemia who developed ataxia and dysarthria following first cycle of chemotherapy, which included ara-C. MRI obtained 3 years later. Sagittal T1-weighted precontrast image shows cerebellar volume loss (*arrow*) with prominence of surrounding cerebrospinal fluid (CSF) spaces and fourth ventricle. Findings compatible with toxicity related to ara-C.

intrathecal MTX a lumbar polyradiculopathy has been described with progressive weakness of the lower extremities, neurogenic bladder dysfunction, and minor sensory deficits. The outcome is variable. MRI findings consist of enhancement of the ventral lumbosacral nerve roots.[61,89,90]

SUMMARY

Traditional and newer agents used to treat cancer can cause significant toxicity to the CNS. MRI of the brain and spine is the imaging modality of choice for patients with cancer who develop neurologic symptoms. It is important to be aware of the agents that can cause neurotoxicity and their associated imaging findings so that patients are properly diagnosed and treated. It some instances conventional MRI may not be able to differentiate posttreatment effects from disease progression. In these instances advanced imaging techniques may be helpful, although further research is still needed.

REFERENCES

1. Stone JB, DeAngelis LM. Cancer-treatment-induced neurotoxicity: focus on newer treatments. Nat Rev Clin Oncol 2015. http://dx.doi.org/10.1038/nrclinonc. 2015.152.
2. Yust-Katz S, Gilbert MR. Neurologic complications. In: Neiderhuber JE, Armitage JO, Doroshow JH, et al, editors. Abeloff's clinical oncology. 5th edition. Philadelphia: Elsevier; 2014. p. 822–44.
3. Magge RS, DeAngelis LM. The double-edged sword; neurotoxicity of chemotherapy. Blood Rev 2015;29:93–100.
4. Nolan CP, DeAngelis LM. Neurologic complications of chemotherapy and radiation therapy. Continuum (Minneap Minn) 2015;21:429–51.
5. Rogers LR. Neurologic complications of radiation. Continuum (Minneap Minn) 2012;18:343–54.

6. Arrillaga-Romany IC, Dietrich J. Imaging findings in cancer therapy-associated neurotoxicity. Semin Neurol 2012;32:476–86.

7. DeAngelis LM, Posner JP. Side effects of radiation therapy. In: Neurologic complications of cancer. New York: Oxford University Press; 2009. p. 511–55.

8. Walker AJ, Ruzevick J, Malayeri AA, et al. Postradiation imaging changes in the CNS: how can we differentiate between treatment effect and disease progression? Future Oncol 2014;10:1277–97.

9. Ruben JD, Dally M, Bailey M, et al. Cerebral radiation necrosis: incidence, outcomes, and risk factors with emphasis on radiation parameters and chemotherapy. Int J Radiat Oncol Biol Phys 2006;65:499–508.

10. Valk PE, Dillon WP. Radiation injury of the brain. AJNR Am J Neuroradiol 1991;12: 45–62.

11. Cross NE, Glantz MJ. Neurologic complications of radiation therapy. Neurol Clin 2003;21:249–77.

12. Soussain C, Ricard D, Fike JR, et al. CNS complications of radiotherapy and chemotherapy. Lancet 2009;374:1639–51.

13. Pena LA, Fuks Z, Kolesnick RN. Radiation-induced apoptosis of endothelial cells in the murine central nervous system: protection by fibroblast growth factor and sphingomyelinase deficiency. Cancer Res 2000;60:321–7.

14. Nordal RA, Wong CS. Molecular targets in radiation-induced blood-brain barrier disruption. Int J Radiat Oncol Biol Phys 2005;62:279–87.

15. Young DF, Posner JB, Chu F, et al. Rapid-course radiation therapy of cerebral metastases: results and complications. Cancer 1974;34:1069–76.

16. Wiesmann M. Hemorrhagic vascular pathologies, II. In: Hodler J, von Schulthess GK, Zollikofer CL, editors. Diseases of the brain, head and neck, spine 2012-2015. Diagnostic imaging and interventional techniques. Milan (Italy): Springer-Verlag Italia; 2012. p. 48–57.

17. Brandsma D, Staplers L, Taal W, et al. Clinical features, mechanisms, and management of pseudoprogression in malignant gliomas. Lancet Oncol 2008;9: 453–61.

18. Wante K, Hager B, Heier M, et al. Reversible oedema and necrosis after irradiation of the brain. Diagnostic procedures and clinical manifestations. Acta Oncol 1990;29:891–5.

19. Kruser TJ, Mehta MP, Robins HI. Pseudoprogression after glioma therapy: a comprehensive review. Expert Rev Neurother 2013;13:389–403.

20. Brandes AA, Franceschi E, Tosoni A, et al. MGMT promoter methylation status can predict the incidence and outcome of pseudoprogression after concomitant radiochemotherapy in newly diagnosed glioblastoma patients. J Clin Oncol 2008; 26:2192–7.

21. Taal W, Brandsma D, de Bruin HG, et al. Incidence of early pseudo-progression in a cohort of malignant glioma patients treated with chemoirradiation with temozolomide. Cancer 2008;113:405–10.

22. Chamberlain MC, Glantz MJ, Chalmers L, et al. Early necrosis following concurrent temodar and radiotherapy in patients with glioblastoma. J Neurooncol 2007; 82:81–3.

23. Young RJ, Gupta A, Shah AD, et al. Potential utility of conventional MRI signs in diagnosing pseudoprogression in glioblastoma. Neurology 2011;76:1918–24.

24. Hein PA, Eskey CJ, Dunn JF, et al. Diffusion-weighted imaging in the follow-up of treated high-grade gliomas: tumor recurrence versus radiation injury. AJNR Am J Neuroradiol 2004;25:201–9.

25. Asao C, Korogi Y, Kitajima M, et al. Diffusion-weighted imaging of radiation induced brain injury for differentiation from tumor recurrence. AJNR Am J Neuroradiol 2005;26:1455–60.

26. Al Sayyari A, Buckley R, McHenery C, et al. Distinguishing recurrent primary brain tumor from radiation injury: a preliminary study using a susceptibility-weighted MR imaging-guided apparent diffusion coefficient analysis strategy. AJNR Am J Neuroradiol 2010;31:1049–54.

27. Kong DS, Kim ST, Kim EH, et al. Diagnostic dilemma of pseudoprogression in the treatment of newly diagnosed glioblastomas: the role of assessing relative cerebral blood flow volume and oxygen-6-methylguanine- DNA methyltransferase promoter methylation status. AJNR Am J Neuroradiol 2011;32:382–7.

28. Hu LS, Baxter LC, Smith KA, et al. Relative cerebral blood volume values to differentiate high-grade glioma recurrence from posttreatment radiation effect: direct correlation between image-guided tissue histopathology and localized dynamic susceptibility-weighted contrast-enhanced perfusion MR imaging measurements. AJNR Am J Neuroradiol 2009;30:552–8.

29. Gahramanov S, Raslan AM, Muldoon LL, et al. Potential for differentiation of pseudoprogression from true tumor progression with dynamic susceptibility weighted contrast-enhanced magnetic resonance imaging using ferumoxytol vs. gadoteridol: a pilot study. Int J Radiat Oncol Biol Phys 2011;79:514–23.

30. Weybright P, Sundgren PC, Maly P, et al. Differentiation between brain tumor recurrence and radiation injury using MR spectroscopy. AJR Am J Roentgenol 2005;185:1471–6.

31. Zeng QS, Li CF, Zhang K, et al. Multivoxel 3D proton MR spectroscopy in the distinction of recurrent glioma from radiation injury. J Neurooncol 2007;84:63–9.

32. Patel TR, McHugh BJ, Bi WL, et al. A comprehensive review of MR imaging changes following radiosurgery to 500 brain metastases. AJNR Am J Neuroradiol 2011;32:1885–92.

33. Stockham AL, Tievsky AL, Koyfman SA. Conventional MRI does not reliably distinguish radiation necrosis form tumor recurrence after stereotactic radiosurgery. J Neurooncol 2012;109:149–58.

34. Greene-Schloesser D, Robbins ME, Peiffer AM, et al. Radiation-induced brain injury: a review. Front Oncol 2012;2:73.

35. Yoshii Y. Pathological review of late cerebral radionecrosis. Brain Tumor Pathol 2008;25:51–8.

36. Pruzincova L, Steno J, Srbecky M, et al. MR imaging of late radiation therapy- and chemotherapy-induced injury: a pictorial essay. Eur Radiol 2009;19:2716–27.

37. Rabin BM, Meyer JR, Berlin JW, et al. Radiation-induced changes in the central nervous system and head and neck. Radiographics 1996;16:1055–72.

38. Wang YX, King AD, Zhou H, et al. Evolution of radiation-induced brain injury: MR imaging-based study. Radiology 2010;254:210–8.

39. Kumar AJ, Leeds NE, Fuller GN. Malignant gliomas: MR imaging spectrum of radiation therapy- and chemotherapy-induced necrosis of the brain after treatment. Radiology 2000;217:377–84.

40. Douw L, Klein M, Fagel SS, et al. Cognitive and radiologic effects of radiotherapy in patients with low-grade glioma: long-term follow-up. Lancet Neurol 2009;8:810–8.

41. Michele M. Cranial radiation therapy and damage to hippocampal neurogenesis. Dev Disabil Res Rev 2008;14:238–42.

42. Wassenberg MW, Bromberg JE, Witkamp TD, et al. White matter lesions and encephalopathy in patients treated for primary central nervous system lymphoma. J Neurooncol 2001;52:73–80.

43. Wong CS, Fehlings MG, Sahgal A. Pathobiology of radiation myelopathy and strategies to mitigate injury. Spinal Cord 2015;53:574–80.

44. Okada S, Okeda R. Pathology of radiation myelopathy. Neuropathology 2001;21: 247–65.

45. Wang PY, Shen WC, Jan JS. Serial MRI changes in radiation myelopathy. Neuroradiology 1995;37:374–7.

46. Nimjee AM, Powers CJ, Bulsara KR. Review of the literature on de novo formation of cavernous malformations on the central nervous system after radiation therapy. Neurosurg Focus 2006;21:1–6.

47. Kolke S, Alda N, Hata M, et al. Asymptomatic radiation-induced telangiectasia in children after cranial irradiation: frequency, latency and dose relation. Radiology 2004;230:93–9.

48. Gaensler EHL, Dillon WP, Edwards MSB, et al. Radiation-induced telangiectasia in the brain simulates cryptic vascular malformations at MR imaging. Radiology 1994;193:629–36.

49. Chan MSM, Roebuck DJ, Yuen MP, et al. MR imaging of the brain in patients cured of acute lymphoblastic leukemia: the value of gradient echo imaging. AJNR Am J Neuroradiol 2006;27:548–52.

50. Fajardo LF. Basic mechanisms and general morphology of radiation injury. Semin Roentgenol 1993;28:297–302.

51. Brant-Zawadski M, Anderson M, DeArmond SJ. Radiation-induced large intracranial vessel occlusive vasculopathy. AJR Am J Roentgenol 1980;135:263–7.

52. Lam WW, Leung SF, So NM, et al. Incidence of carotid stenosis in nasopharyngeal cancer patients after radiotherapy. Cancer 2001;92:2357–63.

53. Shichita T, Ogata T, Yasaka M, et al. Angiographic characteristics of radiation-induced carotid stenosis. Angiology 2009;60:276–82.

54. Nishio S, Morioka T, Inamura T, et al. Radiation-induced brain tumors: potential late complications of radiation therapy for brain tumors. Acta Neurochir (Wien) 1998;140:763–70.

55. Pettorini BL, Park YS, Caldarelli M, et al. Radiation-induced brain tumors after central nervous system irradiation in childhood: a review. Childs Nerv Syst 2008;24:793–805.

56. Harrison MJ, Wolfe DE, Tai-Shang L, et al. Radiation-induced meningiomas: experience at Mount Sinai Hospital and review of the literature. J Neurosurg 1991;75:564–74.

57. Soffietti R, Trevisan E, Ruda R. Neurologic complications of chemotherapy and other newer and experimental approaches. Handb Clin Neurol 2014;121: 1199–218.

58. DeAngelis LM, Posner JP. Side effects of chemotherapy. In: Neurologic complications of cancer. New York: Oxford University Press; 2009. p. 447–510.

59. Mahoney DH Jr, Shuster JJ, Nitchke R, et al. Acute neurotoxicity in children with B-precursor acute lymphoid leukemia: an association with intermediate-dose intravenous methotrexate and intrathecal triple therapy. A Pediatric Oncology Group study. J Clin Oncol 1998;16:1712–22.

60. Rollins N, Winick N, Bash R, et al. Acute methotrexate toxicity: findings on diffusion-weighted imaging and correlation with clinical outcome. AJNR Am J Neuroradiol 2004;25:1688–95.

61. Vazquez E, Delgado I, Sanchez-Montanez A, et al. Side effects of oncologic therapies in the pediatric central nervous system: update on neuroimaging findings. Radiographics 2011;31:1123–39.

62. Ohmoto YY, Kajiwara KK, Kato SS, et al. Atypical MRI findings in treatment-related leukoencephalopathy: case report. Neuroradiology 1996;38:128–33.

63. Oka M, Terae S, Kobayashi R, et al. MRI in methotrexate-related leukoencephalopathy: disseminated necrotizing leukoencephalopathy in comparison with mild leukoencephalopathy. Neuroradiology 2003;45:493–7.

64. Marinella MA, Markert RJ. Reversible posterior leukoencephalopathy syndrome associated with anticancer drugs. Intern Med J 2009;39:826–34.

65. Bartynski WS. Posterior reversible encephalopathy syndrome, part 2: controversies surrounding pathophysiology of vasogenic edema. AJNR Am J Neuroradiol 2008;29:1043–9.

66. Marra A, Vargas M, Striano P, et al. Posterior reversible encephalopathy syndrome: the endothelial hypothesis. Med Hypotheses 2014;82:619–22.

67. Bartynski WS. Posterior reversible encephalopathy syndrome, part 1; fundamental imaging and clinical features. AJNR Am J Neuroradiol 2008;29:1036–42.

68. McKinney AM, Short J, Truwit CL, et al. Posterior reversible encephalopathy syndrome: incidence of atypical regions of involvement and imaging findings. AJR Am J Roentgenol 2007;189:904–12.

69. Grisold W, Oberndorfer S, Struhal W. Stroke and cancer: a review. Acta Neurol Scand 2009;119:1–16.

70. Rogers LR. Cerebrovascular complications in patients with cancer. Semin Neurol 2004;24:453–60.

71. Lee EQ, Arrillaga-Romany IC, Wen PY. Neurologic complications of cancer drug therapies. Continuum 2012;18:355–65.

72. Schutz FA, Je Y, Azzi GR, et al. Bevacizumab increases the risk of arterial ischemia: a large study in cancer patients with a focus on different subgroup outcomes. Ann Oncol 2011;22:1404–12.

73. Fraum TJ, Kreisl TN, Sul J, et al. Ischemic stroke and intracranial hemorrhage in glioma patients on antiangiogenic therapy. J Neurooncol 2011;105:281–9.

74. Yang JC, Haworth L, Sherry RM, et al. A randomized trial of bevacizumab, an anti-vascular endothelial growth factor antibody, for metastatic renal cancer. N Engl J Med 2003;349:427–34.

75. Gordon MS, Margolin K, Talpaz M, et al. Phase I safety and pharmacokinetic study of recombinant human anti-vascular endothelial growth factor in patients with advanced cancer. J Clin Oncol 2001;19:843–50.

76. Johnson DH, Fehrenbacher L, Novotny WF, et al. Randomized phase II trial comparing bevacizumab plus carboplatin and paclitaxel with carboplatin and paclitaxel alone in previously untreated locally advanced or metastatic non-small-cell lung cancer. J Clin Oncol 2004;22:2184–91.

77. Carden CP, Larkin JM, Rosenthal MA. What is the risk of intracranial bleeding during anti-VEGF therapy? Neuro-oncol 2008;10:624–30.

78. Norden AD, Drappatz J, Wen PY. Antiangiogenic therapies for high grade glioma. Nat Rev Neurol 2009;5:610–20.

79. Kieslich M, Porto L, Lanfermann H, et al. Cerebrovascular complications of L-asparaginase in the therapy of acute lymphoblastic leukemia. J Pediatr Hematol Oncol 2003;25:484–7.

80. Feinberg WM, Swenson MR. Cerebrovascular complications of L-asparaginase therapy. Neurology 1988;38:127–33.

81. Baker WJ, Royer GL Jr, Weiss RB. Cytarabine and neurologic toxicity. J Clin Oncol 1991;9:679–93.
82. Winkelman MD, Hines JD. Cerebellar degeneration caused by high dose cytosine arabinoside: a clinicopathological study. Ann Neurol 1983;14:520–7.
83. Pirzada NA, Ali II, Dafer RM. Fluorouracil-induced neurotoxicity. Ann Pharmacother 2000;34:35–8.
84. Watterson J, Toogood I, Nieder M, et al. Excessive spinal cord toxicity from intensive central nervous system-directed therapies. Cancer 1994;74:3034–41.
85. Sherman PM, Belden CJ, Nelson DA. Magnetic resonance imaging findings in a case of cytarabine-induced myelopathy. Mil Med 2002;167:157–60.
86. Garcia-Tena J, Lopez-Andreu J, Menor F, et al. Intrathecal chemotherapy-related myeloencephalopathy in a young child with acute lymphoblastic leukemia. Pediatr Hematol Oncol 1995;12:377–85.
87. McLean DR, Clink HM, Ernst P, et al. Myelopathy after intrathecal chemotherapy: a case report with unique magnetic resonance imaging changes. Cancer 1994; 73:3037–40.
88. Counsel P, Khangure M. Myelopathy due to intrathecal chemotherapy: magnetic resonance imaging findings. Clin Radiol 2007;62:172–6.
89. Rolf N, Boehm H, Kaindl AM, et al. Acute ascending motoric paraplegia following intrathecal chemotherapy for treatment of acute lymphoblastic leukemia in children: case reports and review of the literature. Klin Padiatr 2006;218:350–4.
90. Koh S, Nelson M, Kovanlikaya A, et al. Anterior lumbosacral radiculopathy after intrathecal methotrexate treatment. Pediatr Neurol 1999;21:576–8.

Imaging of Spinal Manifestations of Hematological Disorders

Puneet S. Pawha, MD[a], Falgun H. Chokshi, MD, MS[b],*

KEYWORDS

- Vertebral • Epidural • Cord • Meninges • Lymphoma • Leukemia • Myeloma
- Hematological

KEY POINTS

- Imaging manifestations of hematological diseases and their potential complications are broad, and there may be significant overlap in features of various disease processes.
- Knowledge of appropriate choice of imaging test, pertinent imaging patterns, and pathophysiology of disease can help the reader increase specificity in the diagnosis and treatment of the patient.
- Most importantly, we encourage readers of this review to engage their radiologists during the diagnostic, treatment, and management phases of care delivery.

INTRODUCTION

The imaging of spinal manifestations of hematological disorders are best understood and appreciated by taking an anatomic compartment approach. In this review, we discuss such manifestations by focusing on the imaging appearance in the vertebral body/epidural, dural/leptomeningeal (meningeal), and spinal cord compartments. This review focuses on radiographic imaging, computed tomography (CT), and MRI, and will predominantly discuss vertebral and epidural disease. Where appropriate, details about meningeal and spinal cord involvement are included.

GENERAL IMAGING FEATURES
Vertebral/Epidural Disease

Compared with spinal metastatic disease, hematopoietic malignancies are more likely to be diffuse and less likely to have cortical destruction.[1] As such, MRI is often superior

Disclosures: F.H. Chokshi is an AUR GERRAF Fellow, 2015 to 2017. This work was supported (in part) by an AUR GE Radiology Research Academic Fellowship Award. P.S. Pawha (None).
[a] Department of Radiology, The Mount Sinai Hospital, Icahn School of Medicine at Mount Sinai, New York, NY 10029, USA; [b] Division of Neuroradiology, Department of Radiology & Imaging Sciences, Emory University School of Medicine, 1364 Clifton Road Northeast, Atlanta, GA 30322, USA
* Corresponding author.
E-mail address: falgun.chokshi@emory.edu

Hematol Oncol Clin N Am 30 (2016) 921–944
http://dx.doi.org/10.1016/j.hoc.2016.03.011
hemonc.theclinics.com

to radiography and CT, particularly in visualizing bony lesions that are largely in bone marrow. It is worthwhile discussing a few imaging basics, particularly regarding MRI sequences as they apply to vertebral marrow disease.

T1 spin-echo weighted imaging (T1WI) is essential in bone marrow evaluation. Due to the size and tumbling frequency of fat molecules, yellow marrow normally has a hyperintense (bright) appearance on T1WI due to a short T1 relaxation time. In contradistinction, tumor and most other pathologic processes will have prolonged T1 relaxation times producing hypointense (low) signal that typically stands out sharply against the hyperintense background of fatty marrow.

Younger patients have more red hematopoietic marrow than yellow marrow, making visualization of lesions on T1WI more challenging. Fat suppression should *not* be used for noncontrast T1WI of the marrow, as this will remove the intrinsic contrast. The opposite is true when performing postcontrast T1WI; if fat suppression is not used, enhancing hyperintense lesions will lose their conspicuity against T1 hyperintense marrow. Therefore, fat suppression is essential for postcontrast T1WI when evaluating vertebral disease.

By the same token, routine T2 spin-echo weighted imaging (T2WI) is not ideal for vertebral and epidural evaluation. Pathologic processes are generally hyperintense on T2WI, and can be masked against background T2 signal of normal marrow. For this reason, fat suppression is also essential for T2WI in vertebral and epidural evaluation of the spine. Short tau inversion recovery (STIR) sequences are often used for this purpose, and provide relatively homogeneous fat saturation. Abnormalities on STIR often appear brighter than on routine T2WI, in part due to the change in dynamic range of the image. For this review, however, we use STIR and fat-saturated T2WI interchangeably.

Noncontrast T1WI, fat-suppressed T2WI (or STIR), and postcontrast fat-suppressed T1WI sequences are the bread and butter of vertebral marrow imaging. There are several additional advanced sequences that are touched on later, which can be useful adjuncts, including diffusion-weighted imaging (DWI), chemical shift imaging (CSI), and dynamic contrast-enhanced (DCE)-MRI techniques.

Detection and characterization of an epidural mass is critical in the imaging evaluation of the spine. MRI is generally preferable to CT for this assessment. As an epidural lesion grows larger, it first narrows the thecal sac and effaces the cerebrospinal fluid (CSF) around the cord, then eventually progresses to compress the cord itself, potentially causing cord edema and eventually myelomalacia. At the lumbosacral levels, epidural masses can compress the cauda equina. Epidural extension of vertebral tumor commonly has a bilobed appearance in the anterior epidural space, which has been called the "curtain sign," due to limitation by the posterior longitudinal ligament and attached midline septum.

Posterior epidural masses are seen more commonly in hematologic malignancy compared with metastatic disease.[1] Epidural masses can extend through intervertebral foramina and into the paraspinal regions. Contrast is useful not only in delineating extent of epidural tumor, but also in distinguishing tumor from disc herniation, which may mimic epidural tumor on noncontrast imaging but should not enhance with contrast.

Meningeal and Spinal Cord Disease

MRI is the standard for imaging meningeal and cord manifestations of hematological malignancy and any complications. Fat-saturated T2WI and postcontrast fat-saturated T1WI sequences are essential to evaluate the meninges, thecal sac CSF, spinal cord, and cauda equina. Precontrast T1WI is not vital by itself, but is useful when comparing with postcontrast T1WI if fat saturation was not used. Conventional T2WI (without fat saturation) can complement fat-saturated or STIR images.

Noncontrast CT or CT with intravenous contrast has minimal use in evaluating meningeal and cord disease. CT myelography can be useful in patients having contraindications to MRI. In this technique, iodinated contrast is injected in the thecal sac, usually via lumbar injection.[2] The contrast fills the thecal sac and surrounds the cord and cauda equina, thereby producing an "outline" of these structures and any significant abnormality in their contour. Although CT myelography has some utility in differentiating intramedullary from intradural/extramedullary findings, further characterization of enhancement pattern, intramedullary characteristics, and extradural (outside the dura mater) is extremely limited to not possible.

HEMATOLOGIC MALIGNANCIES
Leukemia

Leukemia is the most common malignancy in children, as well as the ninth most common in adults.[3,4] Acute lymphoblastic leukemia (ALL) and acute myeloid leukemia (AML) subtypes arise from immature leukocytes. Of childhood leukemia cases, approximately 80% are due to ALL and 10% are of the AML subtype.[3] Chronic lymphocytic leukemia and chronic myeloid leukemia (CML) arise from mature cell lines.

Leukemia tends to infiltrate rather than focally replace the bone marrow. A caveat to this is that myeloid leukemias can have focal chloromas, also referred to as granulocytic sarcomas. These occur in 2.5% to 9.1% of patients with AML, and 5 times less commonly in patients with CML, with most younger than 15 years of age.[5] Chloroma may occur before the onset of leukemia and can rarely be multifocal.[6]

Computed tomography and radiography
Vertebral/epidural disease Leukemic infiltration can appear as a permeative or mottled bone marrow appearance, which may be diffuse or regional. Lucent bands ("leukemic lines"), periosteal reactions, and subperiosteal erosions may be seen, although less commonly than in the appendicular skeleton. After treatment, lucent lines generally resolve quickly, whereas other CT and plain film findings may lag or persist.

Focal abnormality may not be evident on plain film or CT, and in many cases only diffuse osteopenia or a normal appearance is seen. Sclerotic foci are rare, and more likely to be encountered after treatment. Vertebral compression fractures are commonly seen (**Fig. 1**). Vertebra plana, complete collapse of a vertebral body, is also occasionally encountered. Chloromas present as focal lytic lesions, with any extraosseous soft tissue components well depicted on CT.

Meningeal/spinal cord disease CT is very poor for evaluation of meningeal and spinal cord disease. MRI is the study of choice and is discussed as follows.

MRI
Vertebral/epidural disease On T1WI sequences, leukemic infiltration of bone marrow often manifests as diffuse homogeneous or speckled T1 hypointensity, and can sometimes be more regional. There is corresponding hyperintensity on STIR sequences, which can vary in intensity and conspicuity. Leukemic lesions enhance on postcontrast T1WI, albeit with high variability.

Approximately 10% of cases will have a normal MRI appearance.[7] In pediatric patients in whom there is a greater fraction of hematopoietic cells, the normal marrow signal may be intermediate to low signal on T1WI. In these cases, detection of leukemic infiltrate can be challenging. Various quantitative MR techniques have

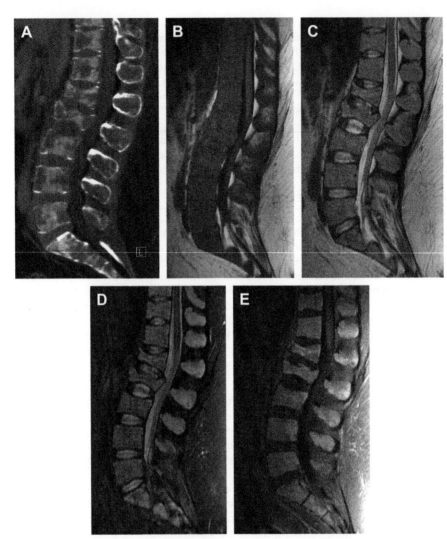

Fig. 1. ALL. CT (*A*) demonstrates a diffuse mixed sclerotic and lytic appearance. There are multiple pathologic compression fractures, most pronounced at L1 and L2. Sagittal T1-weighted MRI (*B*) shows diffusely low signal throughout the marrow. T2WI (*C*) best demonstrates the bony retropulsion at L2 and associated moderate spinal canal narrowing. STIR sequence (*D*) demonstrates subtle diffuse hyperintense signal of the marrow, much better appreciated than on the non–fat-suppressed T2 image (*C*). Subtle patchy marrow enhancement is seen on postcontrast T1WI (*E*).

been described for improving detection, including bulk T1 relaxation measurement and MR spectroscopy.[8–10] CSI also has been used, demonstrating a lower fat fraction within tumor infiltrated marrow. Moore and colleagues[11] demonstrated increased T1 relaxation times in those with active disease. These techniques have been used not only to improve detection, but also to evaluate response to therapy.[12] Early work with DCE-MRI suggests it also may be useful in assessment of disease burden.[13,14]

Chloromas appear as focal T1WI isointense and STIR hyperintense mass lesions. Enhancement is typically homogeneous, although necrotic foci have been reported.[15] Chloromas can be predominantly epidural in location, sometimes without significant bony involvement. Epidural lesions may extend into neural foramina and the paravertebral region, may have multilevel involvement, and are at high risk for cord compression.

Meningeal/spinal cord disease Although not as common, leukemic involvement of meninges can occur (neoplastic meningitis). The typical pattern on MRI is nodular or diffuse enhancement of the leptomeninges and cauda equina and/or diffuse enhancement of the CSF on fat-saturated postcontrast T1WI. Although this finding is not specific for leukemia, it is highly concerning if the patient has a history of the disease. Moreover, a normal MRI does not exclude neoplastic meningitis because MRI is less than 50% sensitive and specific. Therefore, CSF sampling is still highly specific (>95%) for neoplastic meningitis, but not as sensitive ($\sim$50%).[16] Last, leukemia rarely infiltrates the cord; however, a case report described intramedullary involvement by leukemia presenting as transverse myelopathy.[17]

Polycythemia Vera

Vertebral/epidural disease
Polycythemia vera (PV) is a proliferative disorder of stem cells. The process is panhyperplastic, but typically causes pronounced erythrocytosis. PV typically demonstrates T1WI hypointense and STIR hyperintense signal abnormality diffusely involving the marrow. Some cases can have focal involvement.[18] It is considered a low-grade malignant process, and 15% undergo transformation to AML. The imaging appearance is somewhat nonspecific among hematologic disorders, and cannot distinguish which cases have undergone myeloid metaplasia. Many cases eventually progress to myelofibrosis.[7]

Lymphoma

Primary vertebral lymphoma is rare; however, lymphoma metastases to the spine are relatively common, found in 40% of patients with lymphoma in one autopsy series.[19] Bony involvement usually occurs during the course of disease and is uncommon at presentation. Vertebral and epidural involvement is typically seen in advanced disseminated disease. Non-Hodgkin lymphoma (NHL) is 3 times as common as Hodgkin disease,[20] and, accordingly, spinal involvement is more frequently encountered in NHL. In Hodgkin disease, vertebral involvement can occur with extranodal stage IV disease. Bony involvement can occur from local or hematogenous spread, and is typically only seen in late-stage widespread disease. When bony involvement does occur, it is commonly spinal.

Computed tomography and radiography
Vertebral/epidural disease Commonly, a permeative, or "moth-eaten" pattern is seen. Focal lesions may be lytic, sclerotic, or mixed. Sclerotic lesions are somewhat more common in Hodgkin disease. An "ivory vertebra" appearance can be seen on radiographs or CT, a name given to diffuse, relatively homogeneous sclerosis of a vertebral body. A lamellated pattern of periosteal reaction can be seen, more commonly with HD. NHL can rarely have an appearance overlapping with that of multiple myeloma, with multiple focal lytic lesions.[21]

Meningeal/spinal cord disease CT is very poor for evaluation of meningeal and spinal cord disease. MRI is the study of choice and is discussed as follows.

MRI

Vertebral/epidural disease Lymphoma lesions demonstrate focal hypointense signal on T1WI. Lymphoma is more likely to focally replace rather than infiltrate the marrow, as opposed to leukemia. It is often not possible to distinguish the lesions from metastatic disease based solely on MRI features. The lesions enhance on postcontrast T1WI (**Fig. 2**). The lesions may demonstrate isointense to mildly hypointense T2WI signal as well as restricted water diffusion on DWI, reflecting hypercellularity.

When involvement is relatively diffuse, there can be overlap in the appearance of neoplastic and non-neoplastic marrow processes. Some initial work with DCE imaging has demonstrated increased perfusion parameters in cases of diffuse tumor,[22] with a potential to differentiate these from benign disorders.

The "wrap-around sign" of vertebral lymphoma describes the appearance of diffuse vertebral involvement, circumferential paravertebral involvement, and preserved depiction of the intervening vertebral cortex. This sign is useful in differentiating patients with lymphoma, from those with other metastatic disease and multiple myeloma.[23]

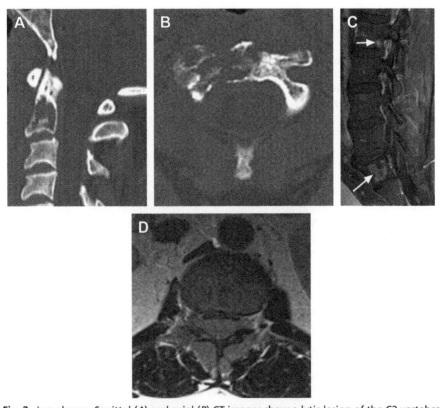

Fig. 2. Lymphoma. Sagittal (*A*) and axial (*B*) CT images show a lytic lesion of the C2 vertebra with areas of cortical destruction. Fat-suppressed postcontrast T1WI (*C*) in a different patient with metastatic NHL shows a discrete homogeneously enhancing marrow replacing lesion in the S1 vertebral body (*long arrow*), as well as a smaller enhancing nodule along the inferior endplate of the L2 vertebra (*short arrow*). Axial T2WI (*D*) from a third patient with NHL demonstrates intermediate signal tumor surrounding the posterior elements, with the epidural tumor component causing severe spinal canal compromise and cord compression.

As with other vertebral tumors, epidural extension can occur with the potential for spinal canal compromise (see **Fig. 2**). Uncommonly, lymphoma may be predominantly epidural without significant vertebral involvement. This may occur by spread from lymph nodes through the intervertebral foramina, and can be seen with both Hodgkin disease and NHL.[20]

Meningeal/spinal cord disease Like leukemia, meningeal involvement of lymphoma can be leptomeningeal (**Fig. 3**). However, dural infiltration can occur both diffusely or focally (masslike). As lymphoma is a great mimicker, its appearance can be heterogeneous and may raise concern for other diseases, such as tuberculosis, sarcoidosis, or metastases from other malignancy. Of note, epidural extramedullary hematopoiesis can be difficult to differentiate from lymphoma, regardless of compartment.[24]

Although rare, intramedullary lymphoma deposits can occur; however, carry a differential diagnosis if a primary diagnosis of lymphoma is not known (**Fig. 4**). This differential diagnosis includes dermoid tumor, astrocytoma, ependymoma, hemangioblastoma, ganglioneuroblastoma, and metastases.[25]

Waldenstrom Macroglobulinemia

Waldenstrom macroglobulinemia (WM) is a type of NHL characterized by infiltration of bone marrow with lymphoplasmacytic cells. It is also considered a plasma cell

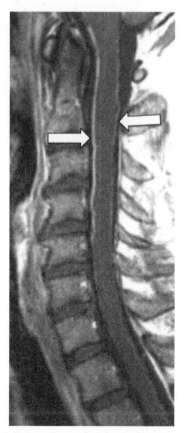

Fig. 3. NHL, leptomeningeal disease. Sagittal T1 postcontrast image shows thin leptomeningeal enhancement (*white arrows*) in this patient with known NHL.

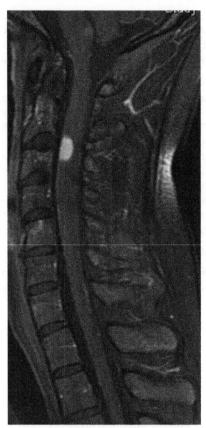

Fig. 4. NHL, spinal cord disease. Postcontrast T1WI shows a well-circumscribed enhancing spinal cord lesion at C2–C3 in this patient with known NHL.

dyscrasia, with monoclonal immunoglobulin M-protein found in serum. Patients also may have lymphadenopathy, organomegaly, and hyperviscosity syndrome among other systemic manifestations. WM is usually an indolent process typically presenting in older patients. Transformation to high-grade lymphoma can occur.[26]

Vertebral/epidural disease
On radiography and CT, studies may appear normal or demonstrate generalized osteopenia. Focal lytic lesions are not typically seen, a differentiating factor from myeloma.[27] MRI often demonstrates diffuse homogeneous or variegated marrow signal abnormality, with hypointensity on precontrast T1WI, hyperintensity on STIR, and enhancement on fat-saturated postcontrast T1WI, which may be patchy. On both CT and MRI, lymphadenopathy may be visualized in the included surrounding soft tissues, such as the retroperitoneum **(Fig. 5)**.[28]

Meningeal/spinal cord disease
Leptomeningeal infiltration of WM is exceedingly rare; however, when it occurs is called Bing-Neel syndrome.[29] MRI can show leptomeningeal and/or pachymeningeal enhancement on postcontrast T1WI.[30] Contrast administration is essential for proper imaging and if findings are present in the setting of known WM, Bing-Neel syndrome should be considered.

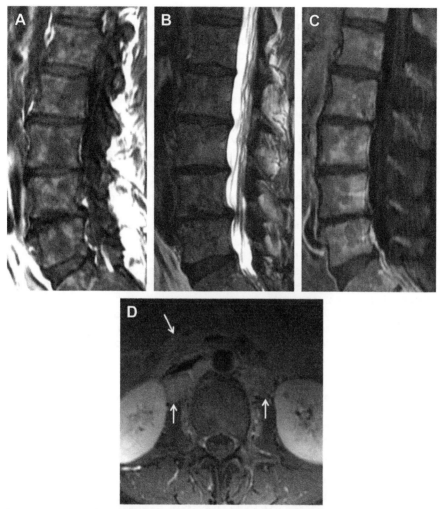

Fig. 5. WM. Sagittal T1WI (*A*) and T2WI (*B*) demonstrate a diffusely heterogeneous signal pattern of the vertebral marrow. Regions of more confluent abnormality are seen to mildly enhance on sagittal postcontrast T1WI (*C*), particularly at L3 and L4. Axial postcontrast image (*D*) demonstrates extensive retroperitoneal lymphadenopathy (*arrows*) including para-aortic and aortocaval regions.

Multiple Myeloma

Multiple myeloma is the most common primary malignancy of bone, and accounts for approximately 10% of hematologic malignancies. Myeloma results from abnormal monoclonal proliferation of plasma cells. It is one of the plasma cell dyscrasias, along with monoclonal gammopathy of unknown site, plasmacytoma, WM, and primary amyloidosis, among others. Myeloma can occur anywhere but does have a predilection for vertebral involvement. Abnormal plasma cells infiltrate the bone marrow in a variety of focal and diffuse patterns.

The International Staging System uses serum Beta^2 microglobulin and albumin to grade disease from I to III. Myeloma also can be characterized from low grade to high grade, according to the percentage of marrow infiltration seen histologically. Durie and Salmon is another commonly used staging scheme, which initially used both plain radiography and clinical/laboratory findings to stage disease from 1 to 3. This system has been adapted to include MRI and FDG-PET findings, both of which are more sensitive for focal lesion detection, termed the Durie-Salmon Plus staging system.[31,32]

Meningeal and spinal cord involvement by multiple myeloma is rare and presents only in the most advanced disseminated cases of this disease. No specific imaging pattern is noted. The following discussion pertains to vertebral/epidural disease.

Computed tomography and radiography

Findings vary from diffuse abnormalities, such as generalized osteopenia or a permeative appearance, to discrete focal lesions. Permeative involvement can be geographic or more diffuse. Focal lesions are generally purely lytic. The abnormal plasma cells strongly stimulate osteoclastic activity; for this reason, bone scintigraphy is of little use in myeloma. The classic appearance is that of a well-circumscribed, ellipsoid, often-subcortical lucency, referred to as a "punched-out" lesion (**Fig. 6**). Untreated lytic lesions will not have a corticated margin. CT can detect lesions when plain radiographs are normal.[33] Even CT, however, may appear normal, particularly with low-grade disease. Multiple compression fractures may be seen, which when coupled with an osteopenic appearance of myeloma, variably mimic benign osteoporotic fractures.

Rarely, sclerotic myelomatous lesions can be encountered, in association with polyneuropathy, organomegaly, endocrinopathy, and skin changes (POEMS syndrome).[34] Bone sclerosis also has more recently been reported after bortezomib therapy, reflecting remineralization of treated lytic lesions.[35]

MRI

Vertebral body disease MRI provides perhaps the best imaging depiction of disease burden. Myeloma can have a variety of MRI appearances, including focal lesions, diffuse involvement, and a variegated heterogeneous appearance. MRI can demonstrate lesions in patients with asymptomatic myeloma.[36] Vande Berg and colleagues[9] demonstrated that presence of MRI lesions in stage I disease are an independent

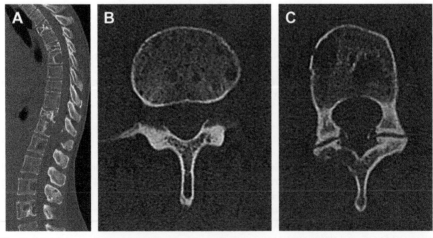

Fig. 6. Multiple myeloma. Axial (*B, C*) and sagittal reconstructed CT (*A*) images demonstrate numerous lytic lesions with a characteristic "punched-out" appearance. Multiple pathologic compression fractures can be seen on the sagittal image.

factor in predicting disease progression. MRI findings in stage III also correlate with disease severity and prognosis.[37] MRI evaluation is often performed with multisequential sagittal MRI spinal surveys covering the entire spine.

Focal lesions are hypointense on T1WI and generally hyperintense on T2WI. On routine T2WI sequences, focal lesions can range from mildly hypointense to hyperintense. Fat-suppressed T2WI is preferable as lesions are more consistently hyperintense and more conspicuous. Focal lesions will enhance postcontrast T1WI (**Fig. 7**). The findings can be indistinguishable from those of metastatic disease. Lesions are often hyperintense on DWI, with corresponding low signal on apparent diffusion coefficient (ADC) maps, indicating hypercellularity of tumor cells causing restricted diffusion of water molecules.

The bone marrow also can show a variegated pattern, which has been called a "salt-and-pepper" appearance. The focal regions of precontrast T1WI hypointensity enhances on postcontrast T1WI. The marrow can alternatively demonstrate a more diffuse pattern of abnormality, which can range from normal marrow signal or mild diffuse heterogeneity in low-grade disease, to diffusely precontrast T1WI hypointense and STIR hyperintense signal in intermediate to high-grade disease. Mild diffuse disease can be difficult to detect and may appear essentially normal on routine sequences. The degree of enhancement in diffuse disease can aid in detecting low-grade involvement, and correlates to grade of disease and microvessel density.[38] Chemical shift and DCE-MRI sequences can also improve detection.[22,39]

Fifty-five percent to 70% of patients with myeloma will develop vertebral compression fractures. Even on MRI, many compression fractures appear benign and similar to osteoporotic fractures. More than 10 lesions or diffuse disease on MRI is a risk factor for future compression fractures.[40]

Epidural disease Epidural tumor typically results from direct extension of vertebral disease, and can cause spinal canal compromise and cord compression. Uncommonly, myeloma lesions of the spine can be entirely extraosseous; these are typically epidural or paraspinal in location. Tirumani and colleagues[41] described 2 patterns of extraosseous tumor in 72 patients: contiguous with bone and noncontiguous with bone; the contiguous lesions were larger and the noncontiguous lesions had a tendency for intermediate or low (rather than hyperintense) T2WI. Extraosseous epidural tumor is associated with a poor prognosis.[42]

Posttreatment appearance After treatment, marrow signal may return to normal; however, often-treated lesions may continue to demonstrate focal precontrast T1WI hypointense and STIR hyperintense signal abnormality. Enhancement will typically resolve or convert from solid to peripheral rim enhancement. Patients with partial response can convert from diffuse signal abnormality on MRI, to a variegated or more focal pattern.[43]

DWI has gained attention in recent years as a way to assess treatment response, particularly with whole-body techniques. Sommer and colleagues,[44] looking at 81 lesions, found that precontrast T1WI and DWI signal within focal lesions did not significantly change after treatment with improvement in serum markers. Although DWI signal did not change, ADC values did increase, reflecting decreased tumor hypercellularity, allowing increasingly facilitated (improved) water diffusion within the lesion. STIR signal increased with improving serum M-protein, reflecting the decreased cellular content of the lesions. The T2WI and ADC components of the diffusion map may effectively cancel each other, highlighting the importance of ADC map and values. Another study showed that clinical responders showed a substantially greater

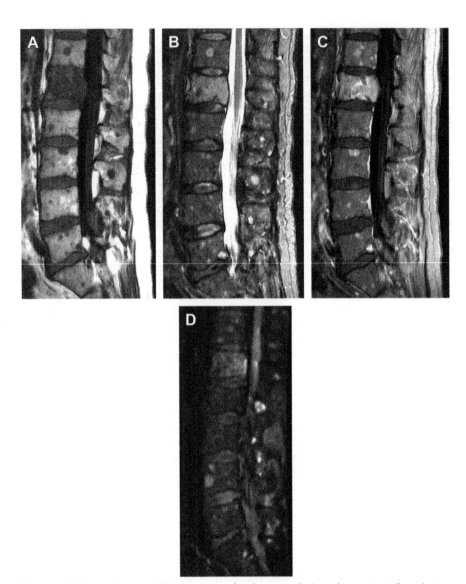

Fig. 7. Multiple myeloma on MRI. Numerous focal marrow lesions demonstrate hypointense signal on T1WI (*A*) and hyperintense signal on STIR sequence (*B*). The lesions enhance with contrast (*C*). At L1, one can appreciate a larger lesion bulging the posterior vertebral margin, indicating epidural extension of tumor. There is only mild spinal canal narrowing, however. The focal marrow lesions are hyperintense on diffusion-weighted sequence (*D*), indicating restricted diffusion.

percentage change in ADC than nonresponders, suggesting the potential of ADC values as a useful biomarker for treatment response.[45]

Other advanced imaging techniques have been proposed to assess treatment response. Avadhani and colleagues[46] evaluated 30 treated patients using DCE imaging, and found that maximal marrow enhancement was significantly higher for poor responders compared with good responders.

Plasmacytoma

Plasmacytoma is a solitary plasma cell tumor without evidence of systemic myeloma. This may in fact be part of the same disease spectrum as multiple myeloma; however, this is not yet fully defined. It is worth discussing separately here, as there can be some characteristic imaging findings. Plasmacytoma can manifest as either solitary plasmacytoma of bone (SBP), which is what is more often seen in the spine, or as extramedullary plasmacytoma (EMP), which is typically seen in head and neck regions.[47]

Meningeal and spinal cord involvement by plasmacytoma is rare and no specific imaging pattern is noted. The following discussion pertains to vertebral/epidural disease.

Computed tomography and radiography

CT and radiography typically demonstrate an expansile lytic solitary bony mass. There may be an extraosseous soft tissue component that would be well depicted on CT. There is no calcification seen within the soft tissue component, differentiating it from several other lesions, including chondrosarcoma and osteosarcoma. On radiography, the extraosseous component is often not appreciated.

Major and colleagues[48] described a pathognomonic appearance of vertebral body plasmacytoma, applicable to both CT and MRI, termed the "mini-brain" appearance. An expansile lytic process replaces the vertebral body, and there are thickened radially oriented platelike bony struts that extend from the peripheral cortex and project centrally (**Fig. 8**). On axial imaging, these are likened to the appearance of sulci radiating into the brain, hence the name "mini-brain."

MRI

One can see the same "mini-brain" appearance on MRI described previously on CT. The thickened bony struts will appear hypointense on all MR sequences, like cortical bone. The signal within the remainder of the lesion will be isointense to hypointense on precontrast T1WI. On STIR, lesions may be homogeneously intermediate to hyperintense in signal. Plasmacytomas will diffusely enhance on postcontrast T1WI. Uniquely, plasmacytomas are more likely to cross the disc space than most metastatic tumors, also appreciable on CT. This is one of a small group of lesions that is more likely to exhibit this behavior, including chordoma, renal cell carcinoma metastases, and aggressive sarcomas.

NON-NEOPLASTIC DISORDERS
Vertebral Marrow Hyperplasia/Reconversion

Hyperplasia or reconversion of the hematopoietic elements of vertebral marrow can be seen with conditions in which hematopoietic demands are increased. This is seen most commonly with anemias, but also may be seen with other conditions, including smoking, obesity, high altitudes, and chronic cardiac failure. Yellow marrow reconverts to red marrow, affecting the axial skeleton first, causing a diffuse decrease in precontrast T1WI signal and hyperintensity on STIR. A similar appearance can also be seen with hematopoietic growth factor therapies such as granulocyte-stimulating factor and erythropoietin analogs. With extensive marrow hyperplasia, there may be expansion of the vertebral medullary spaces. Less commonly, extramedullary hematopoiesis may occur in the spine, manifesting radiographically as ovoid paravertebral masses, typically bilateral. Rarely, this may involve the epidural space and compromise the spinal canal.[49]

Hemoglobinopathies, such as sickle cell anemia and thalassemia, may demonstrate central endplate depressions that have been termed "H-shaped" or "Lincoln log"

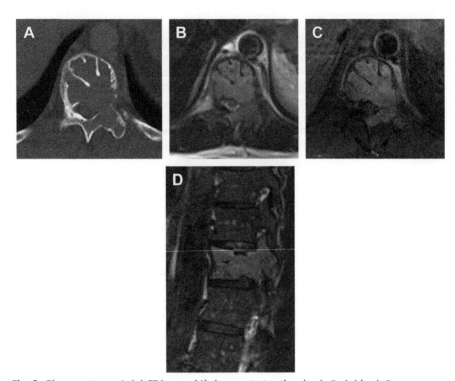

Fig. 8. Plasmacytoma. Axial CT image (*A*) demonstrates the classic "mini-brain" appearance described in vertebral plasmacytoma. There are thickened bony struts radiating inward from the peripheral vertebral cortex. This appearance can also be seen on axial T2 (*B*) and post-contrast (*C*) images in this patient. Note the extension to the left posterior elements and epidural space. Sagittal postcontrast T1WI (*D*) demonstrates diffuse enhancement, mild loss of vertebral body height, and extension into the adjacent neural foramina.

deformities, as a result of microvessel infarction along the endplates. These deformities, in combination, with diffuse homogeneous precontrast T1WI hypointense marrow signal abnormality are characteristic of hemoglobinopathies.

Hemochromatosis

A patient receiving repeated blood transfusions may develop transfusional iron overload, or secondary hemochromatosis. This is not uncommon in patients with hemoglobinopathy, and may add to the previously described imaging picture. Increased iron deposition in the marrow will result in more pronounced diffuse hypointense signal, particularly on T2WI, lower in signal than normal adjacent muscle. Signal loss will be more profound on T2-weighted gradient recalled echo sequences (T2-GRE), which are more sensitive to the presence of paramagnetic material, such as iron and calcium. Axial T2WI of the spine may also reveal abnormal marked signal hypointensity within the included portions of the liver and spleen, but sparing the pancreas, providing additional clues to the diagnosis (**Fig. 9**).

Radiation-Induced Marrow Change

After radiation therapy, red marrow may undergo fatty change, manifest on MRI as pronounced T1 hyperintense signal. This is usually limited to a well-demarcated radiation portal, and may even be seen as a sharply marginated change in signal through

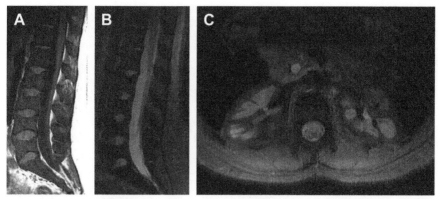

Fig. 9. Sickle cell disease with transfusional iron overload. Sagittal T1WI (*A*) demonstrates diffuse signal hypointensity of the marrow, as well as central endplate depressions. At L2, this takes on a typical "H-shaped" appearance. Sagittal STIR (*B*) demonstrates profoundly T2 hypointense signal indicating increased iron deposition that was related to blood transfusions in this patient. Axial T2 gradient echo image (*C*) also shows the liver, spleen, and renal cortices to be hypointense secondary to increased iron deposition.

the center of a vertebral body at the margin of the radiation field. This geographic region of hypocellularity and fatty change also will be markedly hypointense on fat-suppressed T1WI and T2WI sequences. The depletion of red marrow can be reversible if doses are less than 30 Gy, but often irreversible at doses greater than 36 Gy.[50] A similar but more diffuse appearance can be seen with other marrow-depletion disorders, such as aplastic anemia.

Radiation Myelopathy

Radiation-induced changes of the spinal cord typically occur with radiation doses of greater than 50 Gy and fractionated radiation schedules of greater than 2 Gy.[51] In general, acute radiation myelopathy presents as cord swelling and intramedullary enhancement on both CT with intravenous contrast and contrast-enhanced MRI. Although CT myelography can be used to outline the edematous cord, this procedure should be done *very* cautiously and only if truly necessary to guide management.

Radiation myelopathy should be suspected if the cranial-caudal extent of disease is similar to vertebral body fatty marrow changes due to radiation treatment (radiation port). Postcontrast T1WI enhancement can be ringlike and heterogeneous.[52] A focal area of enhancement usually becomes the center of cord atrophy on subsequent imaging once the inflammation subsides.[53] STIR MRI images show increased signal in and around areas of cord enhancement and areas of ischemia can show cytotoxic edema (restricted water diffusion) on DWI (bright signal) and ADC (low signal).

Myelofibrosis

In myelofibrosis, bone marrow is replaced with connective tissue and progressive fibrosis. On MRI, this results in pronounced low T1WI and T2WI signal, replacing the normal marrow signal. The process is considered a myeloproliferative disorder and typically causes anemia. Extramedullary hematopoiesis is not uncommonly seen, which may manifest as paraspinal masses. Myelofibrosis may be primary or secondary; secondary myelofibrosis may be seen as an end stage of polycythemia vera, or after radiation and/or medical therapy for hematologic or other vertebral malignancy (**Fig. 10**).

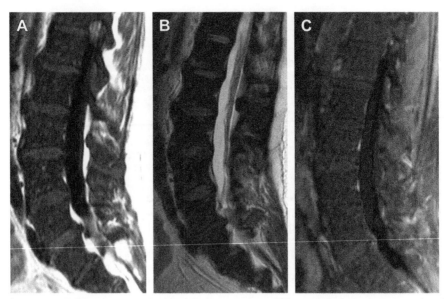

Fig. 10. Myelofibrosis. Sagittal T1WI (*A*) demonstrates diffuse mildly heterogeneous signal hypointensity in this patient who developed myelofibrosis after a history of treated polycythemia vera. Note the pronounced hypointensity on T2WI (*B*) reflecting fibrosis, and the lack of enhancement on postcontrast T1WI (*C*).

Epidural Hematoma

Generally, benign hematologic disorders of the spinal column do not exhibit epidural extension or spinal canal compromise. A notable exception is epidural hemorrhage, which can result from various hematologic disorders, including immune thrombocytopenic purpura, hemophilia, and other bleeding disorders; any marrow replacing or depleting process resulting in thrombocytopenia; and vertebral fractures. They can also occur spontaneously or as a complication of anticoagulation therapy.

Computed tomography

As this is an extraosseous process, a cross-sectional study is needed to make the imaging diagnosis; radiography is of no use. On CT, one will see focal epidural soft tissue causing a variable degree of thecal sac compression. On noncontrast CT, acute blood will often be hyperdense, differentiating from other masses. One caveat is that acute hemorrhage in patients with profound anemia may be isodense to hypodense on CT due to diminished hematocrit. Differentiation from other epidural lesions may be challenging, as density measurements and morphologies may overlap.

MRI

MRI, with its superior ability to differentiate between different tissues, is the imaging test of choice and can often make a specific diagnosis. Larger epidural hematomas are often ellipsoid in configuration. They are generally eccentric and localized, as opposed to subdural hematomas that have a greater propensity to spread concentrically around the thecal sac and in cranial-caudal direction. Thus, an epidural hematoma is more likely to cause significant mass effect on the thecal sac and cord compression, as compared with subdural hematomas. Acute blood will be isointense on T1WI and generally hyperintense on STIR with focal regions of T2WI hypointensity. In the subacute phase, hemorrhage will evolve to hyperintense precontrast T1WI signal, reflecting methemoglobin (**Fig. 11**). The evolving signal of blood products in the spine is somewhat less consistent when compared with intracerebral hemorrhage. T1WI isointensity may persist for several days longer than what is typically seen in the brain, before becoming hyperintense.[54,55] T2-GRE sequences can show regions of magnetic susceptibility manifest as marked signal loss (due to deoxyhemoglobin and hemosiderin). Spotty internal enhancement on postcontrast T1WI has been described in acute epidural hematomas, perhaps reflecting continuous contrast extravasation, and indicating a more active lesion possibly requiring urgent intervention.[56]

Opportunistic Infections

Due to the immunosuppressed (chemotherapy) or immunocompromised (AIDS) status of many patients with hematological disorders, opportunistic infections and their imaging findings are important to consider. Discussion of each microbe is beyond the scope of this review; however, select imaging patterns are discussed. MRI with contrast is the study of choice to image leptomeningitis and myelitis; however, it can be completely normal, thereby warranting CSF sampling.

CT with or without intravenous contrast has little utility. CT myelography can show clumping of nerve roots or nodular contouring of the cauda equina, but is of little use to evaluate any cord-related changes. Inflamed leptomeninges become "sticky" and nerve roots of the cauda equina can clump together (ie, arachnoiditis). When nerve roots stick to the thecal sac wall, an "empty" thecal sac sign is seen.

Pyogenic vertebral discitis-osteomyelitis

For this review, we discuss only pyogenic vertebral discitis-osteomyelitis (VDO), the most common type of VDO. The most common cause of pyogenic VDO is *Staphylococcus aureus* and it infects by both by a hematogenous route (up to 84% of cases of nontuberculous VDO)[57] and via direct inoculation (up to 33%).[58] Patients usually

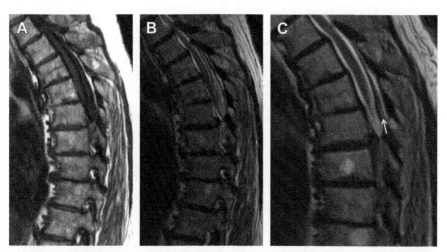

Fig. 11. Epidural hematoma. This dorsal epidural hematoma, located posterior to the thoracic spinal cord, demonstrates isointense T1 signal (*A*) and hyperintense T2 signal. Note the narrowing of the thecal sac and mass effect on the cord (*B*). A follow-up MRI shows the collection to be smaller on sagittal T2WI (*C*), and demosntrates areas of T2 hypointensity (*arrow*) within a the previously predominantly T2WI hyperinense collection in image B, typical of spinal hematoma.

present with back pain and muscle spasm 90% of the time, with only 40% to 50% of patients demonstrating leukocytosis and fever.[59]

Radiography/computed tomography Spine radiography is a poor imaging modality for VDO because it shows signs of demineralization, disc space narrowing, and endplate erosion only after 2 to 8 weeks following the onset of infection and symptoms. CT has limited utility in acute VDO, showing endplate erosion, paraspinal soft tissue enlargement, and vertebral body demineralization earlier than radiographs.[59]

MRI MRI is the study of choice to image VDO. Acute pyogenic VDO shows precontrast T1WI hypointense and irregular STIR hyperintense signal of the endplates, adjacent vertebral bodies, and the infected disc. The endplates are irregular and ill defined. On postcontrast fat-saturated T1WI, there is enhancement of the disc and affected endplates[59] **(Fig. 12)**. Extraosseous spread can extend into the paraspinal tissues, the epidural space (ie, spinal epidural abscess), and the psoas musculature, possibly with abscess formation. MRI appearance can be complicated, especially in immunocompromised or recently immune-reconstituted patients and a CT or fluoroscopic-guided needle biopsy may on occasion be needed for confirmation of VDO.[59]

Spinal epidural abscess Patients with spinal epidural abscess (SEA) associated with pyogenic VDO present with back pain (71%), fever (66%), tenderness, and/or progressive myelopathy or radiculopathy.[60] *S aureus* causes most cases, of which 15% are methicillin-resistant (ie, MRSA).[61,62] Intravenous contrast-enhanced CT can show a

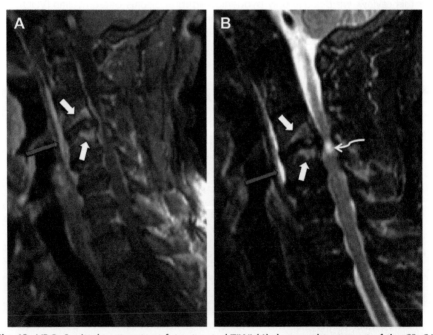

Fig. 12. VDO. Sagittal postcontrast fat-saturated TIWI (*A*) shows enhancement of the C3–C4 endplates (*white arrows*), corresponding to hyperintense T2WI signal (*B*) in the same endplates (*white arrows*), compatible with early VDO. Note incidental myelomalacia of the cord at C3–C4 (*white curved arrow*) due to a degenerated disc. The *red arrows* shows mild prevertebral edema and fluid.

soft tissue mass with tapering edges in the spinal epidural space with mass effect on the thecal sac and spinal cord. *CT myelography should be avoided unless absolutely necessary and only after consultation with neurosurgery AND radiology.*

On MRI, SEA is isointense to cord on precontrast T1WI, and hyperintense to cord on STIR. Postcontrast enhancement can be thin and peripheral, heterogeneous, or diffuse and smooth.[63] SEA carries a mortality of 18% to 30% and is a surgical lesion.[62] MRI can help make the important distinction of phlegmon and SEA, because the latter may require surgical drainage.

Infectious leptomeningitis

Pyogenic leptomeningitis is the most common intradural spinal infection. Precontrast T1WI can be normal appearing or show mildly increased CSF signal, or dural thickening if there is a secondary myelitis. Additional findings include adhesions, nerve

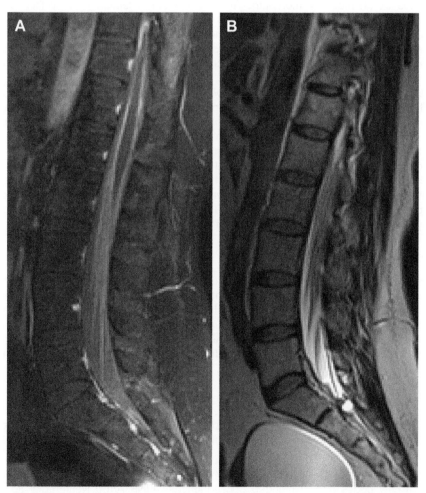

Fig. 13. Bacterial (pyogenic) leptomeningitis. Sagittal postcontrast fat-saturated T1WI (*A*) and T2WI (*B*) show diffuse leptomeningeal enhancement of the lower spinal cord and cauda equina (*A*), with thickened cauda equina nerve roots (*B*) in this patient with pyogenic leptomeningitis.

root clumping, CSF loculations, and poor visualization of the spinal cord–CSF interface. T2WI and STIR images are less helpful due to the intrinsic hyperintensity of the CSF; however, cord enlargement may be present. Postcontrast T1WI may show an inflamed cord-pial surface, dural enhancement and thickening, and abnormal enhancement of the cauda equine nerve roots. Enhancement can be diffuse (smooth), linear, or nodular[64,65] **(Fig. 13)**.

Mycobacterial leptomeningitis tends to have thick nodular thickening of the nerve roots and layering of granulomatous debris at the thecal sac termination, usually at the S2 level of the spine.[66] Such findings will prompt CSF sampling to evaluate the causative organisms(s). Please note that cauda equina nerve root enhancement is a nonspecific finding and can include both infectious diseases and noninfectious processes (eg, Guillain-Barre syndrome, sarcoidosis, carcinomatosis).[67]

Infectious myelitis

Viruses are the most common pathogens to cause cord infection (viral myelitis). MRI findings can range from simple edematous reaction (high T2WI signal and cord expansion) to necrotizing myelitis (heterogeneous, long-segment enhancement, and edema), caused by highly virulent microbes, such as herpes simplex virus 2 and cytomegalovirus.[67] If the patient survives, the cord atrophies and can show persistent high T2 signal, indicating injury (myelomalacia).

Bacterial myelitis is usually due to *Staphylococcus* and *Streptococcus* species. If left untreated or diagnosed late, myelitis progresses to cord abscess, which shows bright DWI and low ADC signal due to the highly viscous pus.[68] Mycobacterial myelitis usually does not progress to abscess, rather continues to spread in a leptomeningeal path.[67] It can also cause cord syringohydromyelia formation due to blockage of the central canal of the cord by mycobacterial granulomas.[67]

Spinal *Cryptococcus*, a fungus, is most commonly seen in immunocompromised patients with human immunodeficiency syndrome/AIDS; however, severely immunosuppressed patients are also susceptible. The fungus causes formation of intramedullary and extramedullary nodular deposits that enhance and are T2 dark on MRI.[69]

SUMMARY

Imaging manifestations of hematological diseases and their potential complications are broad, and there may be significant overlap in features of various disease processes. Knowledge of appropriate choice of imaging test, pertinent imaging patterns, and pathophysiology of disease can help the reader increase specificity in their diagnosis and treatment of the patient. Most importantly, we encourage the readers of this review to engage their radiologists during the diagnostic, treatment, and management phases of care delivery.

REFERENCES

1. Kim HJ, Ryu KN, Choi WS, et al. Spinal involvement of hematopoietic malignancies and metastasis: differentiation using MR imaging. Clin Imaging 1999; 23(2):125–33.

2. Chokshi FH, Tu RK, Nicola GN, et al. Myelography CPT coding updates: effects of 4 new codes and unintended consequences. AJNR Am J Neuroradiol 2016. [Epub ahead of print].

3. Parker BR, Marglin S, Castellino RA. Skeletal manifestations of leukemia, Hodgkin disease, and non-Hodgkin lymphoma. Semin Roentgenol 1980;15(4 Pt 2):302–15.

4. Parker BR, Blank N, Castellino RA. Lymphographic appearance of benign conditions simulating lymphoma. Radiology 1974;111(2):267–74.
5. Guermazi A, Feger C, Rousselot P, et al. Granulocytic sarcoma (chloroma). Am J Roentgenol 2002;178(2):319–25.
6. Pomeranz SJ, Hawkins HH, Towbin R, et al. Granulocytic sarcoma (chloroma): CT manifestations. Radiology 1985;155(1):167–70.
7. Alyas F, Saifuddin A, Connell D. MR imaging evaluation of the bone marrow and marrow infiltrative disorders of the lumbar spine. Magn Reson Imaging Clin N Am 2007;15(2):199–219, vi.
8. Thomsen C, Sorensen PG, Karle H, et al. Prolonged bone marrow T1-relaxation in acute leukaemia. In vivo tissue characterization by magnetic resonance imaging. Magn Reson Imaging 1987;5(4):251–7.
9. Vande Berg BC, Lecouvet FE, Michaux L, et al. Stage I multiple myeloma: value of MR imaging of the bone marrow in the determination of prognosis. Radiology 1996;201(1):243–6.
10. Berg BCV, Schmitz PJ, Scheiff JM, et al. Acute myeloid leukemia: lack of predictive value of sequential quantitative MR imaging during treatment. Radiology 1995;197(1):301–5.
11. Moore SG, Gooding CA, Brasch RC, et al. Bone marrow in children with acute lymphocytic leukemia: MR relaxation times. Radiology 1986;160(1):237–40.
12. Rosen BR, Fleming DM, Kushner DC, et al. Hematologic bone marrow disorders: quantitative chemical shift MR imaging. Radiology 1988;169(3):799–804.
13. Chen B-B, Hsu C-Y, Yu C-W, et al. Dynamic contrast-enhanced MR imaging measurement of vertebral bone marrow perfusion may be indicator of outcome of acute myeloid leukemia patients in remission. Radiology 2011;258(3):821–31.
14. Sun YS, Zhang XP, Tang L. Locally advanced rectal carcinoma treated with preoperative chemotherapy and radiation therapy: preliminary analysis of diffusion-weighted MR imaging for early detection of tumor histopathologic downstaging. Radiology 2010;254:170–8.
15. Seok JH, Park J, Kim SK, et al. Granulocytic sarcoma of the spine: MRI and clinical review. AJR Am J Roentgenol 2010;194(2):485–9.
16. Chamberlain MC, Glantz M, Groves MD, et al. Diagnostic tools for neoplastic meningitis: detecting disease, identifying patient risk, and determining benefit of treatment. Semin Oncol 2009;36(4 Suppl 2):S35–45.
17. Yavuz H, Cakir M. Transverse myelopathy: an initial presentation of acute leukemia. Pediatr Neurol 2001;24(5):382–4.
18. Kaplan KR, Mitchell DG, Steiner RM, et al. Polycythemia vera and myelofibrosis: correlation of MR imaging, clinical, and laboratory findings. Radiology 1992;183(2):329–34.
19. Fornasier VL, Horne JG. Metastases to the vertebral column. Cancer 1975;36(2):590–4.
20. Szekely G, Miltenyi Z, Mezey G, et al. Epidural malignant lymphomas of the spine: collected experiences with epidural malignant lymphomas of the spinal canal and their treatment. Spinal Cord 2008;46(4):278–81.
21. O'Neill J, Finlay K, Jurriaans E, et al. Radiological manifestations of skeletal lymphoma. Curr Probl Diagn Radiol 2009;38(5):228–36.
22. Rahmouni A, Montazel J-L, Divine M, et al. Bone marrow with diffuse tumor infiltration in patients with lymphoproliferative diseases: dynamic gadolinium-enhanced MR imaging. Radiology 2003;229(3):710–7.
23. Moulopoulos LA, Dimopoulos MA, Vourtsi A, et al. Bone lesions with soft-tissue mass: magnetic resonance imaging diagnosis of lymphomatous involvement of the bone

marrow versus multiple myeloma and bone metastases. Leuk Lymphoma 1999; 34(1–2):179–84.

24. Alorainy IA, Al-Asmi AR, del Carpio R. MRI features of epidural extramedullary hematopoiesis. Eur J Radiol 2000;35(1):8–11.

25. Do-Dai DD, Brooks MK, Goldkamp A, et al. Magnetic resonance imaging of intramedullary spinal cord lesions: a pictorial review. Curr Probl Diagn Radiol 2010; 39(4):160–85.

26. Oza A, Rajkumar SV. Waldenstrom macroglobulinemia: prognosis and management. Blood Cancer J 2015;5:e296.

27. Renner RR, Nelson DA, Lozner EL. Roentgenologic manifestations of primary macroglobulinemia (Waldenström). Am J Roentgenol 1971;113(3):499–508.

28. Moulopoulos LA, Dimopoulos MA, Varma DG, et al. Waldenström macroglobulinemia: MR imaging of the spine and CT of the abdomen and pelvis. Radiology 1993;188(3):669–73.

29. Malkani RG, Tallman M, Gottardi-Littell N, et al. Bing-Neel syndrome: an illustrative case and a comprehensive review of the published literature. J Neurooncol 2010;96(3):301–12.

30. Simon L, Fitsiori A, Lemal R, et al. Bing-Neel syndrome, a rare complication of Waldenstrom macroglobulinemia: analysis of 44 cases and review of the literature. A study on behalf of the French Innovative Leukemia Organization (FILO). Haematologica 2015;100(12):1587–94.

31. Durie BG. The role of anatomic and functional staging in myeloma: description of Durie/Salmon plus staging system. Eur J Cancer 2006;42: 1539–43.

32. Durie BG, Salmon SE. A clinical staging system for multiple myeloma. Correlation of measured myeloma cell mass with presenting clinical features, response to treatment, and survival. Cancer 1975;36:842–54.

33. Mahnken AH, Wildberger JE, Gehbauer G, et al. Multidetector CT of the spine in multiple myeloma: comparison with MR imaging and radiography. Am J Roentgenol 2002;178(6):1429–36.

34. Clarisse PD, Staple TW. Diffuse bone sclerosis in multiple myeloma. Radiology 1971;99(2):327–8.

35. Schulze M, Weisel K, Grandjean C, et al. Increasing bone sclerosis during bortezomib therapy in multiple myeloma patients: results of a reduced-dose wholebody MDCT study. Am J Roentgenol 2013;202(1):170–9.

36. Moulopoulos LA, Varma DG, Dimopoulos MA, et al. Multiple myeloma: spinal MR imaging in patients with untreated newly diagnosed disease. Radiology 1992; 185(3):833–40.

37. Lecouvet FE, Vande Berg BC, Michaux L, et al. Stage III multiple myeloma: clinical and prognostic value of spinal bone marrow MR imaging. Radiology 1998; 209(3):653–60.

38. Baur A, Bartl R, Pellengahr C, et al. Neovascularization of bone marrow in patients with diffuse multiple myeloma: a correlative study of magnetic resonance imaging and histopathologic findings. Cancer 2004;101(11):2599–604.

39. Baur A, Stabler A, Bartl R, et al. Infiltration patterns of plasmacytomas in magnetic resonance tomography. Rofo 1996;164(6):457–63 [in German].

40. Lecouvet FE, Malghem J, Michaux L, et al. Vertebral compression fractures in multiple myeloma. Part II. Assessment of fracture risk with MR imaging of spinal bone marrow. Radiology 1997;204(1):201–5.

41. Tirumani SH, Shinagare AB, Jagannathan JP, et al. MRI features of extramedullary myeloma. Am J Roentgenol 2014;202(4):803–10.

42. Hall MN, Jagannathan JP, Ramaiya NH, et al. Imaging of extraosseous myeloma: CT, PET/CT, and MRI features. AJR Am J Roentgenol 2010;195:1057–65.

43. Moulopoulos LA, Dimopoulos MA, Alexanian R, et al. Multiple myeloma: MR patterns of response to treatment. Radiology 1994;193(2):441–6.

44. Sommer G, Klarhofer M, Lenz C, et al. Signal characteristics of focal bone marrow lesions in patients with multiple myeloma using whole body T1w-TSE, T2w-STIR and diffusion-weighted imaging with background suppression. Eur Radiol 2011;21(4):857–62.

45. Giles SL, Messiou C, Collins DJ, et al. Whole-body diffusion-weighted MR imaging for assessment of treatment response in myeloma. Radiology 2014;271(3): 785–94.

46. Avadhani A, Shetty AP, Rajasekaran S. Isolated extraosseous epidural myeloma presenting with thoracic compressive myelopathy. Spine J 2010;10:e7–10.

47. Tong D, Griffin TW, Laramore GE, et al. Solitary plasmacytoma of bone and soft tissues. Radiology 1980;135(1):195–8.

48. Major NM, Helms CA, Richardson WJ. The "mini brain". Am J Roentgenol 2000; 175(1):261–3.

49. Kalina P, Zaheer W, Drehobl KE. Cord compression by extramedullary hematopoiesis in polycythemia vera. Am J Roentgenol 1995;164(4):1027–8.

50. Cavenagh EC, Weinberger E, Shaw DW, et al. Hematopoietic marrow regeneration in pediatric patients undergoing spinal irradiation: MR depiction. AJNR Am J Neuroradiol 1995;16(3):461–7.

51. Rogers LR. Neurologic complications of radiation. Continuum (Minneap Minn) 2012;18(2):343–54.

52. Calabro F, Jinkins JR. MRI of radiation myelitis: a report of a case treated with hyperbaric oxygen. Eur Radiol 2000;10(7):1079–84.

53. Hirota S, Yoshida S, Soejima T, et al. Chronological observation in early radiation myelopathy of the cervical spinal cord: gadolinium-enhanced MRI findings in two cases. Radiat Med 1993;11(4):154–9.

54. Mohazab HR, Langer B, Spigos D. Spinal epidural hematoma in a patient with lupus coagulopathy: MR findings. Am J Roentgenol 1993;160(4):853–4.

55. Fukui MB, Swarnkar AS, Williams RL. Acute spontaneous spinal epidural hematomas. AJNR Am J Neuroradiol 1999;20(7):1365–72.

56. Chang F-C, Lirng J-F, Chen S-S, et al. Contrast enhancement patterns of acute spinal epidural hematomas: a report of two cases. AJNR Am J Neuroradiol 2003;24(3):366–9.

57. Hadjipavlou AG, Mader JT, Necessary JT, et al. Hematogenous pyogenic spinal infections and their surgical management. Spine 2000;25(13):1668–79.

58. Jimenez-Mejias ME, de Dios Colmenero J, Sanchez-Lora FJ, et al. Postoperative spondylodiskitis: etiology, clinical findings, prognosis, and comparison with nonoperative pyogenic spondylodiskitis. Clin Infect Dis 1999;29(2):339–45.

59. DeSanto J, Ross JS. Spine infection/inflammation. Radiol Clin North Am 2011; 49(1):105–27.

60. Reihsaus E, Waldbaur H, Seeling W. Spinal epidural abscess: a meta-analysis of 915 patients. Neurosurg Rev 2000;23(4):175–204 [discussion: 5].

61. Endress C, Guyot DR, Fata J, et al. Cervical osteomyelitis due to i.v. heroin use: radiologic findings in 14 patients. AJR Am J Roentgenol 1990;155(2):333–5.

62. Rigamonti D, Liem L, Sampath P, et al. Spinal epidural abscess: contemporary trends in etiology, evaluation, and management. Surg Neurol 1999;52(2): 189–96 [discussion: 97].

63. Post MJ, Sze G, Quencer RM, et al. Gadolinium-enhanced MR in spinal infection. J Comput Assist Tomogr 1990;14(5):721–9.
64. Lury K, Smith JK, Castillo M. Imaging of spinal infections. Semin Roentgenol 2006;41(4):363–79.
65. Smith AS, Blaser SI. Infectious and inflammatory processes of the spine. Radiol Clin North Am 1991;29(4):809–27.
66. Chang KH, Han MH, Choi YW, et al. Tuberculous arachnoiditis of the spine: findings on myelography, CT, and MR imaging. AJNR Am J Neuroradiol 1989; 10(6):1255–62.
67. Lury KM, Smith JK, Matheus MG, et al. Neurosarcoidosis–review of imaging findings. Semin Roentgenol 2004;39(4):495–504.
68. Thurnher MM, Bammer R. Diffusion-weighted magnetic resonance imaging of the spine and spinal cord. Semin Roentgenol 2006;41(4):294–311.
69. Taber KH, Hayman LA, Shandera WX, et al. Spinal disease in neurologically symptomatic HIV-positive patients. Neuroradiology 1999;41(5):360–8.

Imaging of Bone Marrow

Sopo Lin, MD[a], Tao Ouyang, MD[a], Sangam Kanekar, MD[a,b],*

KEYWORDS

- Imaging • Bone marrow • Anatomy • Techniques • Pathology
- Hematological malignancies

KEY POINTS

- Bone marrow disorders or dysfunctions may be evaluated by blood workup, peripheral smears, and marrow biopsy.
- Noninvasive techniques such as plain radiograph, computed tomography (CT), MRI and nuclear medicine scan may also be used to evaluate bone marrow disorders.
- It is important to distinguish normal spinal marrow from pathology to avoid missing a pathology or misinterpreting normal changes, which may result in further testing and increased costs.

INTRODUCTION

Bone marrow is one of the largest organs of the human body. It serves the essential function of hematopoiesis. Its function is of vital importance for the normal functioning of the body as it continuously replenishes the cells required for oxygen delivery, excretion of waste/toxic material, various defense mechanisms, and maintaining the balance between the bleeding and clotting mechanism of the body. Bone marrow disorders or dysfunctions may be evaluated by blood workup, peripheral smears, and marrow biopsy. They may be also evaluated using noninvasive techniques such as plain radiographs, computed tomography (CT), MRI and nuclear medicine scan (single photon emission CT/PET). MRI, owing to its better soft tissue differentiation and higher spatial resolution, can evaluate marrow changes very early, thus giving a lead to the clinician regarding the undergoing disease process.

It is important to distinguish normal spinal marrow from pathology to avoid missing a pathology or misinterpreting normal changes, either of which may result in further testing and increased health care costs. On imaging, bone marrow pathologies may be classified into focal and diffuse (**Table 1**). In this article, we focus predominately

a Department of Radiology, Hershey Medical Center, The Pennsylvania State University, 500 University Drive, Hershey, PA 17033, USA; b Department of Neurology, Hershey Medical Center, The Pennsylvania State University, 500 University Drive, Hershey, PA 17033, USA
* Corresponding author. Department of Neurology, Hershey Medical Center, The Pennsylvania State University, 500 University Drive, Hershey, PA 17033.
E-mail address: skanekar@hmc.psu.edu

Hematol Oncol Clin N Am 30 (2016) 945–971
http://dx.doi.org/10.1016/j.hoc.2016.03.012
0889-8588/16/$ – see front matter © 2016 Elsevier Inc. All rights reserved.

Table 1
Classification of bone marrow pathologies into focal and diffuse lesions

MR Signal Intensity	Focal Lesions	Diffuse Lesions
T1 hyperintense	Normal variant	Prior radiation treatment
	Focal fatty marrow	Osteoporosis
	Solitary hemangioma	Multiple hemangiomas
	Degenerative disk disease	Spondyloarthropathy
	Paget disease	Anorexia nervosa
	Melanoma metastasis	Chronic malnutrition
	Bone marrow hemorrhage	
	Lipoma	
T1 Hypointensity	Degenerative endplate changes	Hematopoietic hyperplasia
	Osteomyelitis	Neoplasm
	Amyloid	Renal osteodystrophy
	Atypical hemangioma	Sarcoidosis
	Fracture	Spondyloarthropathy
	Malignancy	Myelofibrosis
	Fibrous dysplasia	Mastocytosis
	Metastasis	Hemosiderosis
	Myeloma	Gaucher disease
	Lymphoma	Gout
	Primary bone tumor	
	Fracture	

on the diffuse bone marrow pathologies, because the majority of the bone marrow pathologies related to hematologic disorders are diffuse.

Bone Marrow Anatomy (Composition of Bone Marrow)

Normal bone structure consists of an outer cortex with an interior network of ossicles, referred to as trabecular, spongy, or cancellous bone. Approximately 80% of total bone volume consists of the compact cortical bone, and the remaining 20% is made up of cancellous or trabecular bone. By definition, trabecular bone refers to the structural network that partitions the space enclosed by the cortical bone. Trabeculae are thin and consist of segments formed by parallel lamellae. Bone marrow is a term used to refer to the tissue occupying the cavities between the trabecular bone.

Normal bone marrow is composed of red marrow, yellow marrow, osseous components, and a supporting system. Red bone marrow is the primary organ for the production of mature blood cells, and therefore represents hematopoetically active bone marrow. It is composed of 40% water, 40% fat, and 20% protein (**Fig. 1**). Red bone marrow has a definitive life span, and must be replenished by the body under normal circumstances. Yellow marrow represents hematopoetically inactive bone marrow. It is composed of 15% water, 80% fat, and 5% protein. Very few capillaries are present in the yellow marrow. With aging, there is a decrease in the number of trabeculae in bone, and subsequent conversion of red to yellow marrow.

Progression of Bone Marrow Changes from Childhood to Adult (Conversion)

At birth, red marrow is present throughout the entire skeleton. Normal physiologic conversion of red to yellow marrow occurs gradually from birth, and continues until adult age. As a general rule, marrow conversion first begins in the distal appendicular skeleton, beginning in the hands and feet and continues into the more proximal bones of the skeleton. By 25 years of age, the adult distribution of red marrow persists

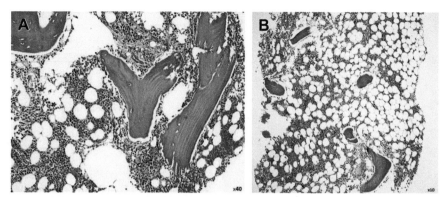

Fig. 1. (*A*, *B*) Adult normocellular marrow with maturing trilineage hematopoiesis. Stain: hematoxylin and eosin.

predominately in the axial skeleton, proximal humeri, and proximal femora. With advancing age, there may be further conversion of red to yellow marrow, including the axial skeleton. Thus, the normal appearance of the bone marrow on imaging widely depends on the age of the patient. It is worth noting that within long bone, red to yellow bone marrow conversion begins first the diaphysis, then in the distal metaphysis, and finally the proximal metaphysis. The epiphysis and apophyses are cartilaginous at birth, and in the adult contain yellow marrow.

IMAGING TECHNIQUES

MRI remains the imaging modality of choice in the evaluation of the bone marrow disorders owing to its excellent soft tissue differentiation and early diagnosis of abnormal conditions compared with the other imaging modalities. Single photon emission CT and PET are sensitive but lack specificity and anatomic resolution in the imaging of the bone marrow.

MRI Techniques

MRI appearance of the bone marrow depends on pulse sequence on which it is being evaluated and the relative composition of the marrow (proportion of proteins, water, fat and cells, ie, the proportion of red and yellow marrow). Commonly used MR sequences for the evaluation of bone marrow disorders include T1-weighted imaging (T1WI), T2-weighted imaging (T2WI), a short-tau inversion recovery sequence (STIR), and fat saturation gadolinium-enhanced T1WI (**Fig. 2**). A T1WI spine echo sequence provides terrific differentiation between the red and yellow marrow components. On T1WI, red marrow will demonstrate decreased signal intensity, lower than subcutaneous fat but higher than disk or muscle. In contrast, yellow marrow demonstrates a hyperintense signal comparable with the subcutaneous fat on T1WI. This is a result of the greater fat content of yellow marrow, which significantly shortens the T1 relaxation time. Owing to longer T2 relaxation of the fat protons, yellow marrow shows high signal intensity on the T2F fast spin echo. Red marrow signal intensity is slightly lower than that of yellow marrow on T2 fast spin echo.

With the STIR technique, the signal from fat is suppressed and the signal from water is preserved, thus providing high tissue contrast, which is very useful in evaluating bone marrow. The STIR sequence produces more homogeneous fat suppression than T2 fast spin echo fat saturation. T2WI spin echo sequences and STIR sequences

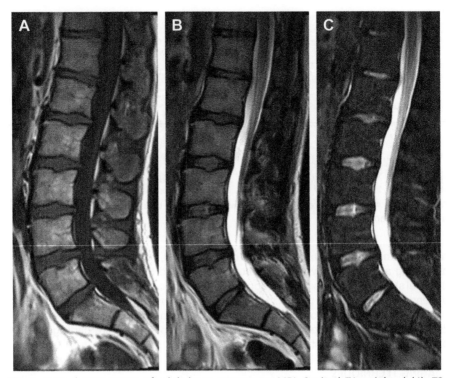

Fig. 2. Normal appearance of adult bone marrow on MRI. Sagittal T1-weighted (*A*), T2-weighted (*B*), and short-tau inversion recovery sequence (*C*) images of the lumbar spine show normal appearance of marrow signal in an adult. Note that marrow signal is hyperintense to disc signal and only slightly hypointense compared with subcutaneous fat on T1- and T2-weighted non–fat-suppressed images and diffusely hypointense on short-tau inversion recovery sequence, a fat-suppressed sequence, because of the high fat content of yellow marrow, which comprises the majority of adult marrow.

are very sensitive for evaluation of bone marrow pathology. T2WI is also very sensitive in diagnosing cord-related pathologies.

Fat saturation gadolinium-enhanced T1WI are used routinely in the evaluation of bone marrow. The basic principle of this technique is to highlight the Gd-related enhancement by suppressing the signal from fat. Contrast-enhanced sequencing is very helpful in confirming neoplastic or infective lesions. It is also very helpful in defining the extent of extramedullary spread in the paraspinal soft tissues and within the canal and in evaluating dural or leptomeningeal metastasis.

Less commonly used MR sequences in the evaluation of the spinal pathologies, which may highlight some of the marrow pathologies include T1 fluid-attenuated inversion recovery, diffusion-weighted imaging–apparent diffusion coefficient and in-phase and out-of-phase imaging sequences. T1 fluid-attenuated inversion recovery optimizes the tissue contrast between fatty marrow and abnormal tissue, thus improving the conspicuity of edema and metastatic lesions in the bone marrow.[1] Diffusion-weighted imaging evaluates the molecular diffusion of the protons. Lesions with higher cellular density shows restricted diffusion that is bright on diffusion-weighted imaging and low signal intensity on apparent diffusion coefficient imaging. This property helps in identifying small primary neoplastic or metastatic disease.

Normal Bone Marrow Appearance on MRI from Infant to Adult

Bone marrow conversion in infant (up to 1 year of age)

From birth, there is a high concentration of red marrow present throughout the entire skeleton (both axial and appendicular). In the long bones, the medullary canals within the diaphysis and metaphysic of the long bones will be composed of red marrow and therefore will demonstrate low T1 signal in these areas. The epiphysis of long bones and apophyseal equivalents are unossified at this age, and will appear as intermediate signal. Once the epiphysis and apophysis ossify, they will contain yellow bone marrow, and therefore appear hyperintense on T1WI. At 1 year of age, red marrow predominates within the axial skeleton, and will appear hypointense on T1WI (**Fig. 3**).

Bone marrow conversion in childhood

In long bones, there is high T1 signal intensity in the diaphysis owing to yellow marrow and intermediate to low T1 signal intensity in the metaphysis. Overall, there is still an abundance of red marrow within the axial skeleton in the first decade of life, and the majority of bone marrow should appear T1 hypointense.

Normal adult bone marrow

By 25 years of age, the majority of normal bone marrow conversion occurs in the appendicular skeleton, with sparing of the proximal femoral metaphyses and proximal humeral metaphysis, which demonstrate intermediate to low T1-weighted signal. Spinal bone marrow has the presence of red marrow throughout life, but the proportions of red and yellow marrow in the axial skeleton vary by age and environmental factors. The marrow conversion pattern in the axial skeleton is less predictable. Several patterns of marrow conversion have been described,[2] including marrow conversion occurring first along the margins of the basivertebral veins, peripheral areas of conversion at the endplates involving the anterior and posterior vertebral body corners, patchy unorganized marrow conversion, or a combination of any of the above. Regardless of the process, there is a gradual decrease in the amount of red marrow in the axial skeleton. Before the age of 40 years, red marrow still dominates in the axial skeleton with only small areas of yellow marrow around the basivertebral plexus. With advancing age, the vertebral bone marrow becomes increasingly replaced with fatty marrow.

IMAGING OF MARROW PATHOLOGIES

Depending on the pathologic mechanism, marrow pathologies are classified into (**Table 2**):

a. marrow reconversion;
b. marrow infiltration;
c. marrow depletion;
d. marrow changes owing to osseous dysplasia and bony abnormalities;
e. marrow abnormalities owing to metabolic disorders; and
f. miscellaneous.

MARROW RECONVERSION

Marrow reconversion refers to replacement of yellow marrow by hematopoietic red marrow, which is a reversal of the normal physiologic conversion of bone marrow. In general, this process occurs as a response when systemic demand for hematopoiesis exceeds the capacity of the existing red marrow stores, for example, in chronic anemia.

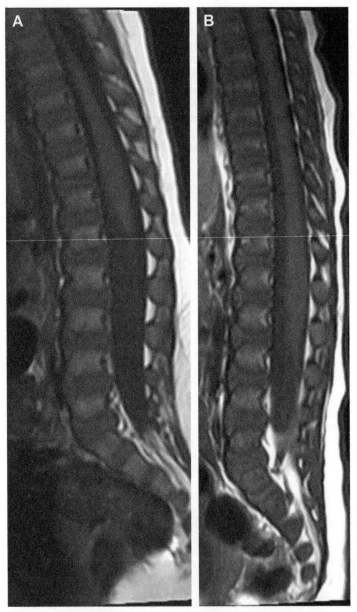

Fig. 3. Normal appearance of bone marrow at age 3 months and 1 year. Sagittal T1-weighted (*A*) image of the thoracolumbar spine of a 3-month-old shows that marrow signal is markedly hypointense compared with subcutaneous fat and closer to that of disc. Sagittal T1-weighted (*B*) image of the spine of a 1-year-old shows similar signal as (*A*).

Reconversion occurs in the opposite pattern of that of normal physiologic conversion. Thus, reconversion of bone marrow begins in the axial skeleton (flat bones of the pelvis and vertebrae of the spine), and progresses to the appendicular skeleton (individual long bones, followed by the distal extremities). Reconversion within individual

Table 2
Classification as per the pathologic mechanism

Pathologic Mechanism	Disorder
Marrow reconversion	Chronic anemia (sickle cell disease, thalassemia, hereditary spherocytosis), neoplastic replacement of normal bone marrow, concurrent administration of granulocyte-macrophage colony-stimulating factor
Marrow infiltration	Lymphoma, leukemia, Chronic myeloproliferative disorders metastasis, multiple myeloma
Marrow depletion	Radiation therapy, systemic chemotherapy aplastic anemia
Marrow changes owing to osseous dysplasia and bony abnormalities	Osteopetrosis, Paget disease, renal osteodystrophy
Marrow abnormalities owing to metabolic disorders	Gaucher disease, iron deposition, and iron overload state
Miscellaneous	Sarcoidosis gout

long bones also follows the predictable pattern of proximal metaphysis, followed by distal metaphysis, and finally the diaphysis.

Common causes of reconversion of bone marrow include states of chronic anemia (sickle cell disease, thalassemia, hereditary spherocytosis), neoplastic replacement of normal bone marrow, concurrent administration of granulocyte-macrophage colony-stimulating factor during chemotherapy treatment, and nonpathologic circumstances, during which an increased oxygen requirement is present, such as rigorous athletic training and high-altitude dwelling.[3–5]

Sickle Cell Disease

Sickle cell disease is a hereditary blood disorder characterized by an abnormality of the hemoglobin molecule in red blood cells, leading to an abnormal "sicklelike" shape of the red blood cells rather than the normal biconcave shape. These sickled red blood cells cause vascular occlusion, which in turn leads to tissue ischemia and infarction. When a patient possesses 2 sickle cell hemoglobin genes (Hb SS), it is called sickle cell anemia. Various other combinations seen include sickle cell trait (Hb SA); HbSC; Hb S-thalassemias, and Hb SD. Hb SS (*sickle cell anemia*) accounts for 60% to 70% of the cases of sickle cell disease in the United States and has the severest clinical manifestations of any of the sickle cell disease variants. The majority of the clinical presentations and complications of the sickle cell disease is owing to infarction and infection.

Anemia in sickle cell disease can be owing to several acute or chronic factors, which include vasoocclusive crisis (obstruction of capillaries by abnormally shaped red blood cells), splenic sequestration (abnormally shaped red blood cells being filtered out by the spleen), and hemolytic crisis (accelerated drops in hemoglobin levels owing to faster rate of breakdown of the abnormal red blood cells). These changes can lead to chronic anemia, which leads to excessive intramedullary and extramedullary hematopoiesis. Another complication is ischemic osteonecrosis owing to vasoocclusion. There is also increased susceptibility to infection in the skeleton and other organs of the body.

MRI is very sensitive in the evaluation of marrow conversion, infarction, and infection of the spine. Because of marrow hyperplasia and reconversion, spine marrow is diffusely T1 hypointense, and is slightly hyperintense on T2 fat saturation/STIR sequences (**Fig. 4**). Widening of osseous medullary spaces leads to osteopenia and thinning of cortical bone, leading to biconcave appearance of the vertebral body and making them vulnerable to pathologic fractures. The central vertebral body compression gives a typical "H-shaped" vertebra, which is seen commonly in thoracic spine and is best appreciated on plain radiograph or reconstructed images of CT (**Fig. 5**).[6–8]

Infarction and osteonecrosis owing to ischemic bone insult are commonly seen in sickle cell disease. These are thought to be owing to impediment of the blood flow secondary to cellular marrow, which enhances stasis, regional hypoxia, and sickling. Infarction is essentially seen in every marrow-containing bone and typically occurs in

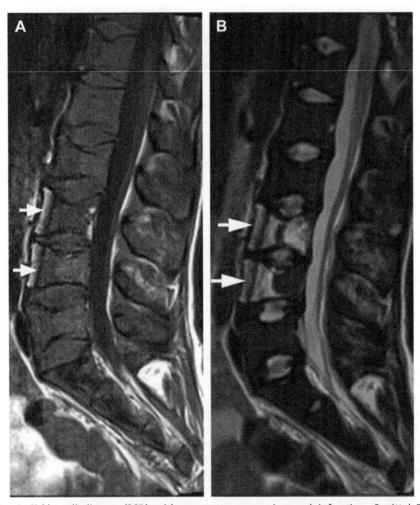

Fig. 4. Sickle cell disease (SCD) with marrow reconversion and infarction. Sagittal T1-weighted (*A*) image of the lumbar spine shows diffusely T1 hypointense marrow signal throughout the vertebrae, consistent with red marrow reconversion. There is, however, abnormal heterogeneous T2 signal in L3 and L4 shown in the sagittal T2-weighted (*B*) image (*arrows*), consistent with infarcts. Note all the visible vertebrae are "H-shaped" which is classic in SCD.

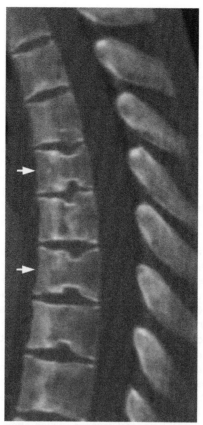

Fig. 5. Sickle cell disease. Sagittal reformatted computed tomography image shows the characteristic H-shaped configuration of vertebrae in sickle cell disease, which are biconcave in shape (*arrows*).

the medullary cavity and the epiphysis. On CT, acute infarct is seen as circular areas of decreased attenuation with disruption of the normal trabecular architecture. Long-standing chronic infarctions show an irregular appearing sclerotic rim along the infarct.

MRI is the most sensitive imaging technique for the diagnosis of bone marrow infarct and can demonstrate abnormalities within a few days of the insult. Acute infarct is seen as an area of hypointensity to hyperintensity on T1WI and high signal on T2/STIR images (see **Fig. 4**). Abnormal T2 hyperintensity may be seen in the periosteal and surrounding soft tissues. As the fibrosis and sclerosis sets in the infarcted area, chronic infarcts show low signal intensity on all the pulse sequences with central area of hyperintensity.

Osteomyelitis is a serious complication of sickle cell disease, most commonly involving the diaphyseal region of the long bones. Infection of the spine is also encountered commonly in these patients. The most frequently encountered organism is *Salmonella*. Signal intensity changes of osteomyelitis are very similar to infarction making it difficult to differentiate between the two. T2WI and contrast-enhanced T1WI are very sensitive in diagnosing and delineating the extent of the paraspinal, psoas, and extradural abscess.

Thalassemias

Thalassemias are autosomal-recessive blood disorders characterized by abnormal formation of hemoglobin. Normal adult hemoglobin is composed of Hb A (98%) and Hb A2 (2%). Hb A hemoglobin in an adult is composed of 4 protein chains—2 α-globin and 2 β-globin chains—whereas Hb A2 contain 2 α-globin chains and 2 δ-globin chains. The thalassemias are classified according to which chain of the hemoglobin molecule is affected. In α-thalassemia, there is a defect resulting in decreased α-globin production leading to an excess of β-chains in adults (γ chains in newborns). The excess β-chains then form abnormal unstable tetramers. β-Thalassemia is characterized by absence or reduced synthesis of the β-globin chains in the red cell and excess of α-chains, which are unstable and precipitate to form intracellular inclusion bodies. These changes lead to accelerated apoptosis of the erythroid precursors and peripheral hemolysis of the erythrocytes. β-Thalassemia is much more common than α-thalassemia. There are 3 different clinical patterns of β-thalassemia, which range from a minor presentation requiring no treatment to severe cases requiring regular blood transfusions.

Anemia owing to an ineffective erythropoiesis state leads to marrow proliferation, marrow reconversion and extramedullary hematopoiesis. Marrow proliferation on CT scan and plain radiograph is seen as expansion of the medulla, thinning of cortical bone, and resorption of cancellous bone resulting in diffuse osteopenia and coarsened trabecular pattern (**Fig. 6**). MRI of the spine demonstrates diffuse T1 hypointensity and mild T2 fat suppression/STIR hyperintensity secondary to marrow hyperplasia and reconversion. Increased hematopoiesis causes widening of the diploic space, with thinning of the outer table and thickening of the inner table giving a "hair-on-end" appearance to the calvarium. Expansion of the facial bones inhibits the pneumatization of paranasal sinuses leading to displacement of the orbits and maxillary protrusion giving a "rodent face" appearance. Extramedullary hematopoiesis is commonly seen in severe thalassemia. They are seen as intermediate T1 and T2 signal intensity and symmetric paravertebral and presacral masses, which show mild enhancement on gadolinium-enhanced scans. These masses may be round, ovoid, or confluent, and can sometimes extend into the spinal canal, causing cord compression and giving rise to myelopathy.

Mainstream treatment of thalassemia is blood transfusion. With chronic transfusions, iron overload occurs in the various systems of the body, including the skeletal system. On MRI, this results in diffuse low signal intensity on T1 and T2 WI, and increased susceptibility artifacts on gradient echo sequences (**Fig. 7**A). MRI of the abdomen may show marked hepatosplenomegaly with signal intensity loss in the liver on T2-wieghted images and T1WI owing to iron deposition in the liver (hemosiderosis; **Fig. 7**B).

MARROW INFILTRATION/REPLACEMENT
Hematologic Malignancies

Lymphoproliferative and myeloproliferative disorders frequently involve the skeletal system. In fact, skeletal involvement is frequently the initial and dominant manifestation of these disorders. Imaging findings are nonspecific; however, in the appropriate context of clinical findings, they can be diagnosed and staged correctly using various imaging techniques.

Lymphomas

Lymphomas refer to a group of blood cell tumors arising from the proliferation of clonal lymphoid cells. They are grouped into 2 main categories: Hodgkin's lymphoma (HL)

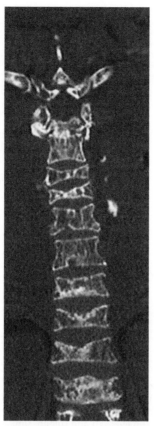

Fig. 6. Thalassemias with marrow proliferation. Coronal reformatted computed tomography image shows diffuse osteopenia, trabecular thickening, and compression deformities of numerous thoracic vertebral bodies.

and non-HL (NHL). NHL is a diverse group of malignant lymphoid tumors that, depending on the cell dominance, is classified into diffuse large B-cell lymphoma, follicular lymphoma, anaplastic large cell lymphoma, lymphoblastic lymphoma, and Burkitt lymphoma. HL is characterized by the presence of Reed–Sternberg cells on histology. Regardless of the type, the distinctive hallmark of lymphoma is the proliferation of clonal lymphoid cells, which typically presents as lymphadenopathy and proliferation of secondary lymphoid tissues.

Lymphoma of the spine may occur as primary lymphoma of bone or as secondary involvement in HL or NHL. Primary lymphoma of the bone is very rare, accounting for less than 5%. The most common route of secondary lymphoma spread to the bone and spine is hematogenous. Diffuse marrow involvement is more common than isolated cortical involvement, owing to the favorable environment for proliferation within the bone marrow. Marrow replacement is more common in NHL than HL.[9] Secondary lymphoma of the spine may be seen owing to direct invasion by adjacent lymphadenopathy (mediastinal in the thoracic and retroperitoneal in the lumbar spine), but this is uncommon.

The radiographic and CT appearance of osseous involvement of HL is variable. Lesions may appear as lytic, sclerotic, or mixed lytic/sclerotic lesions. The lesions usually

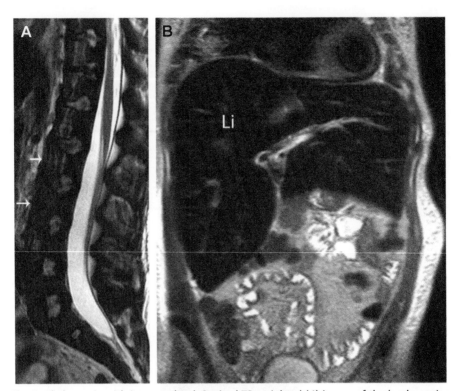

Fig. 7. Thalassemia with iron overload. Sagittal T2-weighted (*A*) image of the lumbar spine shows diffusely hypointense marrow signal (*arrows*) related to iron overload from chronic transfusions. Coronal T2-weighted (*B*) image of the abdomen shows enlargement of and diffusely hypointense signal in the liver (Li) and spleen, similar to the marrow signal, owing to iron deposition in these organs.

show poorly defined borders. In NHL, the axial skeleton is affected more commonly than the appendicular skeleton. Typical imaging appearance in NHL is that of multiple ill-defined lesions (permeative osteolytic destruction) involving multiple vertebral bodies. Periosteal reaction may be present in NHL, but this finding is less commonly seen than in HL.

On T1-weighted MRI of lymphomatous bone marrow, the appearance is similar to that of other infiltrative processes, such as leukemia. This is seen as focal or diffuse hypointense areas on the axial skeleton. However, the corresponding T2 signal may be variable, and may appear heterogeneously hypointense, isointense, or hyperintense (**Fig. 8**). The variability of the T2 signal may be directly related to the proportional content of fibrous tissue. Inversion recovery sequences are often superior to T2 fat saturation sequences when evaluating a large field of view, as is often performed for evaluation of the spine.

MRI is also a valuable tool in evaluating early extension into the adjacent soft tissues and spinal canal, differentiating benign fracture from pathologic, and in the diagnosis of associated infection in an immunocompromised patient. A pathologic fracture is suggested when there is convexity of the posterior cortex towards the spinal canal, and/or when an adjacent epidural mass is visualized, whereas benign fracture would show a normal concavity.

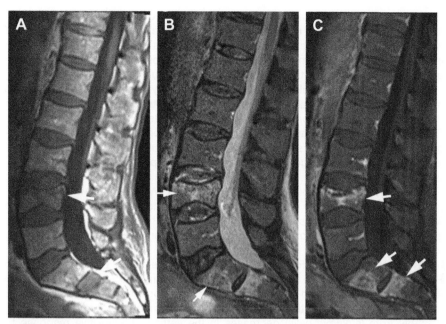

Fig. 8. Lymphoma. Sagittal T1-weighted (*A*) image of the lumbar spine shows focal hypointense areas of marrow signal in the L4 vertebral body as well as the upper aspect of S2 (*arrows*). Note relatively normal marrow signal in the other vertebrae. Sagittal T2-weighted (*B*) image shows abnormally hyperintense marrow in L4 and S2, but also in S1 anteriorly (*arrows*). Note compression deformity of L4 suggestive of pathologic fracture. Sagittal T1-weighted postcontrast fat-suppressed (*C*) image of the lumbar spine reveals enhancement of the lesions in L4, S1, and S2 (*arrows*), consistent with lymphomatous marrow involvement.

One of the limitations of MRI is in the assessment of early response after treatment. PET scan, owing to its cellular imaging properties, is able to distinguish viable tumor from necrotic or fibrotic tissue very early and therefore more widely used to assess the response to treatment. Fluorodeoxyglucose PET provides the best whole body scanning technique for staging and to assess the response in both HL and NHL.

Leukemia

Leukemia refers to a group of cancers involving the bone marrow that result in a pathologically increased number of abnormal white blood cells. Conventionally, they are grouped into acute and chronic forms. Acute leukemias represent defective blast maturation, which in turn leads to an accumulation of immature cells within the bone marrow. Chronic leukemias are characterized by unregulated overgrowth of mature cells within the bone marrow. Both acute and chronic forms may arise from myeloid or lymphoid cell lines, and therefore there are classically 4 types of leukemias (acute myelogenous leukemia, acute lymphatic leukemia, chronic myelogenous leukemia, and chronic lymphatic leukemia).

Acute leukemias are most commonly seen in childhood. The overwhelming majority of acute leukemias are lymphoblasic in origin, with the peak incidence occurring at 2 to 3 years of age. Proliferation and accumulation of immature cells within the bone marrow suppresses the normal function of marrow, leading to anemia, neutropenia, and thrombocytopenia, which are responsible for most of the clinical signs and symptoms. There are several well-described radiographic characteristics of acute leukemia, each of which is a nonspecific finding individually, but the conglomerate of which greatly increases the suspicion for the diagnosis of leukemia. These findings include transverse lucent metaphyseal bands, subperiosteal cortical bone erosions, periosteal reaction, focal lytic osseous lesions, and diffuse demineralization.

In contrast with acute leukemias, chronic leukemias typically present in adults. The myelogenous subtype usually affects middle aged adults from the fourth to the sixth decade, whereas the lymphocytic form typically affects a more elderly population. Chronic leukemias very rarely affect the pediatric population.[10] Generally, radiographic osseous findings are less extensive in chronic leukemias compared with acute leukemias. On plain radiography, leukemic marrow replacement is represented by diffuse osteopenia.

MRI evaluation of leukemia is best performed with T1WI and STIR. Marrow replacement by leukemia typically manifests as diffuse hypointense T1 signal as compared with adjacent skeletal muscle, with a corresponding hyperintense T2 signal. This appearance is shared by other marrow replacement processes and is not specific to leukemia.

MRI is also very useful for evaluating response of leukemic patients to therapy. Patients responding to the therapy will show return of normal T1 signal in the spine (**Fig. 9**). Similarly, relapsed disease will show the reappearance of hypointense T1 signal. It has been shown that the proportion of bone marrow edema present (presumably from leukemic cells) decreases in the setting of a positive response to therapy; thus, the amount of edema seen on imaging may be correlated with disease response. Quantitative chemical shift ("in and out of phase") imaging is a sensitive sequence in differentiating fat and water within marrow and therefore provides an important information regarding response to therapy. In concurrence with a positive response to therapy, the edema component within bone marrow shows sequential decreases on chemical shift imaging. The converse is also true; a nonresponse to therapy would be characterized by low fat signal within the marrow.

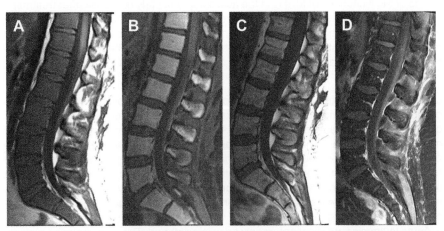

Fig. 9. Leukemia before and after treatment. Sagittal T1-weighted (*A*) and T1 postcontrast fat-suppressed (*B*) images of the lumbar spine show diffusely abnormal marrow signal, which is hypointense compared with muscle on T1 and avidly enhancing. After successful treatment, bone marrow signal returns to normal on sagittal T1-weighted (*C*) and T1 postcontrast fat-suppressed (*D*) images.

Chronic myeloproliferative disorders

Chronic myeloproliferative disorders encompass 3 disorders: osteomyelofibrosis/sclerosis, polycythemia vera, and essential thrombocytopenia, all of which are diseases of myeloid stem cells.

Osteomyelofibrosis/osteomyelosclerosis is a disease that occurs in the sixth to seventh decades of life. Osteomyelofibrosis/osteomyelosclerosis is seen more commonly in association with other malignant bone disorders like leukemia, lymphoma, and multiple myeloma. In the early stages, the bone marrow is hyperplastic, and there is a reduction in the proportion of intramedullary fat. At this point, there is marked T1 and T2 hypointensity, reflective of the diffuse increase in hematopoietic cells and decrease in fat cells. This is followed by a subsequent hypocellular stage, with replacement of marrow with fibrosis and sclerosis. In the late stages, there is persistent T1 and T2 hypointensity; however, this is owing to extensive marrow fibrosis and sclerosis rather than the presence of active hematopoietic cells (**Fig. 10**). There will be corresponding osteosclerosis on CT and radiograph.

Polycythemia vera is a rare neoplasm in which the bone marrow overproduces red blood cells. It may be associated with an overproduction of white blood cells and platelets as well. MRI findings are similar to other myeloproliferative disorders.

Metastatic disease

Metastasis is the most common tumor of the bone. Various primary tumors such as breast, lung, and prostate cancer have a predilection to metastasize to the bones. Because bone marrow does not have a lymphatic system, metastatic disease to the bone marrow is either by hematogenous or contiguous spread. It is thought that the hematopoietic properties and stromal cells of the bone marrow provide a favorable condition for growth and expansion. Osseous metastatic disease begins in the red bone marrow. The thoracic and lumbar spine, along with the pelvis, are statistically the most affected sites, perhaps owing to the role of retrograde flow in Batson's vertebral plexus.

Plain radiography is insensitive for early osseous metastatic disease. Only with extensive destruction of bone and demineralization greater than 50% can plain radiography reliably detect metastatic disease. CT offers a more sensitive imaging modality, because it better assesses trabecular bone loss and cortical destruction. Osteolytic and osteoblastic lesions (**Fig. 11**A) are clearly demonstrated on CT. Additionally, CT is a terrific tool for the assessment of impending pathologic fracture.

Still, because of its ability to visualize early marrow changes owing to high soft tissue contrast, MRI is the most sensitive imaging modality for the detection of metastatic disease. Additionally, tumor infiltration into the adjacent soft tissues and spinal canal can be characterized more easily on MRI. For the purposes of screening of osseous metastatic disease, a combination of conventional T1WI and STIR sequence has proved to be highly sensitive in the ability to evaluate malignant marrow disorders.[11] The majority of metastatic lesions are hypointense on T1 and hyperintense on STIR sequences secondary to increased water content within tumor cells. Osteoblastic metastasis shows hypointense signal on STIR imaging (**Fig. 11**B, C). Intravenous contrast enhancement can occasionally be helpful; osseous metastatic lesions often shows peripheral enhancement.

Diffuse infiltrative metastatic disease of the bone marrow can be difficult to detect. On T1-weighted sequences, the marrow will demonstrate homogeneous hypointensity, with a concurrent increased STIR signal. The signal alterations may be extremely subtle, and given the homogeneity of the signal owing to diffuse infiltration pattern, can

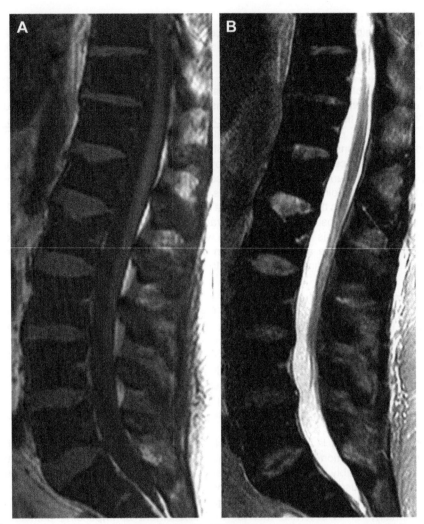

Fig. 10. Myelosclerosis/myelofibrosis. Sagittal T1-weighted (*A*) and T2-weighted (*B*) images of the lumbar spine show homogeneously extremely hypointense marrow signal on both T2 and T2 sequences owing to replacement of cellular marrow and fat by fibrosis.

be very difficult to visualize. The "bright disc" sign is a finding that corresponds with diffuse marrow infiltration of metastatic disease. This finding refers to the higher signal of the intervertebral disc as compared with the pathologic diffuse hypointense signal of the bone marrow on T1-weighted sequences.[12]

MARROW DEPLETION

Marrow depletion refers to a state when there is a failure to increase hematopoiesis even when the overall amount of hematopoietic red marrow is depressed.[13] Histopathology shows hypocellular or acellular marrow on a background of diffuse fatty replacement. Marrow depletion is most commonly seen after radiation or chemotherapy and in aplastic anemia.

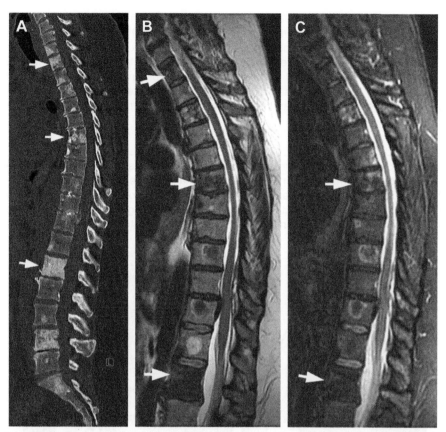

Fig. 11. Osteoblastic metastases. Sagittal reformatted computed tomography (CT) scan (A) of the thoracolumbar spine shows multiple dense foci within the vertebral bodies (arrows), representing sclerotic metastases. Similarly, sagittal T2-weighted (B) and short-tau inversion recovery sequence (C) images of the thoracic spine show that the sclerotic lesions on CT are hypointense on both sequences (arrows).

Radiation Therapy

Therapeutic medical radiation is used for the treatment of cancers. An established side effect of such treatment is marrow suppression. The hematopoietic marrow is more susceptible to radiation damage than is yellow marrow, and is thus injured first. The degree of damage and determination of reversibility depends on the dose of radiation, volume of marrow affected, and the frequency of treatment.[14] Reversible changes in bone marrow may persist for up to 2 years,[15] and generally occurs with a local total dose of less than 30 Gy. A dose of greater than 50 Gy results in complete ablation of the affected marrow.[16]

Marrow changes can be detected on imaging as early as 8 days after the initial insult.[17,18] By 3 weeks, changes will be apparent. The earliest change occurs on T2 fat saturation/STIR images, where the marrow will demonstrate increased signal intensity. The hyperintense signal on fluid-sensitive images is thought to represent edema, although there is possibly a component of hemorrhage and an influx of unaffected cells.[18]

Around 3 to 6 weeks after treatment, the signal intensity on T2 fat suppressed/STIR imaging decreases. Concurrently, the marrow signal on T1 (which has remained normal during this period) begins to increase. This is reflective of an increased concentration of fatty marrow. By 6 weeks, the majority of patients imaged will demonstrate an abnormally hyperintense T1 signal, which may last for up to 2 years (**Fig. 12**).[15,19] The pattern of T1 signal hyperintensity is typical. The hyperintense fatty marrow is usually well-defined with sharp margins, which are reflective of the margins of the radiation field.

Chemotherapy

Systemic chemotherapy, a mainstay of cancer treatment, has the unfortunate side effect of collateral damage to hematopoietic bone marrow. After the initiation of chemotherapy, there will be decreased T1 signal intensity of marrow with a corresponding increase in T2 fat-suppressed/STIR signal intensity, thought to be secondary to marrow congestion. With continued destruction of the hematopoietic elements, there

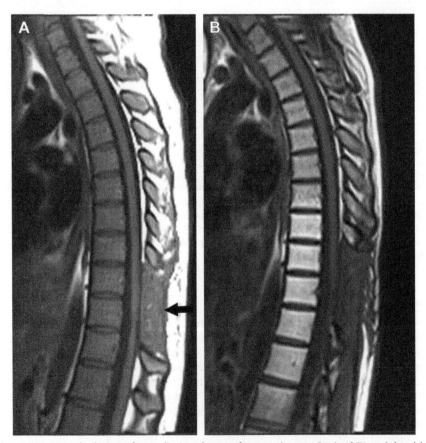

Fig. 12. Marrow depletion after radiation therapy for germinoma. Sagittal T1-weighted (*A*) image of the thoracic spine before radiation therapy shows normal marrow signal, which is hypointense compared with fat and similar to muscle. Note the laminectomy changes in the lower thoracic spine (*arrow*). Sagittal T1-weighted (*B*) image of the thoracic spine after radiation shows diffusely hyperintense marrow signal in the radiation field, essentially isointense of fat.

is increased fatty deposition, and a subsequent increase in the T1 signal of the marrow. Of note, when a chemotherapy regimen includes granulocyte-colony stimulating factor, there may be a pattern of marrow reconversion superimposed. This change may be mistaken for disease relapse or inefficacy of treatment,[20] and therefore careful attention to the clinical history is important during the interpretation of postchemotherapy imaging.

Aplastic Anemia

Aplastic anemia is a rare condition characterized by pancytopenia and hypocellularity of the bone marrow. It is considered a disease of the bone marrow, because it reflects an inherent inability of the hematopoietic stem cells within the marrow to function appropriately. Although the majority of cases are idiopathic, aplastic anemia can be acquired after toxic or chemical exposure, medication exposure, radiation exposure, or chemotherapy treatment. Definitive diagnosis is performed by bone marrow biopsy.

Aplastic marrow is diffusely hyperintense on T1 sequences owing to a predominantly fatty component. This is especially obvious in areas that are normally dominant in hematopoietic marrow (spine and pelvis). It is worth noting that areas of aplastic marrow can seem to be heterogeneous on T1-weighted sequences if there is fibrosis. Treatment of aplastic anemia consists of an immunosuppressive drug regimen. During treatment, myeloid element (red marrow) function may return, which may be represented on MRI by scattered foci of T1 hypointensities within fatty marrow.

PRIMARILY OSSEOUS DYSPLASIAS AND BONY ABNORMALITIES
Osteopetrosis

Osteopetrosis, also known as Albers–Schonberg disease, is a rare inherited disorder resulting in diffuse increase in the density of bone. The disease is attributed to malfunctioning osteoclasts, which results in an imbalance between bone formation and resorption, in the favor of osteoblasts (bone formation). Despite the increase in bone density, the abnormal osteoclast function adversely affects the underlying bone structure, leading to structurally weak bone which is more susceptible to fracture.

On plain radiographs and CT scan, osteopetrosis manifests as uniformly dense bones. Involvement of long bones involves the entire bone—diaphysis, metaphysis, and epiphysis. Cranial vault, skull base, and entire spinal axis are also involved and are responsible for various neurologic symptoms. CT is very sensitive in demonstrating the abnormal remodeling of cranial nerve foramina, which can result in deafness and blindness. In the spine, the "sandwich vertebrae" is a classic descriptor of osteopetrosis, with increased sclerosis seen at the superior and inferior endplates (**Fig. 13**A).

MRI is used primarily to assess the degree of bone marrow involvement. The marrow seems to be hypointense on both T1WI and T2WI owing to diffuse sclerotic bone (**Fig. 13**B). These findings are nonspecific and may be seen in various other disorders such as hemosiderosis, fibrosis, and diffuse blastic metastatic disease.[21] MRI is also useful in the assessment of response to therapy after bone marrow transplant.

Paget Disease

Paget disease, also known as osteitis deformans, is a chronic skeletal disorder thought to be secondary to an imbalance between osteoblast and osteoclast activity. The initial insult is felt to be owing to an increase in the rate of bone resorption in localized areas by osteoclasts. This is followed by a compensatory increase in bone

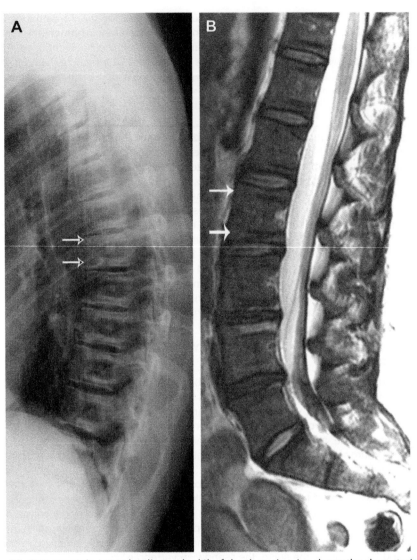

Fig. 13. Osteopetrosis. Lateral radiography (*A*) of the thoracic spine shows the characteristic "sandwich vertebrae," with increased sclerosis seen at the superior and inferior endplates (*arrows*). Sagittal T2-weighted (*B*) image shows hypointensity of the superior and inferior endplates corresponding with sclerosis on radiography.

formation by osteoblasts, which produce lamellar bone quickly and in a disorganized fashion. This results in excessive fibrous connective tissue and hypervascular bone filling in the normal marrow spaces. These cellular changes divide the Paget disease into 3 major phases:

a. A lytic or active phase, during which osteoclastic resorption is the predominant process,
b. A mixed osteoblastic/osteoclastic phase, and
c. A blastic or late inactive phase, during which osteoblastic activity predominates.

The etiology of the Paget disease is debatable. The proposed etiologies include viral, vascular diseases, genetic diseases, an immunologic or metabolic disorder, or a true neoplastic process. After the pelvis, spine is the second most commonly affected site.

Imaging appearance varies widely and depends on the stage of the disease. Imaging is essential for establishing the diagnosis, evaluating the phase of the disease, monitoring the complications, and efficacy of therapy. In the lytic phase, radiography and CT show areas of osteolysis. In the long bone this classically appears as a wedge-shaped or flame-shaped area of radiolucency in the diaphyseal or metaphyseal regions. In the skull, active osteolysis produces areas of lucency, which is termed *osteoporosis circumscripta*. The blastic (late inactive) phase manifests as osteosclerosis. These are seen as areas of increased sclerosis, coarsening of the trabeculae, cortical thickening, and generalized enlargement of the affected bone (**Fig. 14**A). Because of the abnormal structure of the bone, the bone is weakened and is prone to fracture. As the name suggests, the mixed phase will bear a combination of imaging characteristics from both phases. The mixed phase of osseous Paget disease involving the spine appears as a classic "picture frame" vertebra, or "bone within bone" appearance. This is caused by cortical thickening along all 4 margins of the vertebral body cortices.

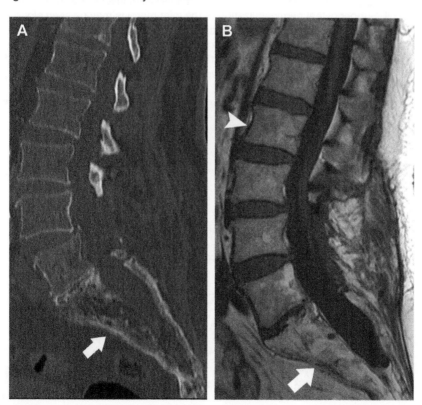

Fig. 14. Paget disease. Sagittal reformatted computed tomography (CT) (*A*) of the lumbosacral spine shows increased sclerosis, coarsening of the trabeculae, cortical thickening, and generalized enlargement of the sacrum (*arrow*), typical of the osteosclerotic phase. Sagittal T1-weighted (*B*) image of the same region shows relatively hyperintense marrow signal in the lumbar vertebrae, indicating fatty marrow (*arrowhead*) and heterogeneous T1 signal in the sacrum (*arrow*).

MRI characteristics of Paget disease are also variable, and reflective of phase of the disease. There are 3 major patterns of Paget disease recognized on MRI.[22] The most common is fat signal intensity within Pagetic bone (**Fig. 14**B): hyperintense on T1WI, with expected corresponding signal drop out on T2 fat-saturated or STIR sequences. The second most common is heterogeneous areas of low T1 signal intensity with corresponding high T2 signal intensity, referred to as the "speckled" appearance. This likely corresponds with the mixed lytic/blastic phase of Paget disease, and is reflective of a mixture of granulation tissue, edema, and hypervascularity. The least common pattern is low signal intensity on both T1WI and T2-weighted images, reflective of fibrous tissue or compact bone during the inactive/blastic phase of Paget disease.

Renal Osteodystrophy

Renal osteodystrophy refers to a bone pathology characterized by deficiency in bone mineralization, which is a direct result of electrolyte imbalances that occur during chronic renal disease. It is thought to be the result of hyperparathyroidism, which is triggered because of hyperphosphatemia and hypocalcemia in the setting of chronic renal failure. The high levels of parathyroid hormone then increase bone resorption.

Radiographic and CT findings of renal osteodystrophy include a combination of osteosclerosis and osteopenia. In the calvarium, this will manifest as a "salt and pepper" skull. Subperiosteal demineralization of the joint margins may be seen along the radial aspects of the second and third digitis of the hands. The classic appearance of renal osteodystrophy in the spine is the "rugger jersey" spine. This term is reflective of the finding of sclerotic bands paralleling the superior and inferior endplates of the vertebral bodies (**Fig. 15**A). These sclerotic bands have poorly defined margins, as

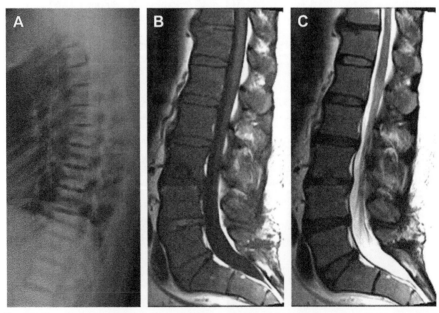

Fig. 15. Renal osteodystrophy. Lateral radiograph (*A*) of the thoracic spine shows the classic "rugger-jersey spine" with sclerotic bands paralleling the superior and inferior endplates of the vertebral bodies. Note that the margins of these sclerotic bands are not sharp, as contrasted with the bands seen in osteopetrosis. Sagittal T1-weighted (*B*) and T2-weighted (*C*) images of the lumbar spine show diffuse hypointensity of the bone marrow.

opposed to the previously described "sandwich vertebrae" of osteopetrosis. On MRI, affected marrow demonstrates focal low T1 signal intensity (**Fig. 15**B) with corresponding high T2 signal intensity (**Fig. 15**C).

METABOLIC DISEASE
Gaucher Disease

Gaucher disease is a lysosomal storage disease. The pathophysiology is defined as a lack of glucocerebrosidease, leading to accumulation of glucocerebrosides within histiocytes called Gaucher cells.[23] The proliferation of these Gaucher cells results in accumulation of glycolipids throughout the reticuloendothelial system. Manifestations include hepatosplenomagaly with associated hepatic dysfunction, neurologic complications, lymphadenopathy, discoloration of the skin, anemia, thrombocytopenia, and skeletal disorders. From a bone marrow standpoint, this results in cellular necrosis and fibrous proliferation.[24]

Radiographically, a classic finding is an "Erlenmeyer flask" deformity of the distal femora bilaterally, which is clinically silent. Other findings include pathologic fractures, vertebral body collapse, and bone infarcts. CT is a great asset for evaluating

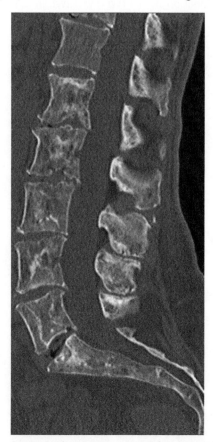

Fig. 16. Gaucher disease. Sagittal reformatted computed tomography image of the lumbar spine shows a mixed lucent and sclerotic appearance of the lumbar vertebrae and sacrum with serpentine sclerotic lines, indicating a mixture of osteopenia, trabecular thickening, and bone infarction.

generalized osteopenia and trabecular coarsening. Osseous involvement of Gaucher disease may also manifest as multiple lytic regions, which seem to be somewhat circumscribed (**Fig. 16**). Superimposed serpiginous pattern of sclerosis may present secondary to bone infarction.

MRI appearance of bone marrow affected by Gaucher disease generally demonstrates hypointense signal on T1, T2 fat-saturated/STIR images owing to glucocerebroside deposition. Early in the disease, signal abnormalities will present as focal lesions that become diffuse during the late phases of the disease. Findings of osteonecrosis may be superimposed. MRI is useful in quantifying disease progression. Patients with Gaucher disease are predisposed to fractures, because there is a weakening of the subchondral bone owing to generalized osteoporosis. Vertebra plana may be seen secondary to fracture.[24,25]

Iron Deposition/Hemosiderosis

Iron deposition and iron overload state can result from increased hemolysis (such as sickle cell anemia, thalassemias, G6PD deficiency), primary disease state (hemochromatosis), or iatrogenic (chronic blood transfusion therapy). MRI demonstrates diffusely hypointense signal on both T1WI and T2WI. In suspected cases, gradient

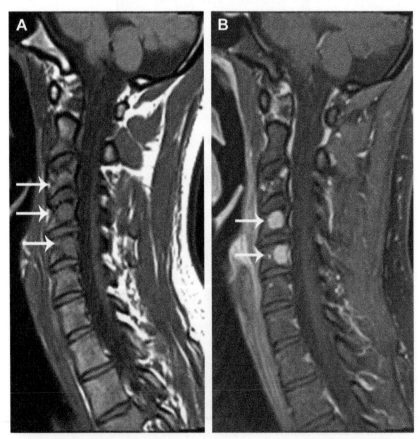

Fig. 17. Sarcoidosis. Sagittal T1-weighted (*A*) imaging of the cervical spine shows areas of slightly hypointense marrow signal in C4 and C5 (*arrows*), which enhance homogeneously on the sagittal T1 postcontrast image (*B*).

echo T2* sequences may be performed, which will demonstrate blooming effect in the vertebrae and in the liver and spleen owing to the presence of excess iron.

MISCELLANEOUS
Sarcoidosis

Sarcoidosis is a multiple system noncaseating granulomatous disorder. The underlying pathologic process is the abnormal accumulation of inflammatory cells

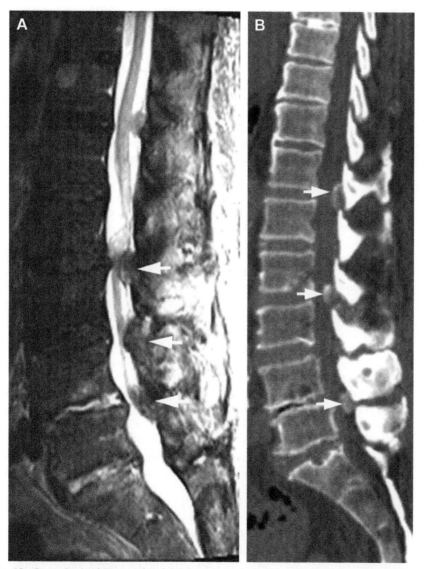

Fig. 18. Gout. Sagittal T2-weighted (*A*) imaging of the lumbar spine shows hypointense marrow signal in the vertebral bodies and hypointense nodules along the posterior margin of the bony canal in the expected region of the ligamentum flava (*arrows*). Sagittal reformatted computed tomography (CT; *B*) image of the same region shows that these ligamentum flavum nodules are hyperdense and partly calcified, likely tophi (*arrows*).

(noncaseating epithelial granulomas) within multiple organs. The granulomas are most often located in the lungs and associated pulmonary lymph nodes, but any organ may be affected. Osseous involvement is rare and is seen in 1% to 13% of the patients.

Radiographically, osseous sarcoidosis can manifest as lytic lesions which may develop sclerotic rim of "healing." Rarely, osseous sarcoidosis can manifest as osteosclerotic lesions. CT correlate will demonstrate multiple lytic lesions within the spine, with healing sclerotic margins. If the spinal cord is involved, cord expansion may be appreciated. On MRI, vertebral marrow affected by sarcoidosis can appear as focal or diffuse signal changes. These areas are hypointense on T1WI and hyperintense on T2WI and show intense enhancement (**Fig. 17**).

Gout

Spinal bone marrow involvement by gout is rare; however, when it does occur, it is not uncommon to see the marrow signal intensity changes in patient with gout. Vertebrae may show focal or diffuse signal intensity changes on MR, which most often manifests as areas of low T1-weighted and variable T2-weighted signal intensity (**Fig. 18**A). Changes are predominately seen in the posterior elements, facet joints and ligament flava. Findings in the vertebral bodies may mimic discitis–osteomyelitis. CT imaging may be helpful in identifying calcifications and tophi formation (**Fig. 18**B).

REFERENCES

1. Melhem ER, Israel DA, Eustace S, et al. MR of the spine with a fast T1-weighted fluid-attenuated inversion recovery sequence. AJNR Am J Neuroradiol 1997;18: 447–54.

2. Ricci C, Cova M, Kang YS, et al. Normal age-related patterns of cellular and fatty bone marrow distribution in the axial skeleton: MR imaging study. Radiology 1990;177:83–8.

3. Fletcher BD, Wall JE, Hanna SL. Effect of hematopoietic growth factors on MR images of bone marrow in children undergoing chemotherapy. Radiology 1993;189: 745–51.

4. Ryan SP, Weinberger E, White KS, et al. MR imaging of bone marrow in children with osteosarcoma: effect of granulocyte colony-stimulating factor. AJR Am J Roentgenol 1995;165:915–20.

5. Shellock FG, Morris E, Deutsch AL, et al. Hematopoietic bone marrow hyperplasia: high prevalence on MR images of the knee in asymptomatic marathon runners. AJR Am J Roentgenol 1992;158:335–8.

6. Vogler JB 3rd, Murphy WA. Bone marrow imaging. Radiology 1988;168:679–93.

7. Moulopoulos LA, Maris TG, Papanikolaou N, et al. Detection of malignant bone marrow involvement with dynamic contrast-enhanced magnetic resonance imaging. Ann Oncol 2003;14:152–8.

8. Kanchiku T, Taguchi T, Toyoda K, et al. Dynamic contrast-enhanced magnetic resonance imaging of osteoporotic vertebral fracture. Spine 2003;28:2522–6.

9. Parker BR, Marglin S, Castellino RA. Skeletal manifestations of leukemia, Hodgkin disease, and non-Hodgkin lymphoma. Semin Roentgenol 1980;15:302–15.

10. Guillerman RP, Voss SD, Parker BR. Leukemia and lymphoma. Radiol Clin North Am 2011;49:767–97.

11. Walker R, Kessar P, Blanchard R, et al. Turbo STIR magnetic resonance imaging as a whole-body screening tool for metastases in patients with breast carcinoma: preliminary clinical experience. J Magn Reson Imaging 2000;11:343–50.

12. Castillo M, Malko JA, Hoffman JC. The bright intervertebral disk: an indirect sign of abnormal spinal bone marrow on T1-weighted MR images. AJNR Am J Neuroradiol 1990;11:23–6.

13. Wang DT. Magnetic resonance imaging of bone marrow: a review – part I. J Am Osteopath Coll Radiol 2012;2:2–12.

14. Sacks EL, Goris ML, Glatstein E, et al. Bone marrow regeneration following large field radiation: influence of volume, age, dose, and time. Cancer 1978;42(3): 1057–65.

15. Ramsey RG, Zacharias CE. MR imaging of the spine after radiation therapy: easily recognizable effects. AJR Am J Roentgenol 1985;144(6):1131–5.

16. Casamassima F, Ruggiero C, Caramella D, et al. Hematopoietic bone marrow recovery after radiation therapy: MRI evaluation. Blood 1989;73(6):1677–81.

17. Stevens SK, Moore SG, Kaplan ID. Early and late bone-marrow changes after irradiation: MR evaluation. AJR Am J Roentgenol 1990;154(4):745–50.

18. Blomlie V, Rofstad EK, Skjønsberg A, et al. Female pelvic bone marrow: serial MR imaging before, during, and after radiation therapy. Radiology 1995;194(2): 537–43.

19. Yankelevitz DF, Henschke CI, Knapp PH, et al. Effect of radiation therapy on thoracic and lumbar bone marrow: evaluation with MR imaging. AJR Am J Roentgenol 1991;157(1):87–92.

20. Ehrlich P. Uber einen Fall von Anamie mit Bemerkungen uber regenerative Veranderungen des Knochenmarks. Charite-Annalen 1888;13:300.

21. Rao VM, Dalinka MK, Mitchell DG, et al. Osteopetrosis: MR characteristics at 1.5 T. Radiology 1986;161(1):217–20.

22. Theodorou DJ, Theodorou SJ, Haghighi P, et al. Distinct focal lesions of the femoral head: imaging features suggesting an atypical and minimal form of bone necrosis. Skeletal Radiol 2002;31:435–44.

23. Cotran RS, Kumar V, Collins T. Robbins pathologic basis of disease. 6th edition. Philadelphia: Saunders; 1999.

24. McAlister WH, Herman TE. Osteochondrodysplasias, dysostoses, chromosomal aberrations, mucopolysaccharidoses, and mucolipidoses. In: Resnick D, Kransdorf MJ, editors. Bone and joint imaging. 3rd edition. Philadelphia: Elsevier Saunders; 2005.

25. Manaster BJ, Disler DG, May DA. Musculoskeletal imaging the requisites. 2nd edition. Saint Louis (MO): Mosby; 2002.

Index

Note: Page numbers of article titles are in **boldface** type.

A

Amyloidosis, systemic amyloid light chain, 845–846
Anemia, imaging of neurologic complications of, 724–725, **733–756**
    aplastic anemia, 742–745
    Fanconi anemia, 745–746
    glucose 6-phosphate dehydrogenase deficiency, 751–752
    hereditary spherocytosis, 742
    imaging modalities, 734
    iron deficiency anemias, 734–737
    paroxysmal nocturnal hemoglobinuria, 741–742
    pyruvate kinase deficiency, 752–753
    secondary causes of, 753–755
        myelodysplastic syndrome, 754–755
        myeloma, 753
        systemic lupus erythematosus, 753–754
    sickle cell anemia, 746–751
    vitamin deficiency anemias, 737–741
Angiography, digitally subtracted, of cortical venous thrombosis, 882
Antithrombin deficiency, imaging of neurologic complications of coagulation
    disorders due to, 774
Aplastic anemia, imaging of bone marrow in, 963
    imaging of neurologic complications of, 742–745

B

Bacterial infection, CNS complications of hematopoietic stem cell transplant
    due to, 890
Blood dyscrasias, imaging of neurologic complications in, **723–731**
    benign hematologic conditions, 723–727
        anemias, 724–725
        disorders of hemostasis, 725–727
    malignant hematologic conditions, 727–729
        leukemia and lymphoma, 727
        plasma cell dyscrasias, 727–729
Bone, imaging of complications of in sickle cell disease, 793–795
Bone marrow, imaging of, **945–971**
    changes in, from childhood to adulthood, 946–947
    composition of, 946
    marrow depletion, 960–963
        aplastic anemia, 963
        chemotherapy, 962–963

Hematol Oncol Clin N Am 30 (2016) 973–986
http://dx.doi.org/10.1016/S0889-8588(16)30070-3
0889-8588/16/$ – see front matter

hemonc.theclinics.com

Bone (*continued*)
    radiation therapy, 961–962
   marrow infiltration/replacement, 954–960
    chronic myeloproliferative disorders, 959
    leukemia, 957–959
    lymphomas, 954–957
    metastatic disease, 959–960
   marrow reconversion, 949–954
    sickle cell disease, 951–953
    thalassemias, 954
   metabolic disease, 967–969
    Gaucher disease, 967–968
    iron deposition/hemosiderosis, 968–969
   miscellaneous, 969–970
    gout, 970
    sarcoidosis, 969–970
   MRI techniques for, 947–949
   normal MRI imaging of, from childhood to adult, 949
   primarily osseous dysplasia and bony abnormalities, 963–967
    osteoporosis, 963
    Paget disease, 963–966
    renal osteodystrophy, 966–967
Bony abnormalities, imaging of bone marrow in, 963–967

C

Cancer treatment. See Oncologic therapy, Chemotherapy, *and* Radiation therapy.
Central nervous system lymphoma, primary. See Lymphoma.
Chemotherapy, imaging of bone marrow depletion with, 962–963
   imaging of CNS complications induced by, 907–915
   for leukemia, neurologic complications due to, 833–835
Coagulation disorders, imaging of neurologic complications of hemorrhagic disorders and, **757–777**
   classification, 759–760
   coagulation cascade, 758–759
   coagulation disorders caused by coagulation factor deficiencies, 771–775
    hemophilia A and B, 771–773
    hereditary thrombophilia, 773–775
    von Willebrand factor, 773
   disseminated intravascular coagulation, 775–776
   hereditary causes, 761–762
   increased vessel fragility, 760–761
   laboratory evaluation, 759
   platelet disorders, 764–771
   secondary causes of vessel wall fragility, 762–764
Computed tomography (CT), of cortical venous thrombosis, 871–873
   CT venography, 873–876
Cortical vein thrombosis, imaging of, **867–885**
CT venography, of cortical venous thrombosis, 873–876

D

Demyelinating disease, as complication of hematopoietic stem cell transplant, 894–895

Diffusion-weighted imaging, of primary CNS lymphoma, 810

Digitally subtracted angiography, of cortical venous thrombosis, 882

Disseminated intravascular coagulation, imaging of neurologic complications in, 726–727, 775–776

Drug-related toxicity, CNS complications of hematopoietic stem cell transplant due to, 888–890

Dural sinus thrombosis, imaging of, **867–885**

Dyscrasias. *See* Blood dyscrasias.

E

Ears, inner, imaging of complications of in sickle cell disease, 791–792

Ehlers-Danlos syndrome, imaging of neurologic complications of, 761–762

Encephalitis, as complication of hematopoietic stem cell transplant, 894

Encephalopathy, posterior reversible syndrome, as complication of leukemia, 835–836

Epidural hematoma, imaging of, 936–937

Extra-axial hemorrhage, as complication of hematopoietic stem cell transplant, 892

F

Factor IX deficiency. *See* Hemophilia B.

Factor V Leiden deficiency, imaging of neurologic complications of coagulation disorders due to, 774–775

Factor XIII deficiency. *See* Hemophilia A.

Fanconi anemia, imaging of neurologic complications of, 745–746

Fungal infection, CNS complications of hematopoietic stem cell transplant due to, 890

G

Gaucher disease, imaging of bone marrow in, 967–968

Glioma, high-grade, as mimic of primary CNS lymphoma, 814

Glucose 6-phosphate dehydrogenase deficiency, imaging of neurologic complications of, 751–752

Gout, imaging of bone marrow in, 970

Graft-*versus*-host disease, as complication of hematopoietic stem cell transplant, 894

H

Head and neck complications, of sickle cell disease, imaging of, 791–795
    bone, 793–795
    inner ears, 791–792
    lymphoid tissue, 793
    orbits, 792–793

Hematologic disorders, imaging of neurologic complications in, 723–971
    anemia, **733–756**
        aplastic anemia, 742–745
        Fanconi anemia, 745–746
        glucose 6-phosphate dehydrogenase deficiency, 751–752
        hereditary spherocytosis, 742
        imaging modalities, 734
        iron deficiency anemias, 734–737
        paroxysmal nocturnal hemoglobinuria, 741–742
        pyruvate kinase deficiency, 752–753
        secondary causes of, 753–755
        sickle cell anemia, 746–751
        vitamin deficiency anemias, 737–741
    blood dyscrasias, **723–731**
        benign hematologic conditions, 723–727
        malignant hematologic conditions, 727–729
    bone marrow, **945–971**
        changes in, from childhood to adulthood, 946–947
        composition of, 946
        marrow depletion, 960–963
        marrow infiltration/replacement, 954–960
        marrow reconversion, 949–954
        metabolic disease, 967–969
        miscellaneous, 969–970
        MRI techniques for, 947–949
        normal MRI imaging of, from childhood to adult, 949
        primarily osseous dysplasia and bony abnormalities, 963–967
    hematopoietic stem cell transplant, **887–898**
        drug-related toxicity, 888–890
        infection, 890–892
        metabolic, 892
        miscellaneous, 894–895
        neoplastic disease after, 894
        vascular, 892–894
    hemorrhagic and coagulation disorders, **757–777**
        classification, 759–760
        coagulation cascade, 758–759
        coagulation disorders caused by coagulation factor deficiencies,
            771–775
        disseminated intravascular coagulation, 775–776
        hereditary causes, 761–762
        increased vessel fragility, 760–761
        laboratory evaluation, 759
        platelet disorders, 764–771
        secondary causes of vessel wall fragility, 762–764
    leukemia, **823–842**
        CNS disease related to secondary effects of malignancy, 827–836
        direct leukemic involvement of CNS, 824–825
        infectious complications, 836–840
        meningeal leukemic infiltration, 825–827
    multiple myeloma, **843–865**

    classification, 844

    IgM, non-IgM, and MGUS, 844–845

    imaging modalities, 849–853

    neurologic complications, 853–863

    solitary plasmacytoma, POEMS syndrome and systemic amyloid light

        chain amyloidosis, 845–846

    staging and risk stratification, 846

    treatment, 846–849

  oncologic therapy, **899–920**

    chemotherapy-induced, 907–915

    radiation-induced, 900–907

  primary CNS lymphoma, **799–821**

    advanced imaging, 808–813

    conventional imaging, 803–808

    mimics of, 813–816

  sickle cell disease, **779–798**

    generalized cerebral volume loss and leukoencephalopathy, 790–791

    head and neck complications, 791–795

    hemorrhage, 787–790

    infarction, 783–787

    management and treatment, 795–797

    posterior reversible leukoencephalopathy syndrome, 790

    vascular disease, 780–783

  spinal manifestations, **921–944**

    general imaging features, 921–923

    in hematologic malignancies, 923–933

    in non-neoplastic hematologic disorders, 933–940

  venous thrombosis, **867–885**

    options for surgical interventions, 883–884

    preimaging planning, 869–870

    technique and assessment of images, 870–882

Hematoma, epidural, imaging of, 936–937

Hematopoietic stem cell transplant, imaging of neurologic complications of,
  887–898

  drug-related toxicity, 888–890

  infection, 890–892

  metabolic, 892

  miscellaneous, 894–895

  neoplastic disease after, 894

  vascular, 892–894

Hemochromatosis, imaging of, 934

Hemoglobinuria, imaging of neurologic complications of hereditary paroxysmal
  nocturnal, 741–742

Hemophilia A, imaging of neurologic complications of, 771–773

Hemophilia B, imaging of neurologic complications of, 771–773

Hemorrhage, extra-axial, as complication of hematopoietic stem cell
  transplant, 892

Hemorrhagic disorders, imaging of neurologic complications of, **757–777**

  classification, 759–760

  coagulation cascade, 758–759

  coagulation disorders caused by coagulation factor deficiencies, 771–775

Hemorrhagic (*continued*)
disseminated intravascular coagulation, 775–776
hereditary causes, 761–762
increased vessel fragility, 760–761
laboratory evaluation, 759
platelet disorders, 764–771
secondary causes of vessel wall fragility, 762–764
Hemosiderosis, imaging of bone marrow in, 968–969
Hemostasis, imaging of neurologic complications in disorders of, 725–727
disseminated intravascular coagulation, 726–727
hemorrhagic disorders, 725
thrombotic microangiopathies, 726
Hereditary hemorrhagic telangiectasia, imaging of neurologic complications of, 761
Hereditary spherocytosis, anemia in, imaging of neurologic complications of, 742

I

Iatrogenic complications, in leukemia, 830–836
direct effect of radiation therapy, 830–831
effects of chemotherapy, 833–835
posterior reversible encephalopathy syndrome, 835–836
radiation-induced secondary neoplasms, 832–833
radiation-induced vascular malformations, 831–832
Imaging, of neurologic complications of hematologic disorders, 723–971
anemia, **733–756**
aplastic anemia, 742–745
Fanconi anemia, 745–746
glucose 6-phosphate dehydrogenase deficiency, 751–752
hereditary spherocytosis, 742
imaging modalities, 734
iron deficiency anemias, 734–737
paroxysmal nocturnal hemoglobinuria, 741–742
pyruvate kinase deficiency, 752–753
secondary causes of, 753–755
sickle cell anemia, 746–751
vitamin deficiency anemias, 737–741
blood dyscrasias, **723–731**
benign hematologic conditions, 723–727
malignant hematologic conditions, 727–729
bone marrow, **945–971**
changes in, from childhood to adulthood, 946–947
composition of, 946
marrow depletion, 960–963
marrow infiltration/replacement, 954–960
marrow reconversion, 949–954
metabolic disease, 967–969
miscellaneous, 969–970
MRI techniques for, 947–949
normal MRI imaging of, from childhood to adult, 949
primarily osseous dysplasia and bony abnormalities, 963–967
hematopoietic stem cell transplant, **887–898**

drug-related toxicity, 888–890
    infection, 890–892
    metabolic, 892
    miscellaneous, 894–895
    neoplastic disease after, 894
    vascular, 892–894
hemorrhagic and coagulation disorders, **757–777**
    classification, 759–760
    coagulation cascade, 758–759
    coagulation disorders caused by coagulation factor deficiencies,
       771–775
    disseminated intravascular coagulation, 775–776
    hereditary causes, 761–762
    increased vessel fragility, 760–761
    laboratory evaluation, 759
    platelet disorders, 764–771
    secondary causes of vessel wall fragility, 762–764
leukemia, **823–842**
    CNS disease related to secondary effects of malignancy, 827–836
    direct leukemic involvement of CNS, 824–825
    infectious complications, 836–840
    meningeal leukemic infiltration, 825–827
multiple myeloma, **843–865**
    classification, 844
    IgM, non-IgM, and MGUS, 844–845
    imaging modalities, 849–853
    neurologic complications, 853–863
    solitary plasmacytoma, POEMS syndrome and systemic amyloid light
       chain amyloidosis, 845–846
    staging and risk stratification, 846
    treatment, 846–849
oncologic therapy, **899–920**
    chemotherapy-induced, 907–915
    radiation-induced, 900–907
primary CNS lymphoma, **799–821**
    advanced imaging, 808–813
    conventional imaging, 803–808
    mimics of, 813–816
sickle cell disease, **779–798**
    generalized cerebral volume loss and leukoencephalopathy, 790–791
    head and neck complications, 791–795
    hemorrhage, 787–790
    infarction, 783–787
    management and treatment, 795–797
    posterior reversible leukoencephalopathy syndrome, 790
    vascular disease, 780–783
spinal manifestations, **921–944**
    general imaging features, 921–923
    in hematologic malignancies, 923–933
    in non-neoplastic hematologic disorders, 933–940
venous thrombosis, **867–885**

Imaging (*continued*)
   options for surgical interventions, 883–884
   preimaging planning, 869–870
   technique and assessment of images, 870–882
Infarction, in sickle cell disease, imaging of, 783–787
 subacute, as mimic of primary CNS lymphoma, 814–816
Infection, CNS complications of hematopoietic stem cell transplant due to, 890–892
Infectious complications, of hematologic disorders, spinal manifestations of, 937–940
 in leukemia, 836–840
  intracranial, 839–840
  sinus, 838–839
Intracraniall myeloma, imaging of, 859
Iron deficiency anemias, imaging of neurologic complications of hereditary, 734–737
Iron deposition disease, imaging of bone marrow in, 968–969

K

Kearns-Sayre syndrome, anemia in, imaging of neurologic complications of, 741

L

Leukemia, imaging of bone marrow infiltration in, 957–959
 imaging of neurologic complications in, 727, **823–842**
  CNS disease related to secondary effects of malignancy, 827–836
   cerebrovascular complications, 827–830
   iatrogenic complications, 830–836
  direct leukemic involvement of CNS, 824–825
  infectious complications, 836–840
   intracranial, 839–840
   sinus, 838–839
  meningeal leukemic infiltration, 825–827
 spinal manifestations of, imaging of, 923–925
Leukoencephalopathy, posterior reversible syndrome of, 790, 835–836
  as iatrogenic complication of leukemia treatment, 835–836
  in sickle cell disease, 790
Lymphoid tissue, imaging of complications of in sickle cell disease, 793
Lymphoma, imaging of bone marrow infiltration in, 954–957
 imaging of neurologic complications in, 727
 primary CNS, neuroimaging of, **799–821**
  advanced imaging, 808–813
   diffusion-weighted imaging, 810
   magnetic resonance spectroscopy, 812
   nuclear radiology imaging, 812–813
   perfusion and permeability, 811–812
   susceptibility-weighted imaging, 812
  conventional imaging, 803–808
   intravascular lymphomatosis, 806
   pattern of recurrence, 806

T-cell lymphoma, 807–808
general characteristics, 800–803
mimics of, 813–816
high-grade glioma, 814
subacute infarction, 814–816
toxoplasmosis, 814
tumefactive demyelinating lesions, 816
secondary CNS, neuroimaging of, 800
spinal manifestations of, imaging of, 925–927
Lymphomatosis, intravascular, neuroimaging of, 806

M

Magnetic resonance imaging (MRI), of bone marrow, 947–949
normal, from childhood to adulthood, 949
techniques, 947–949
of CNS complications of oncologic therapy, **899–920**
of cortical venous thrombosis, 876–880
MR venography, 880–882
Magnetic resonance spectroscopy, of primary CNS lymphoma, 812
Marrow. *See Bone* marrow.
Metabolic disease, imaging of bone marrow in, 967–969
Metabolic issues, CNS complications of hematopoietic stem cell transplant
due to, 892
Metastatic disease, imaging of bone marrow infiltration in, 959–960
Monoclonal gammopathy of undetermined significance (MGUS), 844–845
Morbidity, due to CNS complications of hematopoietic stem cell transplant, 895
Mortality, due to CNS complications of hematopoietic stem cell transplant, 895
Multiple myeloma, imaging of neurologic complications in, **843–865**
classification, 844
IgM, non-IgM, and MGUS, 844–845
solitary plasmacytoma, POEMS syndrome and systemic amyloid light
chain amyloidosis, 845–846
imaging modalities, 849–853
neurologic complications, 853–863
cranial nerve involvement, 859
extramedullary (extraosseous) spinal myeloma, 856–858
hematologic complications, 862–863
immunosuppression and infectious complications, 860–862
metabolic complications, 859–860
skull and intracranial myeloma, 859
spinal myeloma, 853–856
staging and risk stratification, 846
treatment, 846–849
spinal manifestations of, imaging of, 929–932
Myelodysplastic syndrome, anemia due to, imaging of neurologic complications of,
754–755
Myelofibrosis, imaging of, 934
Myeloma, anemia due to, imaging of neurologic complications of, 753
Myelopathy, radiation-induced spinal, imaging of, 935
Myeloproliferative disorders, imaging of bone marrow infiltration in chronic, 959

N

Neoplastic disease, as complication of hematopoietic stem cell transplant, 894
Neuroimaging. *See* Imaging.
Neurologic complications, of hematologic disorders, imaging of, 721–973
    anemia, **733–756**
        aplastic anemia, 742–745
        Fanconi anemia, 745–746
        glucose 6-phosphate dehydrogenase deficiency, 751–752
        hereditary spherocytosis, 742
        imaging modalities, 734
        iron deficiency anemias, 734–737
        paroxysmal nocturnal hemoglobinuria, 741–742
        pyruvate kinase deficiency, 752–753
        secondary causes of, 753–755
        sickle cell anemia, 746–751
        vitamin deficiency anemias, 737–741
    blood dyscrasias, **723–731**
        benign hematologic conditions, 723–727
        malignant hematologic conditions, 727–729
    hematopoietic stem cell transplant, **887–898**
        drug-related toxicity, 888–890
        infection, 890–892
        metabolic, 892
        miscellaneous, 894–895
        neoplastic disease after, 894
        vascular, 892–894
    hemorrhagic and coagulation disorders, **757–777**
        classification, 759–760
        coagulation cascade, 758–759
        coagulation disorders caused by coagulation factor deficiencies, 771–775
        disseminated intravascular coagulation, 775–776
        hereditary causes, 761–762
        increased vessel fragility, 760–761
        laboratory evaluation, 759
        platelet disorders, 764–771
        secondary causes of vessel wall fragility, 762–764
    leukemia, **823–842**
        CNS disease related to secondary effects of malignancy, 827–836
        direct leukemic involvement of CNS, 824–825
        infectious complications, 836–840
        meningeal leukemic infiltration, 825–827
    multiple myeloma, **843–865**
        classification, 844
        IgM, non-IgM, and MGUS, 844–845
        imaging modalities, 849–853
        neurologic complications, 853–863
        solitary plasmacytoma, POEMS syndrome and systemic amyloid light chain amyloidosis, 845–846

staging and risk stratification, 846
treatment, 846–849
oncologic therapy, **899–920**
chemotherapy-induced, 907–915
radiation-induced, 900–907
primary CNS lymphoma, **799–821**
advanced imaging, 808–813
conventional imaging, 803–808
mimics of, 813–816
sickle cell disease, **779–798**
generalized cerebral volume loss and leukoencephalopathy, 790–791
head and neck complications, 791–795
hemorrhage, 787–790
infarction, 783–787
management and treatment, 795–797
posterior reversible leukoencephalopathy syndrome, 790
vascular disease, 780–783
venous thrombosis, **867–885**
options for surgical interventions, 883–884
preimaging planning, 869–870
technique and assessment of images, 870–882
of hematological disorders, imaging of, spinal manifestations, **921–944**
general imaging features, 921–923
in hematologic malignancies, 923–933
in non-neoplastic hematologic disorders, 933–940
Nocturnal hemoglobinuria, imaging of neurologic complications of hereditary
paroxysmal, 741–742
Nuclear radiology imaging, of primary CNS lymphoma, 812–813

O

Oncologic therapy. See also Chemotherapy and Radiation therapy.
imaging of CNS complications of, **899–920**
chemotherapy-induced, 907–915
radiation-induced, 900–907
Opportunistic infections. See Infectious complications.
Orbits, imaging of complications of in sickle cell disease, 792–793
Osseous dysplasia, imaging of bone marrow in, 963–967
Osteoporosis, imaging of bone marrow in, 963

P

Paget disease, imaging of bone marrow in, 963–966
Paroxysmal nocturnal hemoglobinuria, imaging of neurologic complications of
hereditary, 741–742
Plasma cell dyscrasias, imaging of neurologic complications in, 727–729
Plasmacytoma, solitary, 845–846
spinal manifestations of, imaging of, 932
Platelet disorders, imaging of neurologic complications of hemorrhagic disorders
due to, 764–771

POEMS syndrome, 845–846

Polycythemia vera, spinal manifestations of, imaging of, 935

Post-transplant lymphoproliferative disorder, as complication of hematopoietic stem cell transplant, 894

Primary central nervous system lymphoma. See Lymphoma.

Protein C and S deficiency, imaging of neurologic complications of coagulation disorders due to, 774

Pyruvate kinase deficiency, anemia in, imaging of neurologic complications of, 752–753

R

Radiation therapy, imaging of bone marrow depletion with, 961–962

    imaging of CNS complications induced by, marrow change, 934–935

        myelopathy, 935

    for leukemia, neurologic complications due to, 830–833

        direct effects, 830–831

        secondary neoplasms, 832–833

        vascular malformations, 831–832

Renal osteodystrophy, imaging of bone marrow in, 966–967

S

Sarcoidosis, imaging of bone marrow in, 969–970

Secondary central nervous system lymphoma. See Lymphoma.

Sickle cell anemia, imaging of neurologic complications of, 746–751

Sickle cell disease, imaging of bone marrow reconversion in, 951–954

    imaging of neurologic complications of, **779–798**

        generalized cerebral volume loss and leukoencephalopathy, 790–791

        head and neck complications, 791–795

            bone, 793–795

            inner ears, 791–792

            lymphoid tissue, 793

            orbits, 792–793

        hemorrhage, 787–790

        infarction, 783–787

        management and treatment, 795–797

        posterior reversible leukoencephalopathy syndrome, 790

        vascular disease, 780–783

Sinus thrombosis, imaging of, **867–885**

Skull myeloma, imaging of, 859

Spherocytosis, anemia due to, imaging of neurologic complications of hereditary, 742

Spinal manifestations, of hematologic disorders, imaging of, **921–944**

    general imaging features, 921–923

        meningeal and spinal cord disease, 922–923

        vertebral/epidural disease, 921–922

    in hematologic malignancies, 923–933

        leukemia, 923–925

        lymphoma, 925–927

multiple myeloma, 929–932
plasmacytoma, 932
polycythemia vera, 925
Waldenstrom macroglobulinemia, 927–929
in non-neoplastic hematologic disorders, 933–940
epidural hematoma, 936–937
hemochromatosis, 934
myelofibrosis, 935
opportunistic infections, 937–940
radiation myelopathy, 935
radiation-induced marrow change, 934–935
vertebral marrow hyperplasia/reconversion, 933–934
Spinal myeloma, imaging of, 853–856
Stroke, as complication of hematopoietic stem cell transplant, 892–894
Susceptibility-weighted imaging, of primary CNS lymphoma, 812
Systemic lupus erythematosus, anemia due to, imaging of neurologic
complications of, 753–754

T

T-cell lymphoma, neuroimaging of, 807–808
Telangiectasia, imaging of neurologic complications of hereditary
hemorrhagic, 761
Thalassemias, anemia in, imaging of neurologic complications of, 735–739
imaging of bone marrow reconversion in, 954
Thrombocytopenia, imaging of neurologic complications of, 764–771
Thrombophilia, imaging of neurologic complications of hereditary, 773–775
Thrombotic disorders, imaging of neurologic complications in, 725
Thrombotic microangiopathies, imaging of neurologic complications in, 726
Toxoplasma infection, CNS complications of hematopoietic stem cell transplant
due to, 890
Toxoplasmosis, as mimic of primary CNS lymphoma, 814
Tumefactive demyelinating lesions, as mimic of primary CNS lymphoma, 816

V

Vascular complications, of hematopoietic stem cell transplant, 892–894
extra-axial hemorrhage, 892
stroke, 892–894
Vascular disease, in sickle cell disease, imaging of, 780–783
Venography, CT, of cortical venous thrombosis, 873–876
MR, of cortical venous thrombosis, 880–882
Venous thrombosis, imaging of neurologic complications in, **867–885**
options for surgical interventions, 883–884
preimaging planning, 869–870
technique and assessment of images, 870–882
Vertebral marrow hyperplasia, as complication of hematologic disorders,
933–934
Viral infection, CNS complications of hematopoietic stem cell transplant due to,
891–892

Vitamin deficiency anemias, imaging of neurologic complications of, 737–741
    folate, 741
    vitamin B12, 737–741
Von Willebrand factor, imaging of neurologic complications of, 773

W

Waldenstrom macroglobulinemia, spinal manifestations of, imaging of, 927–929

Moving?

Make sure your subscription moves with you!

To notify us of your new address, find your **Clinics Account Number** (located on your mailing label above your name), and contact customer service at:

Email: journalscustomerservice-usa@elsevier.com

800-654-2452 (subscribers in the U.S. & Canada)
314-447-8871 (subscribers outside of the U.S. & Canada)

Fax number: 314-447-8029

Elsevier Health Sciences Division
Subscription Customer Service
3251 Riverport Lane
Maryland Heights, MO 63043

*To ensure uninterrupted delivery of your subscription, please notify us at least 4 weeks in advance of move.

Printed and bound by CPI Group (UK) Ltd, Croydon, CR0 4YY

03/10/2024

01040392-0011